Health Facility
Commissioning
HANDBOOK

Health Facility Commissioning

HANDBOOK

*Optimizing Building System Performance
in New and Existing Health Care Facilities*

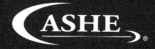

THE AMERICAN SOCIETY FOR HEALTHCARE ENGINEERING
OF THE AMERICAN HOSPITAL ASSOCIATION

CHICAGO

The American Society for Healthcare Engineering
155 North Wacker Drive, Suite 400
Chicago, IL 60606
312-422-3800
ashe@aha.org
www.ashe.org

Dale Woodin, CHFM, FASHE, Executive Director
Patrick J. Andrus, MBA, Director, Business Development
Pamela James Blumgart, Senior Editor
Susan G. Rubin, MPH, Senior Specialist, Marketing & Communications

ISBN: 978-0-87258-902-5

ASHE catalog #: 055383

Cover credits: Vista Award winners from 2011 (an awards program sponsored by ASHE and *Health Facilities Management* magazine), Exterior: SSM St. Clare Health Center, Fenton, Missouri (HGA Architects and Engineers, Milwaukee); Generator: AnMed Health Medical Center, Anderson, South Carolina; NICU: Aspirus Wausau Hospital, Wausau, Wisconsin; Training photo: ASHE; Sample EPA Energy Star dashboard: TME Inc., Little Rock

Printed in the United States of America on archival-quality paper
Book design by www.DesignForBooks.com

Contents

PART 3

Health Facility Retrocommissioning

APPENDICES 277

Foreword

As professionals responsible for the health care physical environment, facility managers and directors are charged with getting the most out of their facilities' performance. The bottom line is that many hospitals do not meet the design performance goals for their building systems, which diverts resources from their institutional mission.

In this era of uncertain revenue streams and shrinking margins, we must take every opportunity to reduce waste in health care and support hospital leadership by bringing solutions to the table. That means providing real value—realized benefits divided by actual costs. Obtaining value is the desired outcome of every health care facility construction or renovation project. But more often than not, actual achievement of value is elusive.

Health facility commissioning (HFCx) makes it possible for an organization to achieve its envisioned results from construction and renovation projects and to operate its facilities effectively and efficiently. So efficiently, in fact, that some health care organizations have used the decrease in utility costs to fund projects that further their mission. HFCx is all about achieving value.

But if undertaking a HFCx effort was a simple decision, every facility project or existing facility would be commissioned or retrocommissioned. To access the benefits of commissioning, it is critical to go beyond an understanding of the commissioning process to the ability to create a business plan that clearly outlines the business value of commissioning to the leaders of a health care organization.

ASHE's goal in publishing the *Health Facility Commissioning Guidelines* and this accompanying document, the *Health Facility Commissioning Handbook*, is to provide a comprehensive set of resources that offers standard language and a clear process for commissioning cost-effective, efficient health care facilities that deliver the desired return-on-investment and can be operated to maintain this cost-effectiveness and efficiency.

ASHE developed the *Health Facility Commissioning Handbook* specifically to support facility managers as they strive to work with project teams and lead their operations and maintenance staffs to optimize the health care physical environment. The HFCx process described in detail in this volume provides a framework and tools to help health care organizations achieve both their envisioned results from design and renovation projects and optimal operation of their building systems over the long term.

Dale Woodin, CHFM, FASHE
Executive Director
ASHE

Preface

Current economics are straining the budgets of U.S. health care facilities. As indicated in Figure A, the average operating margin for U.S. hospitals has declined to near zero. Passage of federal health care reform legislation (the Patient Protection and Affordable Care Act of 2010 and the Health Care and Education Reconciliation Act of 2010) may further aggravate this situation. The legislation (among many other things) expands Medicaid cover-

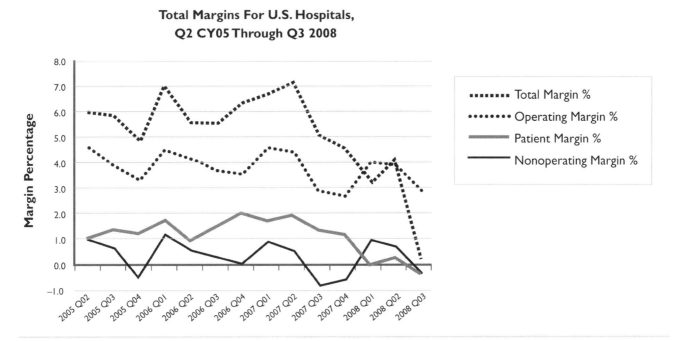

**Total Margins For U.S. Hospitals,
Q2 CY05 Through Q3 2008**

Figure A: Health Facility Operating Margins

Due to a perfect storm of higher costs and capped revenues,
health facility operating margins are razor thin.

age, imposes tax penalties on individuals who do not have health insurance, eliminates Centers for Medicare & Medicaid Services (CMS) reimbursement for medical errors, and reduces CMS reimbursements for hospitals with high readmission rates.

Concurrent with declining margins and the uncertain impact of health care reform, other market forces are driving the need for renovation of, additions to, and construction of new health care facilities:

+ The Hill-Burton Act enacted in 1946 provided grants and loans that led to the construction of more than 6,800 health care facilities in more than 4,000 communities between 1950 and 1975. Most of these facilities have little remaining economic life.

+ Hospital utilization for persons 65 to 74 years old is more than three times that for persons 45 to 54 years old. The number of people in the United States who are 65 years old or older is expected to increase from 35 million in 2000 to more than 70 million in 2030. It has been said that the construction of a new 100-bed hospital each week for the next 10 years would not adequately accommodate the increased demand.

+ The U.S. population continues to move south and west with Texas, Arizona, Florida, and Georgia recently gaining the most. In addition, the population centers of many cities have continued to move to the suburbs. Urban flight has shifted demand from large urban hospitals to smaller primary care facilities located near these bedroom communities. In other cities, however, young professionals are returning to more urban areas.

+ The health care business is continuously changing. Recent trends include family-centered care and evidence-based medicine. Family-centered care typically requires private patient rooms, larger patient rooms, play areas for children, lounge areas, and comfortable in-room sleeping accommodations for family members. Older health care facilities do not typically have these features. Evidence-based medicine recognizes that the health care facility environment can influence outcomes and recovery times. Recent studies indicate that natural light, healing gardens, and reduced noise levels can reduce recovery times. Shorter recovery times reduce costs and increase margins.

+ Medical technology continues to evolve at a rapid pace. Recent advances include archival communication systems, digital imaging, PET scanners, 64-slice CT scanners, and hybrid operating rooms. Hospitals are forced to renovate existing facilities to accommodate these technological advancements, creating larger rooms, reinforcing floors, increasing ceiling height, adding shielding, and upgrading electrical distribution and HVAC equipment.

+ Many health care facilities are planning, designing, and constructing specialty facilities such as cardiovascular and orthopedic hospitals (specialty hospitals typically focus on the most profitable service lines).

+ Compliance with constantly shifting building codes and regulations requires numerous health facility renovations and upgrades.

Current health facility operating margins (let alone those that may result after health care reform) are not sufficient to finance the needed renovations, additions, and new facilities, and health care organizations are under tremendous pressure to improve their margins. Because competition and fixed reimbursements limit their ability to increase revenue, the only means of increasing or restoring margin is to reduce costs. In response, most health care facilities have capped or even reduced their operations and maintenance budgets. Health facility budgets typically range from $7 to $12 per square foot per year (with larger facilities at the low end of the range and smaller facilities at the high end). (Figure B illustrates a typical hospital operations and maintenance budget.)

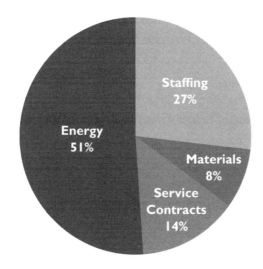

Figure B: Typical Hospital Operations and Maintenance Budget

Since health facility maintenance staffing levels are already too low and material and service contract costs are increasing, health facility managers have no alternative but to reduce energy costs. A 25 percent reduction in energy costs has the potential to double a health care facility's operating margin. Energy costs are the product of energy consumption and energy unit costs. Energy unit costs are volatile and generally on the rise.

As indicated in Figure C, the average retail electricity rate in the United States has increased from 6.64 cents per kWh to 9.89 cents per kWh in the past 10 years. Natural gas rates have also increased significantly. Reducing energy costs in the face of increasing utility rates will require dramatic reductions in energy consumption. Energy efficiency is no longer optional.

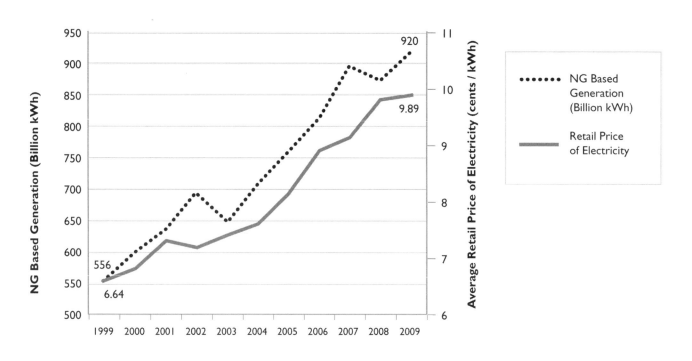

Figure C: Retail Electricity Rates

Health care facilities have conventionally responded to the mandate to reduce energy costs by seeking energy efficiency through LEED certification, standard commissioning, and energy-efficient design. Unfortunately, these methods are not always successful. LEED-certified facilities, which have been commissioned (commissioning is a prerequisite for LEED certification), are not always energy-efficient. Very few new health care facilities are eligible to receive the EPA Energy Star after their first 12 months of occupancy as they often have Energy Star ratings of less than 75.

ASHE believes the conventional status quo methods of optimizing energy efficiency are not foolproof because they do not adequately address the transition from construction to occupancy. This Handbook presents ASHE's response to this void. In this volume, readers will find additional steps needed to reduce health facility energy consumption and costs.

Acknowledgments

ASHE thanks all those listed for contributing their time and knowledge to the ASHE Health Facility Commissioning Handbook Task Force and its development of the *Health Facility Commissioning Handbook*.

Introduction and
Chapter 1 – Predesign Phase

Mark Kenneday, *chair*
Bert Gumeringer
John Fowler
Ken Monroe
Tim Peglow
Purdue University research team
Principal investigators:
   Gregory Lasker
   Phillip Dunston
Research assistant: Chen Chen
Lead student researchers:
   Danielle McGarry
   Lance Garland Moe
   Mitchell Erickson
Student collaborators: Spring 2011
Healthcare Built Environment class
University of Arkansas–Little Rock interns
   Andrew Johnson
   Chris McKenney
   Stephanie Shank

Chapter 2 – Design Phase

Clay Seckman, *chair*
Steve Wiggins
Doug King
Damian Skelton
Mark Thuringer

Chapter 3 – Construction Phase

Rusty Ross, *chair*
Byron Hall
Bart Miller
Gene Hildman
Ari Tinkoff
Jack Limbach

Chapters 4 and 5 development

Leo Gehring, *chair*
Larry Rubin
Paul Raschilla
Keith Shortall
Tim Staley
Brian Cotten

Chapter 4 – Transition to
Occupancy Phase

Ed Tinsley
Tim Staley

Chapter 5 – Warranty Phase

Rusty Ross

Chapter 6 – Retrocommissioning

Ed Tinsley, *chair*
Mike Locke
David Volz
Dale Kondik
Bill Duckett
Tracy Robinson
Yeqiao Zhu
Jonathan Flannery

PART I

Health Facility
Commissioning

Introduction

The commissioning process pertains to all types of building systems, including fire and life safety, heating, ventilation, and air-conditioning (HVAC), plumbing, medical gas, electrical, information technology, lighting, vertical transport, and material-handling systems as well as the building envelope. Most general definitions of the term *commissioning* relate it to a process intended to improve building performance in line with the owner's expectations and the design intent.

Best commissioning practices generally prescribe a process that is collaborative, logical, and thoroughly defined. For the results of this process to be sustainable, however, the commissioning process must include elements to assure that operations and maintenance staff become invested in a positive outcome and to provide them with the training and other resources they need to maintain optimum performance of a facility's building systems.

WHAT IS HEALTH FACILITY COMMISSIONING?

As used in the ASHE *Health Facility Commissioning Guidelines* and this companion handbook, the word *commissioning* embraces the traditional definition, in which the goal is to assure that performance matches the owner's expectations, but expands it to (1) include additional systems critical to health facility operations (e.g., medical gas, nurse call, etc.); (2) assure that all parties, especially operations and maintenance staff, are adequately prepared to operate and maintain the completed project, including sustaining the performance of the systems over time; and (3) provide for development of key documents required by regulatory bodies. In the opinion of the authors of this handbook, these additional outcomes are best achieved for health care facilities through a commissioning process managed by a designated and independent health facility commissioning authority (HFCxA).

Early involvement of the health facility commissioning (HFCx) team increases the effectiveness of the commissioning process.

Commissioning Types

An identifiable subset of terms is broadly recognized within the general category of *commissioning*. These terms differ from each other with respect to the timing and the desired outcome of the processes to which they refer. However, these terms are often misunderstood and used inconsistently. Definitions as used in the ASHE health facility commissioning process are provided here:

The term *retrocommissioning* is applied to existing facilities or systems that have been in operation for some time but were either never commissioned or improperly commissioned at turnover.

The term *recommissioning* indicates that commissioning did occur at turnover, but for various reasons the process needs to be repeated. The goal in these cases is to improve the performance of existing systems.

Another term, *ongoing commissioning*, refers to a process by which building performance is continually optimized over time.

---

*By demonstrating that it costs more **not** to commission a building than it does to commission it using the ASHE HFCx process, the value equation discussion can neutralize resistance to the cost of the commissioning process.*

For optimal outcomes, the HFCx team should be established and engaged at the outset of a project and remain fully involved throughout planning, design, and construction. This early involvement will optimize the effectiveness of the commissioning process. A fully empowered HFCx team can develop value-added solutions that reduce initial cost by providing effective alternatives early in the design process without compromising the owner's project requirements.

DEMONSTRATING THE VALUE OF COMMISSIONING AT THE C-LEVEL

Most successful budgetary requests to the C-level of a health care organization—composed of members of the leadership team whose title generally begins with "chief" (e.g., chief executive officer, chief operating officer, chief financial officer, chief nursing officer)—rely on the principles expressed in this simple value equation:

$$Value = Benefit/Cost$$

Using this equation, commissioning can be shown to increase the value of a project in the following ways:

- Commissioning increases the benefits obtained from the project, thereby increasing the value derived from it.
- Commissioning decreases the cost to complete the project and reduces the operations and maintenance (O&M) costs associated with productive use of the space, thereby increasing its value.
- Thus, commissioning increases the benefits obtained from the project and at the same time decreases both the cost to complete the project and the O&M costs, thereby maximizing the value derived.

To the C-suite, the most convincing argument is the third one, in which benefits are increased while total costs are reduced. The challenge for the HFCx team is to optimize the value equation and maximize the health care facility's return on investment (ROI). There are many variables in this task, which is not a simple exercise, especially for a team anxious to move forward with other aspects of the project. However, those who developed the ASHE HFCx process firmly believe that if this step is not given full attention by the health facility project team, the project commissioning initiative is less likely to receive funding approval and thus the project is less likely to provide the best possible economic value for the owner.

Many C-suite professionals do not fully comprehend the total value or replacement cost of their facilities. Generally, only the chief executive officer (CEO), the chief financial officer (CFO), and the chief operating officer (COO) are fully aware of the investment represented by their buildings and campus, so the first task for the HFCxA is to provide substantive information on replacement cost, life cycle cost, life cycle position, and O&M costs. By demonstrating that it costs more *not* to commission a building than it does to commission it using the ASHE HFCx process, the value equation discussion can neutralize resistance to the cost of the commissioning process.

Most of the many competing requests for capital in health care facilities come from departments that represent the organization's primary mission—to provide the highest level of quality care and customer satisfaction in the delivery of clinical services. For academic medical centers, this responsibility also includes provision of education for health care professionals and sustained growth for centers of excellence for scientific study and translational research. Thus, to frame the discussion of value in the perspective of the C-suite, facility executives must include arguments and justifications that focus on the C-level executives' primary responsibility—support for the mission of the health care organization.

An important point in cost vs. revenue discussions is that revenue-producing projects generally support an institution's core mission. However, revenue must be serviced by overhead, making it a significant challenge to generate even a single dollar to margin. Most health facility projects are funded through a combination of debt, philanthropy, and institutional reserves with the expectation that servicing the debt and replenishing reserves will be a function of mission-based activities once productive use of the space is underway. Regardless of the financing strategy, one thing the HFCxA and HFCx team must remember is that every dollar they take from the cost of project delivery and every solution they provide to reduce O&M costs during productive use go directly to the institution's margin.

Every dollar saved by a well-commissioned, efficient project can be used to support the growth of the institution's patient care, education, and research missions. By presenting the value statement in these terms, the argument clearly speaks to the choice between spending more in the local utility and construction economy or saving energy and eliminating excess construction costs and using those funds to grow the institution's missions. Lowering the

To help C-suite executives understand the role of facilities in strategic thinking, hospital-based facility managers or consultants can demonstrate how every organizational growth strategy requires facility support.

energy intensity rating of a campus can lower the incremental energy cost per unit to deliver mission products. The simple argument is that a reduction in dollars per square foot of operating cost provides immediate margin to support mission outcomes.

In summary, facility executives must frame construction and renovation projects as opportunities to support the health care organization's mission critical strategies. A statement of the value of the commissioning process can help the entire C-suite appreciate how much commissioning contributes to the organization's efforts to achieve strategic planning goals and long-term success. Employing a value statement argument can assure that facility initiatives, including commissioning, will be approved and that, once the C-suite has accepted its value, commissioning will become a standard when they consider future health facility projects.

Balancing the Costs and Benefits of Commissioning

By focusing on the specific benefits derived from properly commissioning a particular health care facility project, the project team can provide a facility executive with the tools needed to develop a funding campaign. Cost can always be debated, but without a proper understanding of the benefits, the argument can become one sided and favor the status quo.

Expanding a facility to support mission growth without proper commissioning almost always results in less than optimal operational outcomes and often in an increase in the institution's overall energy intensity. Although these unfavorable results seem counterintuitive to the outcomes expected from hiring a great architect, engineer, and contractor, they are almost always what is delivered when commissioning is not employed. Case studies document increases in overall cost per square foot in new health facility projects even where premiums were placed on efficient design, efficient systems, and quality construction practices.

To best demonstrate the benefits of commissioning a project, the HFCxA should define all value derived from commissioning from the perspective of the various interest groups in the C-suite. The HFCxA must explain how a well-commissioned health care facility project will provide capital to support their mission-based operations by focusing on the benefits derived from commissioning activities and how they support the individual interests of C-level executives and the institution's mission as a whole. For instance, the chief of staff (COS) and chief nursing officer (CNO) might not see the significance of commissioning a new bed tower, but they will certainly see the significance of commissioning's intended benefits (e.g., improved thermal comfort, HVAC system reliability, life safety, clinical outcomes). By formulating the value statement from the perspective of managing the comfort of patients, the HFCxA can better gain support for a fully commissioned environment.

The actual cost of commissioning is a challenge to compute until the project scope has been fairly well defined. For example, a small project might be mechanically complex or create difficult challenges for the building envelope.

Benefits from engaging in commissioning are traditionally framed like this:

+ The owner and design team are obliged to carefully document the owner's project requirements (OPR).

+ Design reviews are conducted in a manner that identifies the most cost-effective methods for achieving the OPR (frequently resulting in substantial savings).

+ Errors and omissions are caught early, avoiding delays and additional costs.

+ The development and use of pre-functional checklists helps identify installation issues.

+ Required functional performance tests improve system capacity, performance, and energy efficiency, yielding corresponding improvements in thermal comfort, infection control, clinical outcomes, staff productivity, and patient and visitor satisfaction.

+ Postoccupancy tests catch any issues missed during the project delivery process as well as issues previously not readily apparent due to weather conditions.

+ Operator training provided assures operational sustainability.

+ Contractor and owner warranty costs are reduced.

Based on the nature of the specific project, many other benefits can also be assigned to commissioning. To communicate all these benefits in C-suite terms, they should be phrased to focus on mission outcomes. They would be better introduced as the "benefits of the ASHE health facility commissioning process" and described as follows:

+ Optimized collaboration between the owner and design team results in careful documentation of the OPR and in savings derived from selecting appropriate mechanical systems and an efficient building envelope. These savings can be redirected to optimize clinical, education, and research initiatives.

+ The design phase commissioning activities assure use of the most cost-effective methods so the project will achieve the OPR and the ROI expected from investment in high-performance systems and buildings.

+ The commissioning process significantly reduces errors and omissions by diminishing their occurrence and catching those that inevitably occur, thereby avoiding project delays and additional costs.

Presenting the benefits of commissioning in a way that achieves buy-in from members of the C-suite with competing funding requests is critical if commissioning is to become a mainstream practice.

+ Pre-functional checklists are developed to mitigate installation issues before they can cause schedule delays.

+ Functional performance testing is used to assure proper system operation is achieved before occupancy.

+ Postoccupancy tests are conducted to verify optimum system performance and catch previously undetected issues. These tests take into account variations in weather, which previously could only be estimated. The postoccupancy tests typically identify differences between actual operation and design intent, for which additional system adjustments may be warranted. After occupancy, mission activities are evaluated as real-time processes to validate design assumptions.

+ Operations and maintenance (O&M) personnel are trained in the techniques and practices needed to achieve sustainable operation of new spaces and equipment. The transition from design, development, construction, and substantial completion to operational sustainability requires the engagement of O&M personnel from the outset of a project. The HFCxA is responsible for assuring staff fully understand the commissioning agenda, can manage the project outcomes in the manner intended, and can deliver the ROI as defined.

+ Warranty costs are reduced by detecting and resolving problems during project construction instead of after the space has been occupied.

Many other benefits of commissioning a project can also be established, including regulatory compliance, investor value, and patient, staff, and visitor safety.

The greatest opportunity afforded by the *Health Facility Commissioning Guidelines* and this *Handbook* is to assure that every health care facility project is properly commissioned. HFCx offers owners optimal value for their project expense, the most efficient and productive use of their space, and—perhaps most important—the promised ROI.

Lessons Learned

A best practice for documenting both positive and negative outcomes from a health care facility project is to debrief after initial occupancy and productive use. This can be done in a meeting that includes the designer, builder, HFCxA, and owner, including the facility executive, staff who took productive use of the space, and the O&M team that maintains the space. Such sessions can provide a good opportunity to institute an iterative learning process that improves the commissioning process and supports better outcomes with lessons learned. The project team can create a table of values for comparing projects that were and were not properly commissioned. This data can be essential in convincing a C-level executive who is doubtful of the value of the health facility commissioning process.

An important deliverable in a health care facility project is assurance that the ROI projected in the planning phase will be achieved. HFCx supports cost savings over the life of a project. The first opportunity for such savings provided by the HFCx process is to assure the project is designed in accordance with the OPR. This might seem like a small difference from other doctrines, but the outcomes from the development of a proper OPR will ripple throughout the project, bringing savings to the owner at each phase of project delivery. Once the owner has worked with the HFCxA to establish the OPR, the design team has a much better definition of their charge. The OPR development process forces the owner to fully define their expectations at the onset of a project rather than after they see something they don't like. As a result, the basis of design (BOD) document developed by the design team will incorporate the elements of the OPR and avoid processes and systems that would later be value engineered out of the project.

Traditional value engineering (VE) or value analysis (VA) exercises typically reduce the upfront cost of a project, which is often their intended purpose. Reducing the upfront cost, however, can reduce the long-term value of a project by compromising energy efficiency, reliability, longevity, and sustainability. Instead, when properly executed, VE or VA exercises should focus on reducing the life cycle cost of the facility rather than the upfront cost. Shifting the traditional practice from decision-making focused solely on upfront cost to decision-making with due consideration of life cycle costs is a key factor in achieving high-performance buildings.

THE COMMISSIONING BUSINESS PLAN

In writing a business plan, it is best to use a standard format and present your plan with the amount of depth and detail necessary to support the funding request. The level of detail should be correlated to the complexity of the project, but should never be too complex or difficult to understand. Too much information is as counterproductive to success as too little. The attention span of the executives reading the plan is short, and they will quickly move on to the next activity in their busy schedules if a plan is not concise, compelling, and indicative of high value.

The path to securing approval for the funds associated with health facility commissioning is no different from that for other capital budget requests. Managers who spend time developing their argument, support it with a good business plan, and present it in a manner that highlights its support of the organizational mission will have a much higher success rate. Managers must

A key factor in achieving high-performance buildings is shifting from decision-making focused on upfront cost to decision-making that includes due consideration of life cycle costs.

resist the temptation to skip development of a commissioning business plan and jump right into the value argument and funding request.

See Appendix A for a sample business plan for a project to replace out-dated HVAC equipment in an academic medical center. The $23 million project included modifying equipment in the energy plan and installing an electric heat pump chiller to reduce dependence on natural gas by simultaneously producing heating and cooling water. The project utilized the ASHE HFCx process, which was supported by all members of the project team.

SUPPORT INFORMATION IN THE APPENDICES

A wealth of information is provided in the appendices to this handbook. In addition to the sample business plan referenced in the text above are Appendices B and C, described below.

Glossary

As in all disciplines, particular words, acronyms, and phrases convey unique meanings when they are used in association with the commissioning process. See Appendix B for a glossary of these terms that defines them and cross-relates them with the terms used by other societies and trade associations that set standards or otherwise provide relevant support information. Key terms and phrases defined in the body of this handbook are also included in the glossary for the convenience of the reader.

Commissioning Crosswalk: A Comparison of Resources

The commissioning crosswalk in Appendix C is a tool intended to help clarify the differences between the commissioning processes put forward by various organizations. The crosswalk compares the ASHE health facility commissioning process with other commissioning processes published by widely known, credible voices in the building construction and facility management industries.

Commissioning and Sustainability

For the foreseeable future, reduction of energy use will continue to be a major concern in all types of construction processes, including HFCx. Many organizations publish sustainability guidelines or certifications that offer significant value and support to health care facility planning and operations. It is significant that most of these programs recognize commissioning as the guarantor of a successful outcome.

Today many companies and organizations support initiatives that focus on improving the environment. These efforts are motivated by a variety of factors, ranging from better fiscal management through energy conservation to shared attitudes regarding stewardship of our finite natural resources. As an extension of such efforts, health care facilities are electing to employ sustainable design and construction practices in their projects.

A widely recognized proponent of sustainability is the U.S. Green Building Council (USGBC). Among its efforts, the most recognized initiative is the LEED® certification program. LEED is an acronym for Leadership in Energy and Environmental Design. The hallmark of the program is a published rating system that defines sets of energy-saving measures for various building categories such as new buildings and existing buildings and for use types such as schools, office buildings, commercial and retail buildings, and the like. The USGBC introduced LEED for Healthcare in April 2011. The rating system applies to the design and construction of both new buildings and major renovations of existing buildings and can be used for inpatient, outpatient, and licensed long-term care facilities; medical offices; assisted living facilities; and medical education and research centers.

Each rating system ranks individual sustainability measures on a weighted scale based on potential environmental value. If a building accumulates sufficient points, it may qualify for certification at the general, Silver, Gold, or Platinum level. Point categories and criteria are developed by LEED committees using an open, consensus-based process. In addition to meeting the point criteria, a building must satisfy a series of prerequisites before it can be certified.

In recognition of the environmental benefits of commissioning, a minimum level of commissioning activity—referred to as "fundamental commissioning of building energy systems"—is a prerequisite for LEED certification. At minimum, the following energy-related components and systems must be commissioned during fundamental commissioning: HVAC equipment and systems and their associated controls, alternative and renewable energy technologies, domestic hot water systems, and lighting and daylighting controls. More information about these requirements is provided in the ASHE *Health Facility Commissioning Guidelines* and the LEED for Healthcare literature.

However, LEED certification and its fundamental commissioning prerequisite are not sufficient to assure delivery of a high-performance building. Additional steps, including measurement and verification of actual building performance and continuous commissioning are required. Nonetheless, LEED certification does establish a useful set of metrics that defines energy-saving criteria. As a public and open process for improvement, it is constantly being revised and updated to reflect best practices in specific building sectors.

Green Design Does Not Guarantee Energy Efficiency

Health care facilities often seek green building designations, such as the widely recognized LEED certification and the Designed to Earn Energy Star certification from the Environmental Protection Agency. These programs can help designers in their efforts to design buildings that use fewer natural resources both in construction and in operation, and LEED certification requires standard commissioning practices. However, there is a big difference between programs that certify design and construction, like LEED, and programs that influence actual building performance. In fact, a 2009 story in the New York Times, titled "Some Buildings Not Living Up to Green Label," found that buildings can rack up LEED points for things like bamboo floors and native landscaping instead of building features that save energy over the long term. The article cited research from the U.S. Green Building Council, which administers the LEED program, that found a quarter of new certified buildings do not save as much energy as their designs predicted and most do not track energy consumption once in use.

While programs such as LEED are a good base for creating green designs, they do not go far enough. Additional steps must be taken to actually assure energy efficiency once facilities are up and running. Through health facility commissioning, hospitals can turn their green building designs into high-performing, energy-efficient buildings that truly live up to expectations.

PART 2

The Health Facility Commissioning Process

Predesign Phase

1.1 ESTABLISH THE COMMISSIONING SCOPE

The commissioning process begins with the health care facility establishing the commissioning scope. A comprehensive scope for commissioning a health care facility includes the systems discussed in this section.

1.1.1 Systems to Be Commissioned

(1) **Building Envelope**

The design of a building envelope addresses concerns for preserving temperature, moisture, and pressure differentials between the outdoors and the interior of the building.

(a) **Insulation.** The chief function of building insulation is to isolate a building's internal thermal environment from outside temperature variances. Insulation also serves numerous other functions within a building: For example, it can reduce heat transfer from adjacent spaces that may have wide temperature differences and provide noise abatement and fire suppression. The thermal effectiveness of insulation is commonly rated on a relative scale using R-value or U-value qualifiers.

(b) **Glazing.** Glazing (the glass used in buildings) provides structural integrity with respect to sealing, window strength, and safety and offers thermal insulation, sound abatement, and protection from solar radiation. Specialty glazing may be used for skylights and atriums.

(c) **Vapor barriers.** Just as insulation preserves temperature differences between different areas, vapor barriers are designed to impede the flow of moisture between interior and exterior spaces. This function is important for maintaining environmental quality and reducing the growth of mold and bacteria within building walls.

(d) **Exterior building walls.** An exterior building wall is composed of various materials that are combined to separate the conditioned space within the building from the elements outside. Use of special materials and sealants may be required for walls that extend below ground level.

(e) **Roof.** Building roofs include a range of designs and materials. The common concern is proper sealing, including flashing details. Correct procedures must be followed wherever there are penetrations for vents, stacks, antennas and other electrical connections, and fixtures.

(f) **Pressure requirements.** Building pressure testing is critical to occupant safety in health care facilities as it measures the effectiveness of the ventilation of the space tested. Improper pressurization adversely affects the opening and closing of doors and wastes energy.

(2) **Life Safety**

(a) **Fire-rated assemblies.** Building elements required to have fire-resistive ratings include floor-ceiling assemblies, fire window assemblies, fire separations, and the doors and hardware required to achieve a particular rating. The ratings for walls and doors (e.g., 1-hour, 1½-hour, 2-hour, fire-stop) specify the time that materials and assemblies can withstand fire exposure as demonstrated through testing. The fire-resistive rating of an assembly must take into account any pipes, conduits, pneumatic tubes, bus ducts, and cables that penetrate it.

(b) **Smoke barriers.** A continuous membrane constituted of walls and doors or a membrane with protected openings designed and constructed to limit the transfer of smoke. Smoke barriers are generally required to have at minimum a one-hour fire-resistive rating.

(c) **Smoke-tight partitions.** A continuous membrane designed to limit the transfer of smoke. Smoke-tight partitions are not generally required to have a minimum fire-resistive rating.

(d) **Stair pressurization system.** Where required, these systems include controls, fans, and detection devices. When activated, such a system pressurizes a stairwell to maintain a smoke-free environment during evacuation.

(e) **Fire command center.** Where required, this is a designated, fire-rated room that houses fire alarm panels, elevator panels, fire pump notification panels, and sometimes generator-run panels. This room should also house a complete set of life safety drawings for the building. Fire departments must be able to quickly access this area.

(f) **Smoke evacuation system.** Where required, smoke evacuation systems automatically vent smoke and the products of combustion. Smoke evacuation systems may be required for atriums, anesthetizing locations, and other areas within a health care facility.

(3) HVAC Systems

(a) **Air terminals.** These introduce warm or cool air into a space depending on the current temperature needs of that zone. A certain amount of outside air may also be introduced. The main source of the air that passes through an air terminal is an air-handling unit. For larger spaces, several discharge grilles are used to distribute the air evenly.

(b) **Induction units** (also known as chilled beams). Placed in individual rooms, these units recirculate the existing air in a room, blending in a percentage of new air supplied by an air-handling unit. The resulting air mixture passes through coils to add or remove heat from the discharge air. The temperature is controlled by a room thermostat.

(c) **Fan coil units.** These units do not rely on an upstream air-handling unit for an air supply. Instead, each unit has its own fan for air distribution and heats and cools the air as required. Most do not introduce fresh ventilation air, so they are usually used in utility areas such as entryways and electrical and communications closets. When placed on outside walls, they can be used to supplement systems that supply fresh air. These units include thermostatic and fan-speed controls.

(d) **Unit heaters.** These stand-alone systems provide temperature control to areas that specifically call for heating applications, such as entryways, shop spaces, and other utility areas. They are self-contained and usually operate only on demand.

(e) **Air-handling units.** These supply large volumes of air for distribution to individual zone units. Processes in an air-handling system include pre-heating and heating of air, cooling, humidification, exhaust, and introduction of outside air. Units are defined by how they operate—constant volume, variable volume, dual-duct, or multi-zone systems.

(f) **Energy recovery units.** These can both extract the heat present in exhaust air and transfer it to fresh inlet air during the heating season and extract heat from fresh inlet air to cool it during hot weather. These systems may treat temperature alone or temperature and moisture (humidity) combined.

(g) **Exhaust system.** These systems may be part of the air-handling unit or separate, isolated equipment. General exhaust systems serve routine areas such as locker rooms and toilets. Kitchen exhaust systems for grill hoods may include mechanisms to catch grease and prevent accidental fires. Dedicated, specialized exhaust systems are used for surgery and special procedure areas.

(h) **Chilled water system.** These systems refrigerate water that is used as a cooling medium and pumped and circulated throughout a facility to units such as air handlers, fan coil units, etc. Chillers are often located in central plants. In the process of chilling water, a condenser gathers heat, which must be dispersed either through air-cooled coils or by circulating the condenser water through a cooling tower.

(i) **Heating water system.** These systems provide hot water for comfort heating to air-handling coils, fan coils, and terminal reheat coils. The water may be heated directly in hot water-heating boilers or heated by steam boilers via a heat-exchange process.

(j) **Steam systems.** Steam boilers heat water beyond the boiling point to create steam, which may be maintained at multiple pressure ranges (high, medium, and low) by mechanical regulators. Steam is used for heating purposes in air-handling units, but sterile steam may be distributed to humidifiers, sterilizers, and other specialized medical equipment.

(k) **Humidifiers.** These are used to add moisture to indoor air, especially during winter months when air tends to dry out. Central humidifiers are located within air handlers, but zone humidifiers may be placed at terminal units and adjusted to particular space conditions. Various mechanisms are available to convert water or steam into particles small enough to be absorbed by the air stream.

(l) **Fire and smoke dampers.** Placed in specific areas of the ductwork, these dampers can be closed to isolate areas from one another. Depending on where a fire incident is located and whether it is just smoke or an actual blaze, the problem zone and surrounding zones may require different relative pressure states to contain the fire or smoke.

(m) **Special applications**

  (i) *Operating rooms* (anesthetizing locations). Operating rooms have specialized HVAC requirements, including increased or even 100 percent outside air, highly filtered air, special humidity conditions, isolated exhaust systems, pressurization requirements relative to surrounding spaces, and the ability to raise and lower temperatures to extreme conditions.

  (ii) *Airborne infection isolation (AII) rooms.* AII rooms, which often have a room-anteroom arrangement, are designed to prevent the spread of communicable disease into public spaces or other patient rooms. AII rooms are isolated and must maintain a negative air pressure relative to surrounding areas.

  (iii) *Protective environment (PE) rooms.* Sometimes called isolation rooms, PE rooms require maintenance of a positive pressure so as to protect the patient from harmful, incoming contaminants. This may be accomplished by using a room-anteroom arrangement and other construction requirements. The goal is to protect vulnerable patients through institutional infection prevention environments and procedures.

  (iv) *Data center.* Data centers house critical equipment and provide storage for valuable electronic records. Temperature and humidity levels are often maintained by separate, stand-alone computer room air-conditioning (CRAC) units. This keeps heat-generating equipment cool and reduces the chance of damage from the electromagnetic sparking prevalent when air is dry.

  (v) *Pharmacy.* Pharmacies may have both special air requirements (temperature, filtration, humidity, etc.) and pressurization requirements. Mixing certain chemical compounds may require a positive pressure environment. If a laboratory hood is present, room pressures in relation to it must be positive so that contaminants are properly exhausted.

  (vi) *Imaging.* Imaging areas often have equipment that generates a large amount of heat. Accommodating this may require separate or individual cooling of both equipment and surrounding spaces.

(4) Controls

(a) **Workstations.** These front-end computers consolidate multiple data points from various building systems and allow an operator to view information and alter system operations by switching devices on or off or modifying equipment operating parameters. Workstations annunciate alarm conditions in prioritized classifications and provide graphs and reports of data trends over time.

(b) **System graphics and dashboards.** Graphics provide building operators with visual illustrations of multiple data points, often using color and animation to highlight the current state of key values. Dashboards target managerial interests by combining current values with historical and statistical information. The displays often include vertical gauges, dial indicators, and bar graphs.

(c) **Networks.** These are built from physical infrastructure components (switches, cabling, end-of-line termination devices, repeaters, routers, gateways) that transfer data from controller to controller or from the controller to the operator workstations. Building topologies often consist of copper or fiber Ethernet networks designed to move large amounts of data. The control network may also leverage and be incorporated into the building's IT network. At the smaller zone-control level, simpler two-wire networks can be used to pass data from device to device at slower speeds.

(d) **Controllers.** In most of today's systems, controllers are digital devices that receive input signals and can be set to respond to them in a predetermined manner. Controllers may simply monitor and record current input values for information purposes. Or, they may be programmed to respond with notification alarms or measured changes in the controller output signal.

(e) **Sensors.** The accuracy of voltage, current, temperature, pressure, humidity, flow, and level sensors, among others, that communicate with the building automation system (BAS) must be verified.

(f) **Actuators.** The function of actuators on dampers and valves must be verified. Do they fully open, fully close, and modulate properly in response to BAS system commands?

(g) **Meters.** Electricity, water, steam, gas, fuel oil, and other meters must be checked to verify that they are set to the correct range and read accurately and reliably within that range.

(5) **Plumbing Systems. Components of the following plumbing systems must be checked to verify that they perform properly under anticipated conditions.**

(a) **Domestic cold water system.** Proper cleaning and pre-treatment of domestic cold water piping must be verified. Components of the domestic cold water system that must be checked for proper functioning include:

(i) Meter

(ii) Backflow prevention devices

(iii) Booster pumps

(iv) Water treatment equipment (e.g., water softeners, RO/DI, filters, etc.)

It is important to note that the commissioning scope does not typically address water quality.

(b) **Domestic hot water system.** Proper cleaning and pre-treatment of domestic hot water piping must be verified. Components of the domestic hot water system that must be checked for proper functioning include:

(i) Water heaters

(ii) Recirculation pumps

(iii) Storage tanks

(iv) Return balancing valves

(c) **Sump pumps.** Proper operation of the float controls and alarms must be verified.

(d) **Natural gas and propane systems.** Components of these systems that must be checked include:

(i) Pressure-regulating valves

(ii) Meters

(iii) Automatic shutoff valves

(e) **Fuel oil system.** Components of the fuel oil system that must be checked include:

(i) Storage tanks

   (ii) Pumps

   (iii) Pump controls

   (iv) Leak detection equipment

   (v) Automatic shutoff valves

   (vi) Boiler/generator control interlocks

  (f) **Plumbing fixtures.** Plumbing fixture components that must be checked include:

   (i) Trap primers

   (ii) Electronic faucets

   (iii) Electronic flush valves

   (iv) Emergency showers

   (v) Eyewash equipment

   (vi) Clinical sinks

   (vii) Shower and faucet temperature control valves

   (viii) Vacuum breakers

   (ix) Backflow prevention devices

   (x) Flushing rim floor drains

  (g) **Disinfection and sterilization systems.** The following components of these systems must be checked:

   (i) Autoclaves

   (ii) Rack washers

  (h) **Rainwater harvesting and gray water system.** The components of this system that must be checked include:

   (i) Tanks

   (ii) Valves

   (iii) Pumps

   (iv) Treatment equipment

  (i) **Process cooling system.** Proper water treatment should be verified, and the following process cooling equipment must be checked for proper functioning:

   (i) Pumps

   (ii) Filters

   (iii) Automatic valves

   (iv) Sensors

(j) **Sewage systems.** Components of the sewage system that must be checked include:

   (i) Lift stations

   (ii) Acid neutralizing tanks

   (iii) Decontamination shower storage tanks

   (iv) Grease traps

(6) **Medical Gas and Other Specialty Gas Systems**

NFPA 99: *Health Care Facilities Code* requires proper operation of medical gas systems to be verified by an ASSE 6030-certified medical gas verifier. Additional verification by the HFCxA is not typically required or recommended. (ASSE 6030: *Professional Qualifications Standard for Medical Gas Verifiers* is published by the American Society of Sanitary Engineering.)

(7) **Electrical Systems**

Components of the following electrical systems must be checked to verify that they perform properly under anticipated conditions.

(a) **Normal power system.** Components of the normal power system that must be checked include:

   (i) Meters

   (ii) Transformers (primary and step-down)

   (iii) Main switchgear

   (iv) Panelboards

   (v) Power conditioners

   (vi) Power factor correction equipment (capacitors and filters)

   (vii) Grounding, contactors

   (viii) Uninterruptible power supplies (UPS)

   (ix) TVSS (transient voltage surge suppressor) equipment

   (x) SCADA (supervisory control and data acquisition) equipment

It is important to note that the HFCxA does not typically provide arc flash labeling, selective coordination, panel directories, megger testing, receptacle testing, receptacle labeling, and similar functions. The HFCxA should work with the health facility manager to assure that these activities are completed within the confines of the project.

In some cases, the HFCxA may actually provide some of these services under the commissioning scope.

(b) **Essential electrical power system.** Components of the essential electrical system that must be checked include:

(i) Generators

(ii) Paralleling switchgear

(iii) Automatic transfer switches

(iv) Isolated power panels

(v) Uninterruptible power supplies (UPS)

It is important to note that the HFCxA does not typically provide arc flash labeling, selective coordination, megger testing, receptacle testing, receptacle labeling, isolated power center testing, and other similar functions.

(c) **Lightning protection.** The lightning protection system should be visually inspected to assure it has been properly installed.

(d) **Grounding systems**

(8) Fire Alarm System

NFPA 72: *National Fire Alarm and Signaling Code* requires testing of the fire alarm system. Each device must be individually tested, and the installing contractor typically provides this service. The HFCxA typically verifies proper interfaces and functionality between the fire alarm system and other building systems, including the smoke evacuation, elevator control, paging, infant abduction, fire protection, HVAC, and security systems, and smoke and hoistway vent dampers.

(9) Information Technology

Historically, proper operation of most information technology (IT) systems is verified by the installing contractor or vendor. Due to rapid advancements in technology, however, it is not uncommon for the HFCxA to participate in the verification process for selected IT systems on a project-specific basis. In these instances, the HFCxA typically verifies proper interfaces and functionality between systems (e.g., verifies that the infant abduction system automatically closes and locks doors). It is important to note, however, that the HFCxA does not typically verify that the IT systems selected by others are appropriate for the application.

IT systems and equipment that may be commissioned by the HFCxA include these:

(a) Telephone system

(b) Data system

(c) Intercom system

(d) Paging system

(e) Doctor's dictation system

(f) Telemetry system

(g) Security system

(h) Master clock

(i) Dedicated antenna system

(j) Television system

(k) Nurse call system

(l) Infant abduction system

(m) Wireless access points

(n) Cell phone repeaters

(10) Fire Protection System

Proper performance under anticipated conditions of fire protection system components must be verified. These components include the following:

(a) Backflow preventer

(b) Fire pump/jockey pump

(c) Drains

(d) Tamper and flow switches

(e) Zone valves

(f) Fire department connections

(g) Pre-action systems

(h) Standpipes

(i) Sprinkler heads

(j) Clean agent systems

(k) Building automation system (BAS) interface

(11) and (12) Interior and Exterior Lighting

Proper performance under anticipated conditions of interior and exterior lighting system components must be verified. These components include the following:

(a) Lighting controls

(b) Daylighting controls

(c) Occupancy sensors

(d) Lighting contactors

(e) Photocells

(f) Performance lighting

(13) Refrigeration

Proper performance under anticipated conditions of refrigeration system components must be verified. These components include the following:

(a) Food service refrigerators

(b) Food service freezers

(c) Clinical refrigerators

(d) Clinical freezers

(e) Blood banks

Proper operation of the interface between the refrigeration systems and the building automation system must also be verified.

(14) Vertical Transport

Local codes typically require testing of the vertical transport systems (elevators, escalators, dumbwaiters, etc.). The installing contractor typically provides this service. The HFCxA typically verifies proper interfaces and functionality between the vertical transport systems and other building systems such as fire alarm, normal power, essential electrical power, and fire protection.

(15) Materials and Pharmaceutical Handling

Proper operation of the materials and pharmaceutical handling systems (pneumatic tube, linen transport, trash removal, and electronic transportation vehicles) is typically validated by the installing contractor or vendor and should be verified by the HFCxA.

1.1.2 Factors Affecting the Commissioning Scope

The scope of the commissioning effort should be tailored based on a number of factors, including size, complexity, phasing, code requirements, and so on. The size of the project should determine the systems to be commissioned and the tasks to be performed.

A smaller project may need fewer plan reviews than defined in the *Health Facility Commissioning Guidelines* and this *Handbook* and may not require a revision of the utility management plan (UMP). As well, the scope of a small project may not be large enough to significantly impact the maintenance budget or the building maintenance program (BMP), making it unnecessary to modify these documents. The construction scope in a renovation project may not require pressure testing or include fire or fire/smoke dampers.

In a phased project, by contrast, numerous systems will be reconfigured over the course of the project. For example, multiple functional tests of the same system may be needed as it is revised from phase to phase. Temporary system installations in the interim phases of a project (e.g., temporary chilled water system or essential electrical system arrangements), although not part of the final scope, may need to be commissioned.

The scope of some projects may not include all the systems suggested for commissioning in this document. The project scope in each case will determine the systems that require commissioning. Many small projects and renovation projects will have a limited number of the systems listed in Section 1.1.1. Some projects may primarily involve mechanical system additions or renovations; others may be focused on revisions to the essential electrical system.

Code requirements will also impact project scope, with consequences for systems to be commissioned. For instance, some jurisdictions require smoke evacuation in atria areas, some require smoke evacuation in anesthetizing locations, some require isolated power systems, and some require stairwell pressurization for certain projects.

The owner and HFCxA must build a project commissioning scope that meets the demands of the project construction scope.

1.2 SELECT THE COMMISSIONING PROJECT TEAM STRUCTURE

The health facility commissioning team may comprise some or all of the following: the building owner or owner's representative, the health facility commissioning authority (HFCxA), members of the health care facility operations and maintenance (O&M) staff, design professionals, the construction manager, the contractor, and subcontractors.

1.2.1 Building Owner or Owner's Representative

The primary responsibilities of the building owner or owner's representative are to clearly communicate project expectations through the development of the owner's project requirements (OPR) and to support the commissioning process and the overall project team. The owner is responsible for selecting the HFCxA.

1.2.2 Health Facility Commissioning Authority (HFCxA)

This is the entity responsible for managing, coordinating, executing, and documenting the commissioning activities.

1.2.3 Health Facility Operations and Maintenance Staff

These individuals are part of the owner's staff and may include managers, engineers, electricians, plumbers, and other maintenance personnel. By participating in the commissioning process, health facility O&M staff will gain an understanding of the building systems before the building is occupied. They gain knowledge of equipment maintainability and access challenges as well as equipment and system control strategies by participating in the following activities:

(1) Reviewing shop drawings

(2) Touring the construction site with the HFCxA

(3) Witnessing functional tests

(4) Participating in training provided by the contractor and the HFCxA

1.2.4 Design Professionals

Design professionals include the architect, mechanical engineer, electrical engineer, and other specialty consultants. Design professionals develop construction documents, including plans and specifications, for the building to provide the functionality and meet the goals for the project as defined in the OPR.

1.2.5 Construction Managers, Contractors, and Subcontractors

The construction manager or general contractor directs and coordinates the construction effort of the project construction team. Subcontractors include a wide variety of disciplines (e.g., mechanical, plumbing, electrical, and specialty subcontractors, such as nurse call or pneumatic tube installers) responsible for constructing the facility and installing its various systems. Their specific commissioning tasks usually include working with the HFCxA to ensure that commissioning milestones for equipment they install are integrated into the master construction schedule, conducting performance tests on installed systems at the direction of the HFCxA, helping to resolve deficiencies, and documenting system startup. They are also responsible for providing system documentation and training the owner's O&M staff.

Figure 1 depicts a functional health facility commissioning team structure that supports the collaborative interaction required to optimize the health care physical environment.

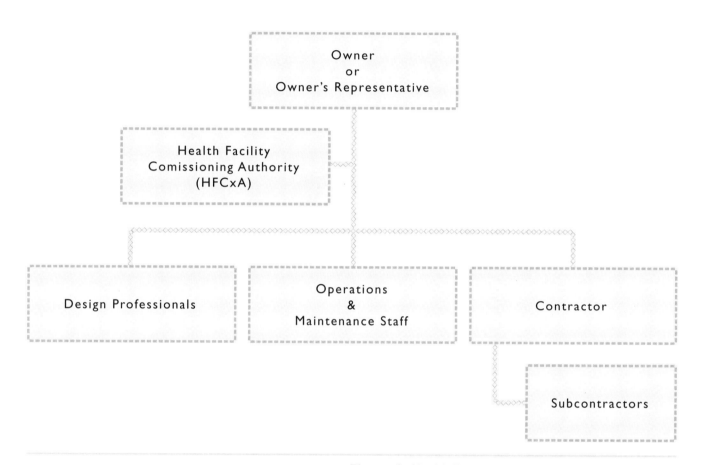

Figure 1: Health Facility Commissioning Team Structure

1.3 SELECT THE HEALTH FACILITY COMMISSIONING AUTHORITY (HFCxA)

1.3.1 Timing

The HFCxA should be selected and engaged at the very outset of a project. Early engagement facilitates timely design reviews by the HFCxA and allows input before the design team has expended extensive effort on a specific design.

Early engagement of the HFCxA also enables the entity or individual to become an active member of the design and construction team who makes positive contributions to the team effort.

The cost-benefit ratio from early engagement of the HFCxA demonstrates major project savings from discovering and addressing issues before the design is complete, budgets are finalized, and the project is under construction.

1.3.2 Qualifications

Commissioning is a professional service. The owner should select the HFCxA based on qualifications, including key personnel; the training, credentials, technical expertise, and demonstrated competence of the personnel on the HFCxA team; references; and similar health care project experience. The qualifications of the HFCxA team should be commensurate with the scope, complexity, and criticality of the owner's project.

The skill set of the HFCxA team is determined by the complexities of the project scope and the desired commissioning scope. The project construction scope may or may not involve significant revisions to the building envelope, electrical systems, IT systems, security systems, elevators, etc. The experience and abilities of the each commissioning team member should be weighted heavily when choosing a firm to provide commissioning services.

1.3.3 Selection Process

The HFCxA can be selected based on a proven and trusted relationship with a qualified HFCxA or through a request for qualifications (RFQ) process. The process for selecting a HFCxA using an RFQ process involves the following steps:

(1) **Establish a selection committee.** The owner appoints a selection committee, which typically comprises three to seven individuals, including the facility manager, the owner's project or program manager, user group representatives, and administrative representatives.

(2) **Develop and issue a request for qualifications.** The selection committee typically initiates the HFCxA selection process by issuing a request for qualifications. In the private sector, an advertisement may be placed in an appropriate forum, such as a newspaper or trade journal, or the RFQ may be sent to a list of potential candidates identified by the selection committee. For public projects, the process generally involves a newspaper advertisement that solicits responses to the RFQ. (Refer to Appendix 1-1 for a sample RFQ.)

Whether for public or private projects, the advertisement provides a general description of the project along with the project budget and schedule, scope of commissioning services being sought, minimum qualifications required of the HFCxA, information that should be included in a proposal (see just below), and the deadline for receipt of the response.

The RFQ should define what is to be included in the submission:

(a) A general description of the commissioning firm. This should include time in business, time offering HFCxA services, areas of expertise offered (various commissioning services as well as services other than commissioning), number of staff—technical and administrative, and location of offices.

(b) An organizational chart for the project team proposed by the HFCxA organization, including resumes of the team members

(c) A list of similar projects completed by (1) the HFCxA organization, (2) key individuals in the HFCxA organization, and (3) the HFCxA organization in conjunction with other members of the project team (designer, contractor, etc.)

(d) A description of the roles and responsibilities the proposed project team members undertook in the completed projects listed as references in the submission

(e) Sample work products, such as commissioning plans, installation checklists, plan reviews, test procedures, and so on. (These are used to assess technical expertise and the degree of detail the HFCxA would provide in project-specific documents.)

(f) The firm's recommended commissioning approach for the defined scope of the project

(3) **Develop a short list of qualified candidates.** The final HFCxA choice may be based solely on a review of RFQ responses, but most often a short list of HFCxA firms for further consideration is culled from the initial response results. The short list can be developed using an analysis matrix (see Appendix 1-2 for an example) to compare the firm's qualifications with the specific project requirements. Send an agenda for the interviews and questions to short-listed HFCx providers so they can prepare their presentation to cover specific issues or concerns.

(4) **Interview HFCxA candidates.** Interviews with prospective HFCxA firms should be face-to-face discussions with those personnel who would execute the process for the project, including the proposed project manager and senior commissioning providers in each area of expertise (mechanical, electrical, low voltage, building envelope, etc.). (Refer to Appendix 1-3 for a sample interview matrix.)

Sufficient time should be allowed for the representatives of each candidate to discuss their firm's qualifications and processes as well as any specific topics the selection committee would like addressed. Each interview should also allow time for questions and answers.

1.3.4 Making the Decision

The HFCxA selection process is most successful when the selection committee bases its choice on the provider's qualifications. A decision-making matrix that highlights the candidates' experience may be used to assist in making the final decision. (Refer to Appendix 1-4 for a sample selection matrix.)

When circumstances require fee to be considered in addition to qualifications, qualifications should remain a key consideration. A more qualified HFCxA can yield significant cost savings in other aspects of the total cost, which will more than offset a difference in fee.

1.4 NEGOTIATE THE HFCXA FEE AND CONTRACT

Once the selection committee has chosen the HFCxA, the selection committee or a committee member designated by the owner should negotiate the commissioning fee. This must represent a fair and responsible process that supports the owner's intent. The HFCxA and the owner should confirm that the scope of services as defined thus far in the selection process is the scope required by the owner or agree that modifications are desired. If modifications are desired, considerations for the size of the project, the number of systems to be commissioned, the number of plan reviews required, the number of meetings that must be attended, the number of phases in the project schedule, and so on, must be elements that define the fee.

The HFCxA should document the final scope in a fee proposal. The two parties should then negotiate and agree that the scope and fee in the pricing proposal are acceptable to both parties. Additionally, agreements must be made concerning what reimbursable expenses (travel, printing, overnight deliveries, etc.) will be acceptable. Will these expenses be reimbursed or included in the fee proposal? Will the HFCxA be required to use a project FTP site or other such Web-based process for accessing and sharing project data, or will paper copies of plans, specifications, and changes be made available at no cost to the HFCxA?

Once a scope has been finalized and a fee agreed upon, the two parties should execute a contract for the HFCx services (refer to the sample contract in the appendix of the *Health Facility Commissioning Guidelines*). The contractual relationship should be directly between the owner and the HFCxA. The HFCxA's role is to be an advocate for the owner, to serve as a representative for the owner independent of the design or construction teams. This cannot be accomplished if the HFCxA's contract is held by the contractor or design team.

Design Phase

In the commissioning process for any project in a health care facility, the design phase is a critical time. At this point, commissioning activities begin to be tailored to the specific project scope and objectives, and generic checklists and templates are adapted to address the identified systems, components, and project phases. It is essential for all project team members to be on the same page in regard to the commissioning process itself, and the absolute need for effective communication during this phase cannot be overstated. It is during the design phase that the foundation for a successful commissioning process is established and integrated into the fabric of the project.

A successful design phase yields a number of important metrics:

+ A common understanding of the commissioning process on the part of all project team members. This understanding must encompass the implications of that process for each team member's scope of work and effort as well as a delineation of the scope of work of the health facility commissioning authority (HFCxA), including the activities or aspects of the project the HFCxA will not be involved with.

+ Early awareness of the tasks and activities needed to achieve a successful commissioning process, with clear timelines and milestones

+ Clearly defined project goals and objectives regarding system start-up procedures, project phasing, shutdowns, energy consumption, and system performance

+ Thorough understanding on the part of the owner's operations and maintenance (O&M) staff of the design intent for the systems and components within the project scope and of the intended operational and performance parameters

+ Provisions in the contract documents for necessary personnel, work effort, and other requirements of the commissioning process (e.g., testing equipment and sequences, meetings, review sessions, and other elements that affect the scope of work of project team members)

The commissioning process for each project is unique and customized in every detail. No two health care facility design and construction projects are alike, and the design phase is a critical time for taking standard commissioning processes and modifying them to fit the needs of the project at hand.

2.1 ORGANIZE AND ATTEND THE PREDESIGN COMMISSIONING CONFERENCE*

The primary objective of the predesign commissioning conference, to be held just before the design phase begins, is to communicate to all project team members the scope of the commissioning process. All participants must have a full understanding of their own role in the process, especially its impact on their scope of work. Although the actual commissioning plan has not yet been fully developed at the beginning of the design phase, the overall project scope and level of commissioning services are generally known and these elements must be communicated to the project team before design gets underway. This knowledge will allow them to make any necessary adjustments in contracts and fees before the project gets too far down the road.

All team members should know what to expect from the commissioning process. Surprising the design team with a peer review or trade contractors with a testing procedure will not foster an atmosphere of collaboration and teamwork, and will likely degrade the effectiveness and value of the commissioning process. Anything required of the project team needs to be identified and discussed up front.

Because the design team should discuss the commissioning process before design begins, it may be necessary to hold two commissioning conferences prior to or early in the design phase, depending on how and when trade contractors and other members of the construction team are selected. To assure the design team receives necessary information early enough, this conference may need to be repeated for those who join the team later, rather than postponed until all contractors are on board. Separate follow-up meetings to review their scope of work with the trade contractors most affected by the commissioning process may also be advantageous.

Setting the agenda for the predesign commissioning conference is crucial. The subheads in Chapter 2 of the ASHE *Health Facility Commissioning Guidelines* are a good starting point for the subjects to be covered in the conference.

*The title of this section in the *Health Facility Commissioning Guidelines* reads "Organize and attend the predesign conference"; the title here has been amended for clarity to read "Organize and attend the predesign commissioning conference."

Sample agenda items:

(1) **Review of project scope, team member roles, and project delivery method.** Review project scope and major milestone events with respect to goals, objectives, schedules, and specific challenges. Review the roles of all project team members as well as the anticipated project delivery method (use of delivery methods such as design-build or integrated project delivery can have a major impact on project team members' roles in the commissioning process).

(2) **Development of project energy efficiency goals.** Discuss desired objectives such as EPA Energy Star or other ratings and indicate implications for the project (e.g., selection of metering systems and exterior envelope construction). Discuss who will perform any required energy use modeling and at what point during the design phase this needs to be done. Review the evaluation process to establish interim goals and metrics for monitoring progress toward achievement of project energy efficiency goals.

(3) **Development of the owner's project requirements (OPR).** Discuss how the OPR will be developed, and identify the key elements already known. (See section 2.3 for more discussion of developing the OPR.)

(4) **Development of the basis of design (BOD) for systems to be commissioned.** Discuss how the BOD will be developed and outline the systems that will be commissioned.

(5) **HFCxA review of the OPR and BOD.** Discuss this review process with the project team. Note especially how the project design will be monitored to assure the owner's requirements and objectives are being met. Discuss timelines for creation and review of these documents and their correlation with the design schedule to minimize the need for redesign and other negative impacts on the project.

(6) **Review of design documents.** Discuss the anticipated design document review process, including schematic design (SD), design development (DD), and construction documentation (CD) phase reviews. Discussion should include:

   (a) Schedule milestones, review periods, turnaround times

   (b) Document formats: hard copy or electronic

   (c) Review session formats: face-to-face, video, etc.

   (d) Comment format

   (e) Response expectations and required follow-up

   (f) Review-comment closure and resolution process

(g) Decision-point milestones for major systems and components

(7) **Development of the commissioning plan.** Discuss how the plan will be developed and the schedule for doing so, and identify any needed input from project team members. Outline the anticipated commissioning process based on the HFCxA scope of services and project scope. Discuss issues such as system training for the owner's staff and reviews of the O&M manuals (including who will provide training, how many training sessions there will be, whether the training will be live and/or recorded video, etc.). This discussion should result in establishment of a schedule of follow-up meetings to review the impact of the commissioning process on all phases of design and construction as they become more fully developed.

(8) **Preparation of the commissioning specifications.** Discuss how the commissioning specifications will be developed and integrated into the project contract documents. Review the effort required to coordinate the commissioning specifications with other, related specification sections (e.g., controls, testing and balancing, systems integration, equipment identification, and O&M manual production) produced by other design team members. This discussion is critical to assure that the trade contractors (mechanical, electrical, controls subcontractors, etc.) meet their responsibilities for the commissioning process and that these are included in their scope of work. For example, confirm who will provide system training and how it is to be carried out. It is critical, while the project specifications are still being developed, to have an understanding of how coordination will occur.

(9) **Update of commissioning plan and specifications.** Discuss how design reviews will affect finalization of the commissioning plan and specifications and how those documents will be coordinated with the final design documents. Establish a review schedule that allows time for issue resolution.

(10) **Development of the utility management plan.** Discuss the process that will be used to develop the utility management plan (UMP), identifying any tasks required of the project team. This might include production of system diagrams, life safety plans, system descriptions, operational sequences, testing procedures, performance certifications, and other information necessary for preparation of the UMP. It is important to use the design and construction process to develop and produce as much of the required UMP material as possible so the facility manager does not have to re-create the material later. (See further discussion in Section 2.13.)

2.2 SET PROJECT ENERGY EFFICIENCY GOALS

The primary reason for setting energy efficiency goals early is to establish the expected energy consumption and utility costs of the completed building when it is occupied, thus estimating their impact on operating costs. The *Health Facility Commissioning Guidelines* provides a clear outline of how to set this goal with a recommended Energy Star target of 75. Early establishment of project energy efficiency goals is also important because these will be key factors in the design of the mechanical, electrical, and plumbing systems as well as in the design, orientation, and massing of the building envelope. In the absence of energy efficiency goals, it is not uncommon for first costs and other emergent project issues to dictate system selection and basic building design, with no consideration given to the effect these have on long-term operational costs.

In addition to considering the EPA Energy Star rating, the project team should discuss to what degree facility energy performance will be linked with ASHE's Energy Efficiency Commitment (E²C) program. This program, described further in Section 5.5 (Benchmark Ongoing Energy Performance) of this handbook, offers benchmarking and sharing of energy performance best practices.

Typically, project teams engage in much discussion about the energy model for a project in terms of who is to develop the model, when it is to be initiated and completed, and to what degree the results of the modeling process are to be used to shape system and facility design. This process should be discussed in detail at the predesign commissioning conference. The energy model is typically developed by either the HFCxA or the engineer of record, depending on their expertise and knowledge of modeling software. One of the major issues to be discussed is the timing of the modeling process, as the model needs to be completed early enough for the results to be fed into the design process, yet late enough for the model to have sufficient building design information to yield accurate energy use predictions (a challenging Catch-22). The project team should also be aware that the cost for developing the energy model is typically not included in standard engineering design fee structures, nor is it necessarily included in the commissioning scope of work, and it can be a substantial figure. Who will develop the model, when it will be developed, and how the information will be applied to development of the project should be decided early.

A design phase energy model is a useful tool for comparing the relative levels of energy consumption that would result from various design options for system type, exterior skin, glazing, orientation, shading, and other features that impact energy consumption. The model is not, however, necessarily intended to be a definitive estimate of actual energy costs. Budgeting for actual utility costs should include input from other sources such as industry benchmarks and data from relevant facilities of similar scope, size, and location.

The entire project team should have a basic understanding of what an energy score is and how it is established. Questions inevitably arise about the initial costs required to achieve energy efficiency goals, and the team must be able to answer them and defend its decisions.

2.3 FACILITATE DEVELOPMENT OF THE OWNER'S PROJECT REQUIREMENTS (OPR)

The OPR and BOD are key documents that establish what the HFCx team will focus on. The OPR communicates in essence "what we want to do" and the BOD "how we want to do it." These documents establish clear goals and plans as a general reference and for use in the commissioning process to determine if the final product ("what we actually did") has accomplished the project objectives.

2.3.1 Team Participation

The owner should provide representatives from all stakeholders in the health care organization to participate in development of the OPR. Often, representation is limited to facility management leadership and department heads. However, it is important to include plant O&M, information technology, security, environmental services, and other staff who will have a stake in operating and maintaining the facility. The OPR development process offers the owner an opportunity to begin fostering the awareness, knowledge, and buy-in on the part of the facility staff that is needed for a successful project life cycle.

There are many ways to facilitate development of the OPR (one process is described in the *Health Facility Commissioning Guidelines*), but the key element is the collaboration of all participants. The HFCxA should assure that no individual dominates the discussion and that ideas are received from and discussed by everyone to assure achievement of a balanced set of requirements.

2.3.2 Developing Key Elements of the OPR

Some information about developing the key elements of the owner's project requirements is provided below.

(1) Background—It is helpful to develop a document that covers the broad scope and context for the project for use as a starting point in developing the commissioning process. This narrative description, usually developed by the design team, provides an overview of the primary purpose of the project, program needs and objectives in terms of departmental and functional gains, operational requirements, the flexibility needed in the project program, future expansion requirements, and other important project features that could affect the commissioning work.

(2) Objectives—It is critical to assure that the project team and the commissioning team learn of all objectives the owner has for a project as soon as possible. Often, the owner's goals are presumed to be known and therefore overlooked or taken for granted. To avoid this, be purposeful about documenting what the owner hopes to gain from the project. Often, the process of doing so prompts questions, and the ensuing discussion helps start the project off on the right foot. Typical objectives refer to first cost, volume of change orders, life cycle cost, energy efficiency, infection rates, patient and visitor satisfaction scores, staffing requirements, maintenance costs, services, capacity for future growth, and schedule.

(3) Functional program—The owner, architect, planner, or a collaboration of these entities typically develops this document, which establishes the specific size, quantity, purpose, and use of each space in the health care facility. The functional program should also include any specific requirements for design of each space, such as security, safety, comfort range, energy consumption, maintainability, utility requirements, specialized ventilation and environmental control features, and so on. Authorities having jurisdiction (AHJs) use the functional program to determine applicable codes and regulations.

(4) Life span, cost, and quality—From the wide range of possible owner's objectives for a project, it is important for the project team to have a clear understanding of the owner's goals for the life span of systems and components, the cost of construction, and the level of quality desired. To clarify these expectations, discuss the balance between construction cost and overall life expectancy of system components and equipment. From these discussions should come a definition of the level of reliability expected from the equipment, the level of automation and flexibility expected from building systems, any preferred technologies and manufacturers, and other specific desires.

(5) Performance criteria—These should be minimum acceptable performance benchmarks for various aspects of the facility and might include these elements:

  (a) Temperature and humidity requirements for critical spaces such as operating rooms, cath labs, etc

  (b) Specialized ventilation, filtration, and pressure relationships for spaces such as trauma, burn, protective environment, and airborne infectious isolation rooms

  (c) Expectations for allowable interruptions in service due to equipment failure, maintenance downtime, or other predictable situations

(d) Expectations for ambient noise levels

(e) Energy consumption expectations, including consideration of adopting an Energy Star rating as a goal and linking facility performance to the ASHE E^{2}C program

(f) Finish and surface durability

(g) Expected building performance in the event of a natural or man-made disaster, depending on the particular threat possible (hurricane, earthquake, bio-weapons, etc.), including required levels of standby power, fuel, water, and supplies

(6) Maintenance requirements—A description should be compiled to delineate how the facility will be operated and by whom as well as the level of training needed for the O&M staff. Specific aspects of the systems design should be specified, including dashboards and associated meters and sensors, commissioning tools used to query the automatic temperature control system, and other system components. Maintenance training requirements will depend on both the level of knowledge of the current O&M staff and the complexity of the proposed systems; any significant gap between the two must be addressed.

(7) Training goals and criteria—These should be established as early as possible in the project schedule and included in the OPR document. Clear definitions of the following will help assure the success of the training efforts:

(a) The purpose of the training

(b) A list of equipment and systems for which training should be provided

(c) A list of personnel to be included in the training process

(d) Definitions of the levels of training for different owner personnel

(e) Schedules for training to be provided during each phase of the project

(f) A plan for documenting training effectiveness

(g) A list of training deliverables

(h) Requirements for archiving training documentation for future reference

For more details, see the accompanying sidebar on training plan components.

Training Plan Components

Following is a detailed outline of the training plan components that should be included in the OPR:

A statement of the purpose for the training program. For example, the document might state, "The purpose of providing training for this project is to ensure the owner's staff understands how to operate and maintain the building and associated systems after initial occupancy. The training program should be developed to provide building occupants and the O&M staff with the functional knowledge necessary to sustain comfort, productivity, air quality, environmental quality, reliable operation, equipment longevity, optimal energy performance, code compliance, and warranty compliance."

A list of the equipment and systems for which training is to be provided. Reference Section 1.1.1 of the *Health Facility Commissioning Guidelines* for a possible list of equipment and systems for which training should be provided. In addition, consider training on the following topics:

- Design intent

- Project sustainability initiatives such as LEED, *Green Guide for Healthcare*, etc.

- Project energy performance goals

A list of personnel to be included in the training process. The OPR document should identify the owner's personnel for whom training should be provided, including these:

- Management and/or leadership, including plant operations directors, chief mechanics, facility directors, and others who will manage the O&M process going forward

- O&M personnel, including IT and audiovisual staff

- Representatives of future building occupants or user groups

- Safety and security personnel

- Night and weekend shift personnel

- Environmental services staff

- Local emergency response personnel

- Local utility personnel

- Outsourced or contract personnel, including vendors and suppliers

Definitions of the levels of training for different owner personnel. The OPR document should address the level of training to be provided for different kinds of personnel. For example, HVAC and building automation system staff should receive detailed training on system operation, maintenance, and troubleshooting, while staff responsible for overseeing systems to be maintained by outsourced service contracts may not need such a detailed level of training.

Schedules for training to be provided during each project phase. A training schedule matrix is useful in communicating this information. There should be a clearly articulated training schedule for the following project phases.

- Predesign phase

- Design phase

- Construction phase

- Commissioning and initial occupancy phase

- Warranty phase

- Ongoing and/or follow-up training

A plan for documenting training effectiveness. The OPR document should make clear the owner's intent to measure the effectiveness of the training programs. Multiple options are available for this, including:

- Testing the owner's staff before and after training to quantify the amount of knowledge acquired. (See Section 4.2.2 in Chapter 4 for more details.)

- Surveying staff about the training to solicit their comments and suggestions for improvement. Surveys are typically distributed to attendees at the end of a training class.

- Administering oral tests at the end of the training session

A list of training deliverables. The list of training deliverables to be provided by the contractor should be specified in the OPR. The HFCxA should carefully review this list to assure the appropriate systems are covered and the level of detail is sufficient. These training deliverables can include the following:

- Access to various online resources for training support

- Access to phone numbers or help desks for training support

- Provision of training materials such as books, papers, presentations, DVDs, CDs, etc.

- Audio recordings of the training sessions for future reference and training programs

- Video recordings of the training sessions for future reference and training programs

- Physical samples or spare parts to be used for future training programs

The OPR should clearly state the form in which the owner wishes to obtain training information and deliverables—hard copy and/or electronic format. If necessary, include the number of copies of different materials the owner would like to receive.

Other training information to include in the OPR. The OPR document should clearly identify:

- Any training that will be provided by the owner

- Any follow-up training the owner will require after project occupancy

- The training venues desired by the owner (e.g., on-site training with a group of staff; on-site, one-on-one training with staff; classroom-style training; on-site vendor training; and off-site vendor training)

2.4 FACILITATE DEVELOPMENT OF THE BASIS OF DESIGN FOR SYSTEMS TO BE COMMISSIONED

The basis of design (BOD) is developed by the designer, owner, and HFCxA before schematic design begins and will shape the project design. With the OPR as a mandate for facility performance and operations, the BOD specifies criteria, requirements, and objectives that will influence selection and definition of most basic project features, including the building systems to be commissioned. Most of the BOD development effort is driven by the design team as part of its early conceptual work, so the HFCxA's role is to serve as a facilitator and catalyst for the process.

The BOD must be written so it provides clear direction for the design process. And it is important to develop it early enough for major project concerns to be identified and addressed before significant design work is done. Issues that typically arise include installation and maintenance space requirements for different types of HVAC systems, trade-offs between the cost and performance of exterior glass and its impact on building heat gain, emergency power provisions required for various systems and equipment, and so on.

The information in a detailed BOD is exceptionally valuable to the commissioning team as they evaluate the ability of a design and its components to meet the owner's project requirements. Material from the BOD documentation is seldom included in the drawings and specifications included in the construction documents as contractors generally do not need such information to meet their obligations. It is also different from the design or pricing narrative frequently used in the industry as a basis of design.

The objective of preparing detailed BOD documentation is to provide information that supports an understanding, at every phase in the project, of the underlying thinking that led to the selection of specific components, assemblies, systems, and methods for system integration. A design narrative that provides an overview of assemblies and systems in a verbal format is usually an integral element of the BOD.

2.4.1 BOD Content

Key elements of the basis of design are listed below:

(1) Applicable codes and standards

(2) Outdoor design conditions (e.g., geography, weather)

(3) Indoor design conditions (e.g., temperature, relative humidity, number of air changes)

(4) Expected building occupancy for all building uses (including nights, weekends, holidays, special events, etc.)

(5) Allowances for miscellaneous power loads for all building occupancies

(6) Illumination levels and controls for all building occupancies

(7) Allowances for other internal loads

(8) Ventilation, pressure relationships, and general indoor air quality requirements for all building occupancies

(9) Building pressurization requirements

(10) Anticipated maintenance management program

(11) Maintenance and service requirements for all commissioned systems

(12) Emergency situation performance criteria

(13) Acoustics criteria for the HVAC system

(14) Life safety criteria (fire protection, fire alarm, and smoke control)

(15) Sustainable design elements

(16) Energy conservation measures

2.5 REVIEW THE OPR AND BOD

The basis of design and owner's project requirements are dynamic, living documents that are continually updated throughout a project.

Meeting the OPR is the "definition of success" for a project, so it is important to review it in great detail. This document must be edited as the project proceeds to conform to changes in the owner's expectations for success. For example, if financial concerns impact the project scope and that fact changes the owner's expectations, those altered expectations must be reflected in the OPR.

The OPR should guide the commissioning scope of work and the intensity of the commissioning process for each system. Before schematic design begins, the HFCxA reviews the OPR to verify that it clearly communicates the owner's requirements to the design team and that it has been provided in a format that facilitates comparison with the BOD document the design team will develop and submit during the design phase. The HFCxA should also verify that the scope of work for the commissioning team matches the level of intensity required by the OPR with respect to the systems included in the project.

Ultimately, the HFCxA is responsible for comparing the BOD to the OPR to verify that the design team has met the owner's requirements and to identify any inconsistencies between the two documents. If inconsistencies are found, the HFCxA is responsible for resolving them by either changing the design (provided the designer agrees to the change) or changing the OPR (provided the owner agrees to change that document).

2.6 REVIEW THE DESIGN DOCUMENTS

Note: This section applies to the *Health Facility Commissioning Guidelines* sections on reviewing schematic design (2.6), design development (2.9), and construction (2.11) documents.

Intermediate milestone reviews of the design documents are critical to verify that the intent and direction of the OPR and BOD are being captured in the actual project documents that will go to the construction team. These reviews allow the HFCxA to assess whether individual project components, assemblies, distribution, controls, and equipment sizes and specifications are aligned with the goals and objectives of the OPR and BOD. At each stage of review, the HFCxA should evaluate whether the actual design meets those requirements.

For example, if the OPR and BOD include requirements for facility operation under emergency conditions (loss of utilities), the review at design milestones should verify provision of standby fuel and water, emergency utility connections, protection of equipment from airborne debris, provision of emergency power to critical components, and other elements needed to fulfill the goals stated in the OPR and BOD.

2.7 DEVELOP THE COMMISSIONING PLAN

The commissioning plan is the first deliverable required from the HFCxA. It must be detailed and completely describe the entire commissioning process, providing a step-by-step outline that assures the owner's project requirements are met during the construction process.

2.7.1 Development of the Plan

The commissioning plan begins with a table of contents that includes appropriate sections for the main phases of the commissioning process and any appendices that are needed. An introduction should provide a description of the scope of work for the project and describe in general terms the scope of commissioning services, focusing on the systems to be included in the commissioning process. If the intensity of the commissioning scope varies from system to system, that variation in intensity must be clearly communicated.

The systems to be commissioned for the project are identified in the commissioning plan. At the beginning of the design phase, the depth of detail will be very limited, and you may only be able to list the systems at the discipline level, such as HVAC, normal power, emergency power, and so on.

The commissioning plan should specify the members of the commissioning team, provide their contact information, and develop a task/responsibilities matrix for the group. Each step of the commissioning process should be listed in sequential order, and each team member's responsibilities during that step should be identified.

> **Sampling Inappropriate for Health Facility Commissioning**
>
> ASHRAE Guideline 0: *The Commissioning Process* permits "sampling" of commissioned systems and equipment, but this approach to systems commissioning should be avoided for health care projects because of the critical nature of building systems in health care facilities. When sampling is employed as part of a project, the level of system or equipment failure that would be acceptable must be identified in the OPR. In other words, if you choose to sample equipment of a given type, you must specify the percentage of failed tests that will be acceptable. If your answer is zero, then this system or type of equipment should not be tested using sampling.

A typical matrix of design phase commissioning responsibilities and tasks is included in Appendix 2-1 as an example.

The devices or forms to be used by the commissioning team to expedite communications should be set in the commissioning plan. These will vary according to the size and complexity of the project and the makeup of the commissioning team and should follow the communication protocol established for the project.

Often, the HFCxA uses a log of commissioning issues or action items as the primary means of communicating with the commissioning team. Such logs are used at different phases of a project to flag issues in design submittals that may require discussion and resolution.

Review all the tasks outlined in the commissioning plan with the design team as the project progresses through the design phase. Make sure these tasks support and are coordinated with the OPR. In the design phase section of the commissioning plan, specify the tasks the commissioning team will undertake during this phase. Commissioning team personnel may change and expand during the design phase, and any new team members need to be identified and added to the roles and responsibilities matrix for this phase. The HFCxA will develop the schedule for commissioning activities during the design phase and distribute it to the team for review and comment. The action item log may be continued, or a new log specific to this phase may be started.

2.7.2 Commissioning Plan Components

The following should be included in the commissioning plan:

(1) Overview

(2) List of equipment and systems

(3) Team roles

(4) Management and communication

(5) Deliverables

(6) Commissioning milestones

(7) Start-up

(8) Installation checklists

(9) Functional testing

(10) Training

(11) O&M manuals

(12) Opposite season testing and warranty reviews

2.8 PREPARE THE COMMISSIONING SPECIFICATIONS

2.8.1 Preparation of the Specifications

The design team may or may not prepare commissioning specifications for a project. If they do, the HFCxA will need to review the commissioning specifications to confirm they meet the needs of the specific project. If they do not, the HFCxA provides project-specific commissioning specifications for the design team to incorporate into the contract documents.

The commissioning specifications must clearly communicate the commissioning scope of work for the project and the contractors' responsibilities during the commissioning process. At a minimum, they should clearly state that contractors will participate in the commissioning process and delineate specific expectations for their participation.

To avoid confusion, the commissioning specifications must be carefully coordinated with all other specifications. The design team must review the commissioning specifications provided by the HFCxA and identify and resolve any discrepancies with the design specifications.

2.8.2 *Commissioning Specifications Elements*

At minimum, the following should be included in the commissioning specifications:

(1) Commissioning team involvement

(2) Contractor's responsibilities

(3) Submittals and submittal review procedures for HFCxA process/ systems

(4) Operation and maintenance documentation/systems manual requirements

(5) Number of project meetings related to commissioning and which commissioning team members are obligated to participate

(6) Construction verification procedures

(7) Start-up plan development and implementation

(8) Functional performance test procedures

(9) Acceptance and closeout procedures

(10) Training requirements, including development of a training plan

(11) Warranty review site visit

2.9 REVIEW THE DESIGN DEVELOPMENT DOCUMENTS
(Refer to Section 2.6 in this chapter.)

2.10 REVIEW THE HVAC OR BAS CONTROL SYSTEM SEQUENCES OF OPERATION

The building automation system (BAS) is the most critical and difficult system to commission because it must interface accurately with numerous building systems (e.g., HVAC, lighting, fire alarm, security, and fire protection systems) and therefore its installation must be coordinated with the work of multiple trade contractors.

The commissioning review of the BAS should verify control sequences for all components and systems to be commissioned as well as integrated functional operations between other systems such as the fire alarm, essential electrical power, and security systems.

Critical to proper BAS operation are the sequences of operation, which are typically developed by the BAS contractor in response to a performance-level BAS specification provided by the design engineer. The sequences must be developed so the system operation meets the intent of the OPR and the BOD.

To assure building energy efficiency targets and operational requirements are met, the detailed sequences of operation must address all factors affecting intended performance, including adjustable setpoints, non-adjustable setpoints, weekly schedules, alarms, warnings, trends, and energy-efficient processes. The HFCxA should carefully review these sequences and make certain they contain adequate detail and will result in the desired system performance.

Later in the commissioning process, BAS functional testing will include verification of all control sequences for equipment and systems being commissioned, including verification of sample control points as well as of the functional operations of systems with integrated functions.

2.11 REVIEW THE CONSTRUCTION DOCUMENTS

(Refer to Section 2.6 in this chapter.)

2.12 UPDATE THE COMMISSIONING PLAN AND COMMISSIONING SPECIFICATIONS

Initial development of the commissioning plan and specifications is usually done early in the design phase of a project. At that point, the scope of the overall project may be fairly well defined, but the exact scope of each system to be commissioned could still be generic and abstract in nature. As a result, the initial commissioning plan and specs will likely include generic checklists and test procedures based on the general system type expected without much detail.

As an example, early information about the HVAC control refrigeration system may only state that the project will use water-cooled centrifugal chillers, with no detail as to the quantity and capacity of the chillers, piping arrangement, control methodology, or component location. As the design is developed and those details are defined, the commissioning plan and specs should be continually updated and modified to reflect the required work. For instance, as a generic HVAC refrigeration system becomes further defined, it is determined whether its distribution will be of a primary/secondary type, a variable primary type, or another type, each of which requires a different pre-functional testing and start-up procedure.

Events that frequently prompt updates to the commissioning plan and specifications include these:

(1) **Development of project phasing.** Whether the project is all new construction, renovation, or a combination of both, the exact sequential phasing of construction frequently evolves along with the design. This evolution can have a huge impact on the commissioning process. Systems that need to be shut down for modifications and then restarted

have unique commissioning requirements and, depending on project scope, some systems might have to be shut down more than once over the course of the project. In other situations, a system may need to be put into service to serve an early phase of the project and would therefore have to be commissioned early. That system might also serve areas built in subsequent phases, so the commissioning process would have to be repeated. To serve the early phase, the system might have to run at a partial or low load level, which would require a different approach to commissioning than the one appropriate for running the system at normal load levels.

(2) **Value engineering or analysis effort.** Value engineering or other management efforts intended to reconcile discrepancies between estimated costs and the budget can lead to changes in system components (vendor, style, type, etc.) or layout (location, distribution, or access), and these changes affect the commissioning process. As such modifications are considered and decisions made, the commissioning plan and specs must be updated to keep them coordinated with the current system design, start-up procedure, and operations.

(3) **Determination of exact location and quantities of components.** The commissioning plan and specs must address each individual component in terms of pre-functional testing, start-up procedure, and operation. Systems often have multiple components (e.g., reheat/variable volume terminals, fire/smoke dampers, medical gas alarm stations) that must be individually verified for proper operation. As these components are identified, sized, and located in the project, the commissioning plan must be updated to accommodate each component.

Typically, the commissioning plan and specs should be 90 percent complete early in the construction documentation phase. The availability of system schedule sheets (for equipment specifications, capacities, and quantities), control system sequences of operation, and component locations are critical to final development of these documents.

2.13 FACILITATE DEVELOPMENT OF THE UTILITY MANAGEMENT PLAN

During the development of the ASHE *Health Facility Commissioning Guidelines*, there was much discussion and debate as to whether a section on development of a facility utility management plan (UMP) should be part of that document. To some degree, this task would seem to be outside the purview of the commissioning process. However, it was finally decided that effective development of the UMP involves the entire design and construction team and thus, to the degree the HFCxA is part of that team, UMP development should be part of the health facility commissioning process. This inclusion is not intended to imply that the HFCxA leads this process. Rather, it was included to present a best-practice approach and to show HFCxA involvement in a support role.

2.13.1 Purpose of the UMP

To qualify for reimbursement from the Centers for Medicare & Medicaid Services (CMS), hospitals and other health care facilities must comply with the CMS Conditions of Participation (for an explanation of this, see Section 2.13.1 in the *Health Facility Commissioning Handbook*). The Joint Commission and several other organizations accredit health care facilities, deeming that they are in compliance with CMS requirements. In the *2011 Joint Commission Comprehensive Accreditation Manual for Hospitals*, facilities are required to have a comprehensive utility management plan.

The entire project team should be aware that the project is likely to be subject to an accreditation survey within weeks or even days of initial occupancy, which means an effective UMP must be in place simultaneous with occupancy.

2.13.2 Process for Development

(1) Take advantage of early development opportunities. In many projects, the opportunity is missed to leverage information readily available during the standard design and construction process for use in developing a utility management plan. When this happens, the facility manager is left with the difficult task of trying to re-create, duplicate, or retrieve information during the initial occupancy of a new facility or expanded or renovated areas in an existing facility.

For example, one element of an UMP might be testing and certification documentation for fire/smoke dampers, medical gas outlets, or elements of the fire protection system. The installing contractor for these systems, as part of the normal course of construction and testing, is required by the contract documents and the commissioning plan to submit test data. If those contractors were instructed to follow test procedures and document results in a format that meets the requirements of relevant deeming authorities (the Joint Commission, etc.), this information could be incorporated in the UMP, relieving the facility manager of one task that must be accomplished prior to initial occupancy.

The same opportunity might be available to satisfy requirements for system riser diagrams, locations of emergency shutoff valves and emergency backup connections, and the delineation of areas served by various systems. The design team often develops these types of documents as a matter of course during the design process, and if they could be tailored to meet regulatory requirements, the facility manager would not be forced to re-create them after construction.

Other examples of material developed during the design phase that can be used later to save time and effort for the facility staff include:

(a) The commissioning plan could be used as a starting point for identifying system components that need to be documented in the written inventory of building systems in the UMP. The plan already identifies each equipment component and specifies its start-up/test procedures. This information could provide a head start for the facility manager to begin building a preventive maintenance or computerized maintenance management system (CMMS).

(b) Documentation developed for training sessions could be used to build the written descriptions of operating procedures, both normal and emergency. As the owner's staff is trained to operate each system and its components, this information could be used to meet system operational and management documentation requirements for the UMP.

(c) Development or modification of the facility life safety plan could be coordinated with design work needed to maintain required occupancy separations, fire resistive-rated partitions, smoke barriers, suite separations, exit passageways, and corridor walls.

(2) The process. For a new facility, the UMP will have to be created from scratch, while for an expansion or renovation project the existing UMP can be modified or updated. At the outset of the design phase, the project team should determine what needs to be done and how the necessary elements will be produced. The process could include these steps:

(a) Start with an UMP matrix, and revise the elements in accordance with the scope of the project.

See Appendix 2-2 for a sample UMP matrix.

(b) Identify which member of the project team will be responsible for each element.

(c) Decide on target dates for when intermediate and final documentation will be drafted, reviewed, and submitted.

(d) Develop a sign-off confirmation procedure to assure that each element has been completed.

(e) Assign responsibility for monitoring the progress for each element to assure timely completion.

This process should be discussed in the predesign commissioning conference to assure that each team member's scope of work includes the task assigned to him or her. To achieve optimum clarity, this documentation also needs to be coordinated with the commissioning plan and specifications.

(3) The HFCxA's role. To repeat, the HFCxA might not have a lead role in this process, but he or she should be able to provide beneficial input and oversight. The owner can decide on a project-by-project basis the degree to which the HFCxA will be involved with UMP development.

2.13.3 UMP Components

See Section 2.13.3 in the *Health Facility Commissioning Guidelines* for a list of UMP components.

2.14 ATTEND THE PRE-BIDDING CONFERENCE

The pre-bidding conference is the primary opportunity for the construction team to review the scope of the commissioning process with the construction team, including the construction manager, general contractor, and primary trade contractors such as mechanical, electrical, controls, test and balance, and others who may be involved with the commissioning process.

Not all projects are bid per se—some are negotiated, in some construction team members are selected through a process like GMP (guaranteed maximum price) pricing, and some use an integrated project delivery approach. No matter what the project delivery approach calls for, however, the HFCxA should conduct a conference similar to a pre-bidding conference prior to final establishment of the builder's scope of services and cost. A pre-bidding conference is intended to assure that construction team members fully understand the commissioning process prior to establishing their bid, and this goal is the same no matter what project delivery method is used. However, different project delivery methods may require different modes to communicate the intended commissioning process.

As mentioned above, a central purpose of the pre-bidding conference is to convey the scope of the commissioning process to the construction team. This scope is usually summarized in the commissioning plan and specifications, both of which should be complete at this stage of the project. The HFCxA should review those documents with the contractors and answer any related questions. Minutes of the meeting should be kept and distributed, as they will note any clarifications made to the commissioning requirements.

The pre-bidding conference should, at minimum, accomplish the following:

(1) Clarify the scope of the commissioning process.

(2) Provide the construction team with a thorough overview of the commissioning process before their contract terms have been finalized.

(3) Review in detail the expectations and responsibilities of the various trade contractors.

(4) Identify the specific parts of the contract documents that refer to the commissioning plan and specifications and their requirements.

Construction Phase

3.1 CONDUCT THE COMMISSIONING CONFERENCE

After the bidding or other pricing of the construction documents is complete and before construction starts, the health facility commissioning authority (HFCxA) organizes the commissioning conference. This meeting is chaired by the HFCxA and attended by appropriate representatives from the owner, contractor, subcontractors, and design team. Its purpose is to review the commissioning plan and specifications to make certain all parties fully understand the commissioning process and their roles and responsibilities in it. The HFCxA presents a review of how the commissioning process will be integrated into the overall construction process and discusses milestone activities and the sequence for commissioning tasks. The commissioning conference should specifically address the process for submittal review and approval that is described in the project manual and commissioning specifications.

3.1.1 Scheduling the Commissioning Conference

The HFCxA coordinates the meeting schedule with the project team. The meeting should occur before the project reaches the stage when shop drawings of equipment to be commissioned are submitted. Often it is scheduled to coincide with a regularly scheduled OAC (owner, architect, and contractor) meeting.

The HFCxA invites the owner's representative, the architect's construction phase administrator, and lead design representatives from the mechanical, electrical, IT, life safety, and other disciplines included in the commissioning scope of work. The HFCxA works with the construction team to ensure attendance by project managers and superintendents from the trades installing the systems to be commissioned. In some cases, a vendor may be invited to attend.

Invitees should include representatives responsible for design, construction, installation, and testing of the following building elements:

(1) Mechanical systems

    (a) Building automation system (BAS)

    (b) HVAC system

    (c) Testing, adjusting, and balancing (TAB) of air and hydronic systems

(2) Electrical systems

    (a) Lighting controls

    (b) Emergency generator

    (c) Paralleling switchgear/automatic transfer switches

    (d) Fire alarm

    (e) IT—Nurse call, paging, security, etc.

    (f) Others as needed

(3) Plumbing systems

    (a) Domestic hot and cold water systems

    (b) Reverse osmosis/deionization (RO/DI)

    (c) Fuel oil

    (d) Medical gas

    (e) Pumping systems such as storm and sanitary pumps

(4) Fire protection system

(5) Vertical transport system

(6) Building envelope elements

(7) Others as needed

3.1.2 Agenda for the Commissioning Conference

The HFCxA prepares an agenda and distributes it to the attendees prior to the meeting. At a minimum, the agenda should include the following:

(1) A general discussion that recaps the scope of commissioning for the project

(2) Roles and responsibilities of each team member (documented in a responsibility matrix)

(3) Integration of the commissioning process into the project schedule

    (a) Items in the schedule to be integrated include:

       (i) Natural gas service

      (ii) Water service

    (iii) Electrical service

    (iv) Commissioning items as indicated in Section 3.5 of this chapter

  (b) Closely monitoring the building service progress—particularly the permit process—is critical for timely project completion. Without utility service, equipment cannot be started, which directly affects the schedule for TAB work and functional testing.

(4) Anticipated commissioning meeting frequency

(5) Anticipated means of disseminating communications about commissioning to the project team

(6) Reviews the HFCxA will be conducting

  (a) Documentation and processes to be reviewed may include these:

       (i) Shop drawings

      (ii) Record drawings

    (iii) Pressure testing

    (iv) Cleaning and flushing

     (v) Start-up procedures

    (vi) Training process

   (vii) Testing, adjusting, and balancing (TAB)

  (viii) Certifications (fire alarm system, medical gas)

    (ix) O&M manuals

  (b) Discuss review procedures:

       (i) How the information should be forwarded to the HFCxA

      (ii) How the review comments from the HFCxA will be distributed to the team

    (iii) How the project team will address review comments

(7) Milestone activities. The HFCxA should discuss what will occur during these key phases of the project and how the project team will work together to support these activities. Milestone activities include:

  (a) Shop drawing phase

  (b) Site visits by the HFCxA

       (i) Installation documentation (pre-functional checklist execution)

       (ii) O&M staff tours during construction

  (c) Start-up of systems, including the use of building systems for temporary heating and cooling (if planned)

  (d) Owner training

  (e) HVAC testing, adjusting, and balancing

  (f) BAS system calibration and point-to-point verification

  (g) Functional testing

  (h) Integrated systems testing

  (i) Project turnover

       (i) Final report

       (ii) O&M manuals

       (iii) Systems manual

       (iv) Dashboards

       (v) HVAC trends

       (vi) Measurement and verification (M&V)

  (j) Opposite season testing

  (k) End-of-warranty period review and meetings

(8) Commissioning deliverables. The HFCxA should discuss all commissioning deliverables to be provided during the commissioning process and the distribution requirements for these items. The deliverables include:

  (a) Reports from reviews listed above

  (b) Meeting minutes

  (c) Site visit reports, including issues log

  (d) Functional testing and integrated systems testing documentation

  (e) Commissioning progress reports

  (f) Final report

  (g) Systems manual

See Appendix 3-1 for a sample commissioning conference agenda.

(9) Resolution of incomplete items from the issues log. The meeting should address expectations for how deficiencies will be resolved and how responses to questions that require action by various members of the project team will be coordinated.

3.1.3 Meeting Wrap-Up

Before closing the meeting, the HFCxA should review near-term objectives in the commissioning process. The schedule for the next commissioning meeting should be discussed in relation to the near-term objectives and milestones. The HFCxA assures that attendance is documented for the meeting and prepares and distributes meeting minutes.

3.2 DEVELOP AND MAINTAIN THE ISSUES LOG

During the course of design, construction, and postoccupancy activities, the HFCxA creates and maintains a log of all identified issues and concerns that affect the commissioning process.

3.2.1 Purpose of the Log During Project Delivery

The purpose of the log is to track items that require resolution by the design team, the construction team, the owner, or the commissioning team to assure they are resolved before they affect the overall project schedule.

The log documents issues related to the design, construction, and commissioning efforts. Each entry includes the following:

(1) A description of the issue

(2) The date the issue was identified

(3) A proposed corrective plan

(4) The party responsible for responding

(5) The date of anticipated resolution

(6) Current status of the item

The log should be addressed at each commissioning meeting and included in the meeting minutes. It should also be included as an attachment to each site visit report and each project commissioning status report. If items require immediate attention or are not addressed in a timely manner, it may be necessary to call a meeting of part or all of the commissioning team or to bring the issue before a regularly scheduled OAC (owner, architect, and contractor) meeting.

3.2.2 The Log as a Record

At the completion of the project, the issues log documentation provides a comprehensive list of all commissioning-related issues and how they were resolved; it must be included in the final commissioning report as a record of this activity. The log can be used to organize the items the commissioning team noted during the commissioning process into categories such as energy

See Appendix 3-2 for a sample
issues log.

concerns, life safety issues, missing equipment, design clarifications, and so on. It serves as a concrete illustration of the return on investment (ROI) realized from the commissioning process.

3.3 REVIEW SUBMITTAL DATA AND SHOP DRAWINGS

3.3.1 Equipment Selection

The process of reviewing all submittal documents related to the commissioned systems is very important to the O&M team because it is the last opportunity to identify acceptable manufacturers before the project team commits to equipment purchases.

The design team frequently includes in the specifications several manufacturers and/or equipment models that would be acceptable choices for a particular product or service; however, selection of an unspecified "approved equal" is often allowed. Based on past experience, the O&M staff may determine that such unspecified "approved equal" products and services are less than equal in quality, features, durability, maintainability, access to vendors, and so on. Thus, the HFCxA performs a crucial function by introducing insight from the O&M staff to help the project team judge the suitability of a proposed product or service.

3.3.2 Sample Review Criteria

Criteria the O&M staff consider in reviewing products and services may include the following:

(1) Cost difference

(2) Cost deviation from the owner's group purchasing agreement

(3) Performance

(4) Parts availability

(5) Service in the area (availability, response time)

(6) Availability of experienced, factory-trained service team

(7) Reliability record of the product

(8) Length of product life cycle

(9) Compatibility with other equipment in the hospital

(10) Owner's preference

3.4 REVIEW OPERATIONS & MAINTENANCE MANUALS

If the specifications do not require the O&M manuals to be submitted for approval immediately after approval of the shop drawings, the HFCxA should work with the contractor and commissioning team to assure they are submitted as soon as possible after the shop drawing process. This timing makes these essential reference manuals available to facility staff prior to the O&M training process and allows any needed corrections to be made before training takes place.

The HFCxA and O&M staff review considers whether the manuals contain the information and guidance needed for effective operation and maintenance of the commissioned systems and equipment. The HFCxA prepares a written list of comments generated by their collective review and forwards them to the design team. The design team incorporates these comments into the design team review or provides an explanation as to why they were not included. Comments and concerns not incorporated into the formal review by the design team are discussed and resolved by the project team.

3.5 CONDUCT COMMISSIONING MEETINGS

During construction, the HFCxA conducts meetings to facilitate commissioning activities. These commissioning meetings are part of the process defined in the initial commissioning conference described in Section 3.1 above.

At a minimum, milestone meetings should be held at the beginning of each commissioning phase to review requirements for team activities during the upcoming phase. Key milestones include:

(1) Shop drawing submittals

(2) Equipment installation and pre-functional checklists

(3) Equipment start-up

(4) BAS calibration verification

(5) HVAC system testing and balancing

(6) Functional performance testing and integrated systems testing

(7) Submission of O&M manuals

(8) Owner training

(9) Project closeout and postoccupancy activities

See Appendix 3-3 for a sample commissioning milestone meeting agenda.

3.5.1 Shop Drawings and Other Submittals

This meeting should occur before shop drawings and other submittal documents have been submitted for review. The project construction team should develop a register that identifies the shop drawings and other submittals to be reviewed, including when the team will submit them for review. This schedule should be discussed, and the HFCxA should identify which submittals are related to the commissioning scope of work and will require review by the HFCxA and the O&M staff. Agreement should also be reached as to how the shop drawings and submittals will be distributed to the HFCxA (i.e., whether they will be provided electronically, posted to a project website, or in paper copies).

A timeframe for the reviews should be determined. Generally, shop drawing reviews must be conducted early enough to allow timely procurement of equipment and systems. Sometimes initial submissions to design team members are not found acceptable and resubmission is required. Therefore, it is important that the HFCxA and O&M staff only review submissions that have already been approved by design team professionals.

At this milestone meeting, the HFCxA and the O&M staff should determine ways to coordinate their review—including turnaround times and frameworks for incorporating their comments—that add to the efficiency of the overall process. As well, the meeting should address how the project team will resolve any issues that arise if the design team discounts or does not respond to concerns expressed by the HFCxA and O&M staff.

Additional meetings may be required to address all commissioning concerns related to this milestone. For example, critical submissions such as the BAS controls, essential system load precedence sequences, and fire alarm sequences often require separate meetings to coordinate sequences of operation.

3.5.2 Equipment Installation and Pre-Functional Checklists

Before equipment is installed, the process for executing and documenting installation should be discussed at a milestone meeting. Unlike some commissioning standards, the ASHE health facility commissioning process requires confirmation of installation in phases, as the installation occurs. Therefore, the HFCxA should describe how progress reports on installation will be distributed and the process by which any deficiencies will be resolved. Plans for maintaining a log of the overall progress of installation of the various systems should also be presented.

Interim meetings may be required to discuss installation progress or deviations and to review expectations for completion. Generally, installation of systems and execution of items on pre-functional checklists should be completed prior to equipment start-up and functional testing. Completion of pre-functional checklist items should be emphasized to all parties as a prerequisite to the testing process.

3.5.3 Equipment Start-Up

This milestone meeting should occur well before start-up actually takes place to initiate preparations for both starting the equipment and maintaining it after start-up. The meeting should focus on requirements for developing and submitting the start-up plan and for executing it. O&M staff should be invited to attend this and follow-up meetings on equipment start-up as well as to witness the start-up process.

Additional meetings should be scheduled to plan the actual start-up of systems after the start-up plan has been approved. These meetings should include discussions related to the flushing and cleaning of hydronic systems; filtration and protection of air-side systems; protection of sensitive equipment such as variable frequency drives (VFDs) that will be operating in a construction environment; chemical treatment of hydronic systems; and the maintenance and monitoring of system operations, including defining minimal safety requirements to protect the systems while they are not operating under full automatic control. Standards should be established for monitoring and documenting that equipment and systems are properly maintained and operated until turnover to the owner. For example, chemical water treatment records should be maintained for boilers, cooling towers, and closed hydronic systems. As well, meters on equipment sensitive to frequent starting and stopping (e.g., chillers, boilers) should be used to monitor the number of starts.

3.5.4 HVAC System Testing, Adjusting, and Balancing

The HVAC system testing, adjusting, and balancing (TAB) process is a critical prerequisite to functional performance testing. The TAB process documents that HVAC loads are being properly served by the HVAC equipment, while the functional testing process verifies that HVAC systems function as intended by the designers. It is critically important to conduct functional tests only after the TAB process has confirmed the equipment is loaded per design. The TAB process thus must be organized and planned to assure that functional testing can be properly scheduled into the overall project timetable.

The TAB milestone meeting should occur before the TAB process begins so it can address the coordination needed between the TAB process and the commissioning process to assure that functional testing is integrated into the construction schedule before project completion.

Additional coordination meetings may be required as the TAB effort progresses through the facility.

3.5.5 Building Automation System

A plan should be implemented to monitor the progress of the installation, calibration verification, and programming of the BAS system. Any steps in the plan that have a direct effect on functional performance testing should be entered into the project schedule and the schedule updated on a regular basis. The main items of concern are power to the controls, a point-to-point check, sensor calibration, and confirmation from the BAS contractor that the sequences of operation have been pretested successfully. This work must be accomplished and confirmed in writing before functional testing is performed.

3.5.6 Functional Testing and Integrated Systems Testing

A systems functional testing plan should be developed to define when and in what order (where applicable) systems will be tested. Produced by the HFCxA in conjunction with the commissioning team, the testing plan should focus on the interdependence between completion of the systems; testing, adjusting, and balancing; and completion of the building elements.

This milestone meeting should focus on scheduling functional testing and identifying the team members needed to support the process and schedule defined by the testing plan. Additional meetings will be required to refine the testing process as it progresses and to address resolution of any deficiencies discovered.

Once functional testing is complete, integrated systems testing (IST) can proceed. This involves multiple systems—HVAC controls, fire alarm and fire protection systems, the essential electrical system, the security system, vertical transport, and so on. Similar to the process followed in planning and executing functional testing, an IST plan should be developed and meetings should be held to plan and review integrated systems testing. All testing must be coordinated with ongoing construction completion progress and, at times, with the owner's need to ready the facility by moving in furniture, stocking the facility, and making other preparations for occupancy.

Functional tests that require outdoor temperatures to be within a certain range must be scheduled when climatic conditions allow (i.e., testing of humidifiers, preheat coils, and water-side and air-side economizers). Often these tests are conducted after construction is complete and months after owner occupancy, but they should be conducted before the end of the one-year warranty period. The planning for conducting these tests will require preparatory meetings.

3.5.7 Submission of Operations and Maintenance Manuals

During the construction phase, a milestone meeting should be held to review when the O&M manuals are required to be completed and submitted, what their format should be, and how they will be reviewed—first, in submitted form, by the design team; then, in approved form, by the HFCxA.

3.5.8 Owner Training

A milestone meeting should be held to discuss training for the facility staff and to initiate planning for this training. Requirements for the training plan and its submission and approval process should be reviewed. This meeting should occur during the construction phase and significantly before training is to begin. Additional meetings will be required to plan the training and to coordinate it with O&M staff schedules and commitments.

3.5.9 Project Closeout and Postoccupancy Activities

Near the end of the construction phase, a milestone meeting should be held to discuss the project closeout process and the postoccupancy activities of the commissioning team. Initial plans should be discussed for these postoccupancy requirements, which include opposite season testing, end-of-warranty review of performance and maintenance issues related to the commissioned systems, measurement and verification (M&V), BAS trending, and development of maintenance dashboards.

3.6 ATTEND SELECTED PROJECT MEETINGS

In addition to commissioning meetings, the HFCxA should periodically attend regular project team meetings—often referred to as OAC (owner, architect, and contractor) meetings—where the status of the commissioning process may be briefly discussed. Although attendance at every OAC meeting is unnecessary, the HFCxA should attend these meetings with some minimum degree of regularity.

The HFCxA should review project team meeting agendas and be alert to the presence of items that would impact the commissioning scope, project schedule, or commissioning process. As well, the minutes from every meeting should be reviewed for items that may impact commissioning. As the project progresses toward completion, the HFCxA should attend more of the project team meetings. When feasible, the HFCxA should coordinate site visits to coincide with OAC meeting dates.

A clear understanding between the owner and the HFCxA about the HFCxA's responsibility to attend OAC meetings should be defined in the commissioning scope.

3.7 LEAD O&M STAFF CONSTRUCTION SITE TOURS

An important factor in achieving a successful project is involvement of O&M staff, including providing them with regular access to the project site. The HFCxA therefore must plan regular site tours for facility staff and coordinate these with their schedules, the number of shifts, and the areas of expertise of the O&M staff. These tours expose staff to various stages of completion, such as rough-in, above ceiling, start-up, and functional performance testing. Staff members gain knowledge of the location of various building elements that will be concealed by finishes as construction progresses. They also gain an understanding of how the building systems are designed to operate through descriptions of the elements of the OPR and sequences of operation provided by the HFCxA during the tours.

During site tours, the HFCxA also listens to and documents the staff's comments and concerns. Using the standard issues log format, the HFCxA maintains a list of staff comments and concerns and works with the contractor and design team to respond to them. The commissioning team often gains significant insight from the staff about the systems to be commissioned. Issues that are raised may need to be addressed by the HFCxA or by the entire commissioning team.

Another goal of the tours is to facilitate the maintenance staff's involvement in and commitment to a positive construction outcome. Staff who consider themselves stakeholders in a project are better equipped to carry out their responsibilities as the commissioning process continues into the postoccupancy period.

3.8 COMPLETE PRE-FUNCTIONAL CHECKLISTS AND INSPECTIONS

The HFCx process uses pre-functional checklists (PFCs) to document whether commissioned equipment and systems have been installed in accordance with the requirements of the design documents. These checklists, based on the requirements of the plans and specifications, combine and classify by category all installation requirements for a particular piece of equipment. The checklists are created during the design phase and must be updated during the construction phase to reflect any modifications that occur as a result of shop drawing reviews or scope revisions. Once these updates have been incorporated, the PFCs are executed in phases as the work progresses (e.g., equipment installation, piping rough-in, electrical rough-in, controls rough-in, and feeder and load side termination for electrical systems).

See a sample pre-functional checklist in Appendix 3-4.

If it is not feasible for the HFCxA or the owner to perform the PFCs, this task can be carried out by other members of the commissioning team, including the contractor or the design team. However, when pre-functional checklists and inspections are executed by the contractor or design team, the HFCxA should periodically review a random selection of representative completed PFCs to assure consistency and quality.

3.8.1 Integration into Construction Schedule

The execution of the PFCs must be integrated into the overall construction schedule, and the HFCxA must work with the project team to assure that key installation milestones are included in the construction schedule. Site visits to document installation must be scheduled to correspond with the phases of installation for all systems.

3.8.2 Mechanical and Plumbing Equipment

The checks listed below are to be defined for each piece of mechanical and plumbing equipment included in the pre-functional checklists. Project-specific requirements are compiled when the PFCs are created in the design phases and updated if revisions occur during the shop drawing phase.

(1) **Equipment installation.** Review installed equipment for access, maintainability, and coordination with other equipment in the space. Confirm equipment has been installed as designed and submitted. Obtain equipment nameplate data such as model numbers, motor horsepower and efficiency ratings, pump impeller sizing, pump nameplate performance criteria, and so on. Confirm equipment is mounted as required, with specified inertia bases, housekeeping pads, vibration isolation on chillers, and so on. Document that terminal boxes, in-duct humidifiers, reheat coils, etc. have been installed where required and are accessible.

(2) **Pipe and duct rough-in.** Confirm that elements in the piping are as specified for valving, hydronic specialties, balancing devices, and so on and that these elements are arranged as specified in the contract documents for items including, but not limited to, these:

   (a) Coil headers

   (b) Pumps

   (c) Cooling towers

   (d) Chillers

   (e) Heat exchangers

   (f) Steam pressure-reducing stations

   (g) Humidifiers

   (h) Boilers

   (i) Deaerators

   (j) Domestic hot water heaters and recirculating systems

   (k) Medical air compressors

   (l) Vacuum pumps

  (m) Water softeners

   (n) Backflow prevention equipment

Document that specialty devices such as hydronic gauges and thermometers are readily observable from the equipment room floor. Confirm that piping arrangements allow for ready access and maintainability for coil pull or service to equipment such as chillers and heat exchangers. Document that ductwork is configured as required for efficient system operation, plenums have been constructed as specified, filters are accessible and arranged as shown on the design documents, and dampers (e.g., return, relief, and outside air dampers) are arranged as shown on the design documents and are accessible. Confirm by spot checks that the return, supply, and exhaust ducts are made of the specified material in the specified metal thickness or gauge.

(3) **BAS device rough-in.** Confirm that safeties such as freezestats and duct high-limit sensors have been installed where shown on the design documents and that sensing elements are of the type specified and have been installed to protect the equipment as intended. Confirm that smoke detectors have been installed where shown on the design documents, and as required by the manufacturer, and that access is provided to service devices that require servicing. Verify that sensing devices such as flow meters, airflow-measuring stations, and temperature and pressure sensors are of the type specified and have been installed as required by the design documents.

(4) **Insulation and labeling.** Document that the insulation used is the type that was specified (foamglass, fiberglass, calcium silicate), that the vapor barriers are as specified, and that both have been installed where required. Confirm that elements in the piping system (valve bodies, thermometer welds, strainers) are insulated as specified and that, if accessibility is required for service, such access is provided. Confirm that all labeling devices such as pipe labels, equipment tags, valve tags, VFD labels, and electrical disconnect tags are as specified and that the nomenclature used is correct. Verify that the labels are secured as required. If color coding is required, document that it has been used as specified.

3.8.3 Electrical Equipment

The checks listed below are to be defined for each piece of equipment included in the PFCs. The project-specific requirements are compiled when the PFCs are created in the design phases and updated when revisions occur during the shop drawing phase.

(1) **Equipment and can installation.** Confirm that equipment layout conforms to design requirements and electrical working clearances are being maintained. Document that housekeeping pads have been installed as required.

(2) **Feeder and circuit rough-in and termination.** Spot-check feeder sizing and document that feeders are being pulled in place properly. Confirm by spot-checking that specified materials (insulation type, lug nut sizing, and conductor type) have been used. Review termination procedures for proper torque. Confirm that feeders are being color coded properly. Spot-check branch circuit sizing and color coding. Confirm proper separation of circuits by voltage and by normal or essential system.

(3) **Final rough-in review prior to energizing.** For unit substations, switchgear, paralleling gear, and so on, review final installation of feeders, grounding, conduit termination, waterproofing, sealing, etc. before gear is energized with permanent power. Document that adjustable settings in switchgear are as required by the electrical coordination study. For generators, document the discharge plenum installation, outside intakes, control dampers, fuel oil piping arrangements, day tank configuration, etc.

(4) **Labeling and directories.** Confirm that all labeling devices such as equipment tags and individual tags for devices in motor control centers are as specified. Document that the nomenclature (i.e., the naming systems for the various branches of the essential system) is correctly used and that the labels are secured as required. Document that any required color coding is used as specified. Document that the panel directories have been provided and installed in the format required. Confirm that the degree of detail required for identifying each load is specific rather than generic (e.g., "receptacles in space XYZ" instead of "receptacles").

3.8.4 Site Visit Protocol

Site visits should be scheduled to complete a specific phase of the scope such as review of equipment installation, ducting or piping of equipment, or installation of electrical distribution equipment prior to energizing switchgear. Site visits should be scheduled with the project team to accommodate any team members who want to participate and to allow the owner's O&M staff to observe.

(1) **Pre-visit coordination.** Before making a site visit, the HFCxA should confirm with the project team that the state of installation is far enough along to allow the desired checks to be made during the visit.

(2) **Exit debrief meeting.** Before leaving the site, the HFCxA should review the findings from the visit with the project team members present. This should be a verbal debriefing of what will be documented in the site visit report. This debrief meeting should address whether

the HFCxA was able to accomplish the mission of the visit, and items found to be installed in accordance with the requirements should be generally discussed. Any items that may require the HFCxA to obtain an interpretation from the design team or owner's representative for later resolution should be mentioned, and items that will be added to the issues log should be reviewed. The HFCxA should discuss a schedule for correcting any deficiencies noted during the visit with the construction team. Before subsequent site visits are scheduled, the construction team should document that all items on the issues log have been corrected.

(3) **Site visit reports.** A report should be written to document the findings of each site visit. This should summarize the purpose of the visit and state whether it was achieved. The report should identify the major elements of the commissioning scope of work that were completed during the visit, cite any major deficiencies discovered, and list action items for follow-up. Any items that deviate from design requirements but are deemed acceptable by the design team and the owner should be noted. Some deviations may be acceptable to the design team but not to the owner, and resolution of such items must be documented. The report should discuss the short-term schedule for future site visits to execute PFCs and assess the overall completion of installation versus the overall project construction schedule. Each site visit report should include a current issues log. Photographs should be used to document items of significant concern.

3.8.5 Completion of Pre-Functional Checklists

The installation of all elements of a piece of equipment or a system should be finished before functional testing occurs. Installations that are not complete when functional testing begins are a deficiency to be added to the master issue logs. Completed PFCs become a part of the commissioning record and are included in the final commissioning report. Installation items not completed before functional testing should be specifically noted in the final report.

3.9 REVIEW BUILDING AUTOMATION SYSTEM PROGRAMMING

Frequently, the way the sequence of operation for a building system or piece of equipment is described in text format in the design documents differs from the way the actual control program is written by the design engineer. One cause for this disparity is that the original text format sequence often lacks the clarity and detail a control system programmer needs to write a program. When this is the case, the BAS programmer should contact the design engineer to obtain the additional information needed. The original text format sequence should then be revised and incorporated into the final approved control system submittal. Too often, this revision does not occur, and the original text format sequence appears in the approved control system submittal without clarifying details.

The failure to communicate sufficient detail in the original text format sequence can result in the programmer misinterpreting the designer's intent or making assumptions regarding the designer's intent in order to meet the project schedule. This communication gap needs to be addressed before the program is written in order to avoid unexpected delays and costly reprogramming during the commissioning process.

To mitigate the effects of such communication gaps, the HFCxA, design engineer, and control system programmer should meet and review the actual set of process control algorithms residing in the controllers to confirm that the algorithms meet the design engineer's intent, match the sequence of operation contained in the approved submittal, and are compatible with the functional performance test written for the system. Since there are almost as many programming languages as there are control companies, the HFCxA and design engineer will almost certainly need the assistance of the control system programmer in deciphering the program's algorithms or steps.

Often this detailed review of a sequence of operation program will raise questions regarding the clarity and completeness of the approved sequence of operation and whether the actual process control program can implement the design intent. When these kinds of issues arise, they should be added to the HFCx issues log to assure they are addressed and so their resolution can be tracked.

Another goal of the BAS programming review is to provide the facility with clear and detailed sequences of operation that not only conform to the designer's intent, but also accurately describe the control process the programs use to implement the sequences of operation. Sequences of operation that meet this goal serve as a valuable reference for the facility and a useful training tool for staff. Verifying that the record design documents and control submittal meet this goal is the responsibility of the HFCxA.

3.10 WITNESS EQUIPMENT AND SYSTEMS START-UP

3.10.1 Planning for Start-Up

The start-up process is an important aspect of protecting and maintaining equipment and systems in like-new condition until a facility is turned over to the O&M staff. The subcontractor responsible for purchase, installation, and start-up of a system provides a start-up plan, which is developed by the installing contractor and the vendor. The plan must be prepared, submitted for review, and approved by the commissioning team prior to start-up. The

See Appendix 3-5 for a sample start-up plan.

HFCxA monitors the development of the start-up plan and assures it is prepared and submitted at the appropriate time.

(1) The start-up plan must include these procedures:

    (a) Start-up procedures. The plan should cover detailed start-up procedures from equipment manufacturers and provide checkout procedures using standard field checkout sheets. This documentation should include checklists and procedures with specific boxes or lines for recording and documenting inspections of each piece of equipment.

    (b) Maintenance procedures. The plan should also include maintenance procedures to follow while the systems are operated prior to turnover to the owner. These procedures should include at least the following:

        (i) Provisions for chemical treatment

        (ii) Filtration

        (iii) Protection of the equipment from exposure to construction

        (iv) Cleaning of the equipment

        (v) Monitoring of systems during operation

        (vi) Schedules for servicing such as pulling strainers and replacing filter

        (vii) A plan for addressing activated alarms such as high static or freezestats that protect the equipment from damage

(2) The start-up plan should be organized and submitted in discipline-specific notebooks, each of which includes the following:

    (a) A cover sheet. Each start-up plan should have an individual, discipline-specific title (e.g. Mechanical Start-Up Plan: Volume 1, Electrical Start-Up Plan: Volume 1, etc.).

    (b) A table of contents

    (c) A separate divider for each piece of equipment (tagged by specification section), including all relevant start-up checklists

    (d) A separate divider for the documentation of each test

3.10.2 Scheduling for Start-Up

The start-up process is scheduled by the subcontractor responsible for the equipment and the systems being started, and it must be coordinated with the commissioning team. The subcontractor prepares an overall schedule of start-up activities for the team to review. The HFCxA witnesses start-up of major equipment and systems and ideally coordinates the schedule to allow the O&M staff to witness the process as well.

3.10.3 Execution of Start-Up

The subcontractor executes equipment start-up according to the start-up plan and provides the HFCxA with a signed and dated copy of completed start-up plan documents. Only individuals with direct knowledge that a task was actually performed may initial or check off that task on the field checkout sheets.

The subcontractor must notify the HFCxA in writing within two working days of any outstanding items from the initial start-up process. The HFCxA should enter these items in the issue log so their resolution can be tracked and recorded. Outstanding items must be satisfactorily addressed and documented within two weeks of initial start-up.

All start-up procedures must be satisfactorily executed before functional testing begins and before the equipment is operated, even temporarily.

3.10.4 Documentation of Start-Up

The HFCxA reviews the documentation of the executed start-up plan and monitors its inclusion in the data to be turned over to the O&M staff. This documentation may be included as an appendix to the final commissioning report.

3.11 REVIEW TAB REPORT

The HFCxA must review the testing, adjusting, and balancing (TAB) report compiled by the contractor, prepare a written response, and distribute it to the owner, contractor, and design team.

3.11.1 Project-Specific TAB Requirements

Prior to reviewing the TAB report, the HFCxA should become familiar with the TAB requirements defined in the section on testing, adjusting, and balancing in the project specifications. The HFCxA should determine whether the specifications require the firm conducting the TAB effort to be a member of a nationally recognized TAB organization such as the Associated Air Balancing Council (AABC), the National Environmental Balancing Bureau (NEBB), or the Testing, Adjusting, and Balancing Bureau (TABB). If so, the HFCxA should become familiar with the national organization's standards, which the member TAB firm must follow during testing and preparation of the TAB report. The TAB firm is obligated to comply with the standards of its certifying organization, but these are to be regarded as supplemental to the project specifications, even when (as sometimes happens) they are more comprehensive and stringent.

3.11.2 Review of the TAB Report

The HFCxA's review of the TAB report should verify or assure the following:

(1) The report's approval and certification requirements comply with the project TAB specifications (e.g., the technician who prepared the report is certified by a national organization, or the report has been approved by a TAB engineer certified by the TAB contractor's certifying organization).

(2) The testing and reporting standards of the national TAB organization were adhered to (if the specifications required the TAB firm to be certified by a national organization).

(3) If required by the specifications or by the certifying organization, the TAB firm performed periodic site reviews of installed systems and provided the HFCxA with copies of site visit reports as they were issued. (Any deficiencies noted in these site visit reports are added to the HFCxA's action item list and tracked until resolution.)

(4) TAB results for all equipment and systems covered in the specifications are included in the TAB report.

(5) Actual flow rates were adjusted to the design values plus or minus specified tolerances.

(6) The procedure used to balance systems with diversity is adequately described.

(7) The control system static pressure sensor setpoint required to supply design airflow to the most hydronically remote component has been documented.

(8) The report clearly states how total system airflows were measured (e.g., duct traverse, sum of outlets/inlets, etc.).

(9) The data in the equipment test forms comply with the specification requirements or the standards required by the TAB contractor's certifying national organization, whichever requirements are more comprehensive.

(10) The report includes a list of test instruments that cites model, manufacturer, serial number, and calibration date for each.

(11) The report discusses any testing, adjusting, or balancing activity that failed to produce the required result.

(12) The report includes measurement data from any sensor calibrations required by the specifications.

(13) A static pressure profile of the system or equipment tested is provided

if required by the project specifications or the relevant TAB certifying organization.

(14) If required, the report includes data related to critical areas such as spaces that must be either negatively or positively pressurized. If this is not required by the specifications, the HFCxA should at minimum spot-check critical spaces for compliance.

3.11.3 Deficiencies

The HFCxA should follow up with the project team on deficiencies noted in the TAB report by the TAB subcontractor and by the HFCxA during the TAB report review. These deficiencies should be added to the HFCx issues log and tracked until resolution.

3.11.4 Verification of Report Accuracy

The HFCxA should verify the accuracy of the TAB report by randomly sampling the air and water readings noted in it. Consideration should also be given to verifying static pressure profile data.

(1) The extent of the sampling to be undertaken should be defined in the commissioning services agreement between the HFCxA and the facility.

(2) The scope of the TAB verification process should be defined in the project specifications.

(3) The HFCxA should coordinate the sampling after functional performance testing is complete and before occupancy.

(4) The HFCxA should note any deviations greater than the tolerance specified in the TAB specifications (+/-10%, for example).

(5) Deviations noted should be corrected and documented by the TAB subcontractor.

(6) If the total number of sampled readings that deviate beyond specified tolerances exceeds 10 percent, the HFCxA should recommend further sampling.

3.12 WITNESS FUNCTIONAL PERFORMANCE TESTS

The HFCxA directs comprehensive equipment and system testing and documents all testing performance. This testing is conducted using functional performance test (FPT) procedures.

The purpose of the functional performance tests is to assure the systems perform in accordance with the design intent.

3.12.1 FPT Procedures

Based on contract document requirements, a set of procedures is compiled for each piece of equipment, system, and integrated system to be commissioned. These procedures establish the testing process and performance expectations and include testing of the following:

(1) Temperature controls

(2) Humidity controls

(3) Safeties and alarms

(4) Air volume control

(5) Operation of equipment and systems on normal and emergency power

(6) Operation during transfer of power

(7) Normal and emergency power distribution

(8) Interface of the HVAC system with the fire alarm system, smoke evacuation system, elevators, fire sprinkler system and fire pump, security system, nurse call system, etc.

Functional test procedures are developed during the design phase and updated during construction to reflect modifications that occur as a result of shop drawing reviews or scope revisions.

The test plan should note all prerequisites that must be completed prior to conducting a functional performance test. These prerequisites include all elements of equipment and system installation, calibration, and balancing—including pre-functional inspections and checklists, equipment start-up, testing and balancing, HVAC controls programming and calibration, and contractor testing. The HFCxA should verify with the team that all these tasks have been completed before functional performance testing begins.

3.12.2 Testing Plan

The HFCxA should work with the commissioning team to develop a testing plan for FPTs that is integrated with the overall project schedule. The plan is used to coordinate FPT efforts and to schedule the appropriate personnel for each test.

The commissioning team members required to participate in each test are noted in the testing plan. Simple tests may require only the HFCxA and the controls subcontractor, but integrated systems tests require additional participants such as the mechanical, electrical, fire alarm, security, and TAB subcontractors, among others.

As the construction team completes various areas of the facility, the HFCxA schedules functional testing of the systems that serve them. In this way, functional performance testing follows completed construction throughout the facility.

The sequence in which FPTs are carried out is developed according to interdependencies between systems. Thus, the testing plan starts with testing subsystems and progresses to systems tests and then to integrated systems testing. An example of this order of precedence is as follows:

(1) Terminal boxes

(2) Zone humidification

(3) Air-handling units (AHUs) serving the terminal boxes

(4) Exhaust fans serving that AHU zone

(5) Pressurization testing for isolation systems (ORs, etc.)

(6) Progress through all AHU systems similar to 1 through 4 above

(7) Hydronic, heating hot water, and chilled water systems

(8) After all of the above have been tested on utility power, spot-checking for functionality on emergency power

(9) Integrated testing of air-side HVAC systems with the fire alarm system

In this example, individual systems must be balanced on both air and water sides before testing. Hydronic systems do not have to be balanced until the testing process progresses to the hydronic system itself, although hydronic systems do need to deliver required water flows at design temperature setpoints when terminal boxes and AHUs are tested.

Dependencies within systems also need to be considered when developing sequencing for a testing plan. For example, testing of an air-handling unit progresses in the following order:

1. Document sample sensor calibration accuracy.

2. Document that safeties and alarms are functional.

3. Document setpoints.

4. Test all sequences of operation under both partial load and full load conditions.

5. Confirm that all BAS graphics are accurate and complete.

Testing of systems related to multiple disciplines can be scheduled simultaneously, but due consideration must be given to how testing of some systems can affect other functional testing and/or ongoing construction. For example, essential electrical system testing will affect functional testing of all systems and ongoing construction, and testing of vertical transportation limits access to areas served by elevators. To address these concerns, functional testing of some systems requires coordination with the entire project team.

Some equipment and systems function independently, such as unit heaters, fan coil units, domestic hot water systems, RO/DI (reverse osmosis/ deionization) systems, and nurse call systems. Testing of these types of systems must be included in the overall commissioning schedule, but its timing does not depend on the schedule for construction completion or functional testing of other systems.

The testing plan should be shared with the owner's O&M staff to allow them to determine whether O&M personnel should witness certain tests.

3.12.3 Equipment and Subsystem Functional Testing

See Appendix 3-6 for a sample functional performance testing plan.

The functional testing process begins with testing of basic elements and individual pieces of equipment, which can be tested at any time after their installation is complete. These include:

(1) HVAC zone equipment such as these items:

    (a) Fan coil units

    (b) Individually mounted reheat coils

    (c) Blower coil units

    (d) CRAC units

    (e) Individual pieces of equipment such as exhaust fans, vent fans, etc.

(2) Plumbing equipment such as the following.

    (a) Domestic booster pumps

    (b) Hot water heating systems

    (c) Lift stations

    (d) Sump pumps

    (e) Medical gas vacuum pumps and air compressors

    (f) RO/DI systems

(3) Electrical equipment such as this:

    (a) Unit substations and switchgear (M-T-M arrangements and Kirk Key arrangements)

    (b) Switchboards

    (c) Shunt trips

    (d) Nurse call systems

    (e) Paging systems

(f) Generators (including batteries, battery chargers, fuel oil day tanks, etc.)

Testing of some individual pieces of equipment relies on limited functionality of other systems (e.g., fan-powered boxes and terminal boxes depend on at least partially functional AHUs and hot water heating system). All equipment and subsystem testing should be successfully completed before testing of any related systems begins.

See Appendix 3-7a for a sample functional performance test matrix for an emergency generator.

3.12.4 Systems Testing

Systems testing is an integrated testing process that tests the controls of the various elements within a system. Several systems and some of the elements that would be tested for them are listed here as examples:

(1) Chilled water systems may include testing for:

    (a) Chillers

    (b) Chilled water pumps

    (c) Cooling towers

    (d) Condenser water pumps

    (e) VFDs

    (f) Heat exchangers

    (g) Chemical treatment systems

    (h) Water filtration systems

(2) Air-handling unit system testing can involve these elements:

    (a) Chilled water coils

    (b) Heating coils

    (c) Unit mounted humidifiers

    (d) In-line coil pumps

    (e) VFDs

    (f) Separate return air or outside air fans

    (g) Air-side or water-side energy recovery systems

(3) Hot water heating system testing can involve:

    (a) Heat exchangers

    (b) Steam systems

    (c) Steam condensate systems

    (d) Pumps

(e) Hot water boilers

(4) Essential system testing that focuses on the functionality of electrical equipment alone may include testing of this equipment:

(a) Normal switchgear

(b) Paralleling switchgear

(c) Switchboards

(d) Generators

(e) Transfer switches

See Appendix 3-7b for a sample functional performance test matrix for an emergency power system.

All system testing should be successfully completed before integrated systems testing is undertaken.

3.12.5 Integrated Systems Testing

In integrated systems testing, the operation of various levels of systems that interact (e.g., a fuel oil system that simultaneously serves boilers and generators) is assessed. Three examples of integrated systems testing are described here:

(1) **Fire alarm system testing.** This assesses reliance on interfaces with elevators, the security system, the building automation system, and HVAC equipment as well as shunt trip functions serving elevator equipment or kitchen appliances, etc.

(2) **Black site testing.** In a black site test, all electrical power is turned off and then restored to test essential system functionality, priority loads, load shed, the fuel oil system, and the functionality of all loads connected to the essential electrical system during both the transfer to emergency power and back to normal power once utility service has been restored.

See Appendix 3-8 for a sample integrated systems testing procedure matrix.

(3) **HVAC system load testing.** The ability of the chilled water system or hot water heating system to serve the collective loads throughout the facility is tested.

3.12.6 Site Visits for Functional System Testing

Plan and coordinate each site visit with the project construction team. Each visit should have a minimum goal of testing completion for a system or group of integrated systems (e.g., testing AHUs 1-x through 2-y).

Before each site visit, the construction team should verify that the systems scheduled for testing are complete, the prerequisites listed in the testing plan have been successfully accomplished, and the construction team has pretested the systems. In addition, the construction team and the HFCxA should confirm which support personnel are required to assist in demonstrating functionality (these subcontractors and vendors should be identified in the testing plan).

As testing progresses from subsystem to system to integrated systems, greater planning and coordination are required to schedule site visits. Each site visit schedule should be shared with the owner, and the O&M staff should be invited to witness all testing.

3.12.7 Exit Debrief Meetings

Before leaving the site, the HFCxA should review the findings from the site visit with the project team members present. This should be a verbal debriefing of what will be documented in the site visit report. Items the HFCxA should cover include these:

(1) Whether the mission of the visit was accomplished

(2) Which items were found to function in accordance with the requirements

(3) Any test results that may require the HFCxA to obtain an interpretation from the design team or owner's representative for later resolution

(4) Items that will be added to the issues log

(5) A general schedule for correcting deficiencies

Before subsequent site visits are scheduled, the construction team should document that all deficiency items have been corrected.

3.12.8 Site Visit Reports

The report written to document the testing results from a site visit should accomplish the following:

(1) Summarize the purpose of the testing and state whether it was achieved.

(2) Identify the major elements of the commissioning scope of work that were completed during the visit.

(3) Cite any major deficiencies discovered.

(4) List action items for follow-up.

(5) Document the resolution of any items previously found to deviate from design requirements and deemed acceptable by the design team but not by the owner.

(6) Discuss the short-term schedule for future site visits to execute functional performance tests.

(7) Assess the overall completion of the testing process versus the overall project construction schedule.

(8) Provide a current version of the issues log.

Photographs should be included in the report to document significant issues that must be addressed.

3.12.9 Completion of Functional Performance Tests

Functional performance testing should be completed prior to reviews by authorities having jurisdiction (AHJs) and building occupancy. Functional testing or integrated systems testing that is not complete as of occupancy or before AHJ reviews becomes a deficiency to be added to the issues log. In such cases, it is critical to identify when such deficiencies will be corrected and available for testing. Should testing be required after occupancy, close coordination must include operations personnel and staff as well as the commissioning team.

Completed FPTs become a part of the commissioning record and are to be included in the final commissioning report. Any elements of functionality not completed or incorporated into the project should be specifically noted in the final report. If FPTs or portions of FPTs remain incomplete because additional testing is specified for the opposite season, this should also be noted in the final report and carried as an open item.

3.13 FACILITATE PRESSURE TESTING

3.13.1 Code Requirements

Current codes require controlled pressure relationships between critical health care spaces such as operating rooms, procedure rooms, airborne infection isolation (AII) rooms, and protective environment (PE) rooms and adjacent spaces. Differences between supply and return/exhaust airflow rates, frequently referred to as offsets, create these pressure relationships. The amount of offset required to create a specific pressure relationship is a function of the effective room leakage area. Figure 3 illustrates the relationship between effective room leakage area, offset, and pressure difference.

As indicated in Figure 3, the airflow offset required to create a 0.01 in. w.g. (inches water gauge) pressure difference with an effective room leakage area of 1.50 square feet is 400 CFM (cubic feet per minute). The actual amount of effective room leakage area is a function of building and room construction and is difficult to predict in advance. Since an increase in effective leakage area increases the required offset, which in turn increases system airflow and fan energy consumption, a higher than expected effective leakage area adversely affects energy costs.

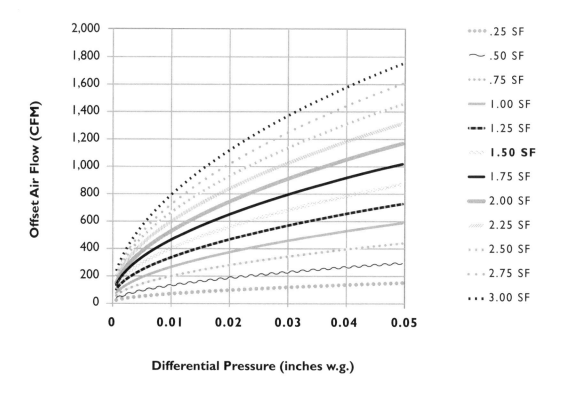

Figure 3: Relationship between Airflow Offsets, Differential Pressure, and Effective Leakage Area

3.13.2 Steps for Positive Pressure Rooms

To ensure proper system operation and limit energy costs, the commissioning process should include pressure testing of all areas requiring controlled pressure relationships (e.g., AII and PE rooms). The recommended pressure testing process for positive pressure rooms includes these steps:

(1) Close all doors to the room.

(2) Seal off exhaust/return air grilles.

(3) Increase the supply air terminal airflow set point until the room differential pressure is equal to the desired value.

(4) Record the supply airflow and the room differential pressure.

(5) Determine the amount of effective leakage area using the relationship shown in Figure 3.

(6) If the amount of effective leakage area is higher than anticipated, the contractor should identify and seal leaks.

(7) The testing and sealing process is then repeated until the effective leakage area is acceptable.

3.13.3 Steps for Testing Negative Pressure Rooms

The recommended pressure testing process for negative pressure rooms includes these steps:

(1)   Close all doors to the room.

(2)   Close the supply air terminal damper.

(3)   Seal off the supply air diffusers.

(4)   Increase the exhaust air terminal airflow set point until the room differential pressure is equal to the desired value.

(5)   Record the exhaust airflow and the room differential pressure.

(6)   Determine the amount of effective leakage area using Figure 3.

(7)   If the amount of effective leakage area is higher than anticipated, the contractor should identify and seal leaks.

(8)   The testing and sealing process is then repeated until the effective leakage area is acceptable.

3.13.4 Steps for Testing the Building Envelope

Controlling building pressure is also critical to efficient and comfortable building operation. The building pressure relative to the outdoors at the main entry should be very close to neutral. The amount of outside air in excess of the building exhaust required to create an appropriate building pressure depends on the integrity of the building envelope. To assure the building envelope is properly sealed, the commissioning process should include building pressure testing.

The recommended pressure testing process for the building envelope includes these steps:

(1)   Close all doors and openings to the building.

(2)   Verify that all exhaust fans are operating at the proper airflow.

(3)   Increase the air-handling unit outdoor airflow until the building pressure relationship is positive 0.01 in. w.g. The building pressure relationship should be determined using a properly installed building pressure transmitter that measures the average differential pressure at the ground-level entrances to the building.

(4)   Record the outdoor airflow, building pressure, and outdoor air temperature.

(5)   If the outdoor airflow is excessive, the contractor should identify and seal envelope leaks.

(6)   The testing and sealing process is then repeated until the amount of outdoor airflow is acceptable.

3.14 REVIEW RECORD DRAWINGS

The HFCxA should review the record drawings regularly throughout the course of the project to confirm that the subcontractors involved in the commissioning scope are documenting all changes to reflect as-built conditions that deviate from the construction documents and result from change orders, field changes, and responses to requests for information (RFIs).

The HFCxA should report the status of the record drawing process to the commissioning team in each site visit report. In addition, the HFCxA should prepare a list of differences between the record drawings and as-built conditions related to commissioning activities and periodically forward them to the owner, contractor, and design team for incorporation into the record documents.

Transition to Operational Sustainability

4.1 FACILITATE THE DEVELOPMENT OF OPERATIONS AND MAINTENANCE DASHBOARDS

Health facility maintenance staffing levels have declined by more than 40 percent, from an average of 104 hours/1,000 sq. ft./year (20,000 SF/FTE) to 62 hours/sq. ft./year (33,000 SF/FTE), over the past 20 years. As a result, the number of skilled crafts and trades (e.g., electricians, plumbers, HVAC technicians, and control instrument technicians) employed by health care facilities is shockingly low. Despite this, low margins will likely lead to further staffing reductions in the future. In today's economic climate, health care facility managers can no longer rely solely on qualified staff to maintain complex equipment and systems. Rather, they must depend on technology to automatically detect inefficient equipment operation and provide guidance for optimizing facility operations.

Dynamic operations and maintenance (O&M) dashboards created for the automatic temperature control system are well-suited to this purpose. Such dashboards have color-coded gauges (red—alarm, yellow—warning, and green—acceptable) to identify problems, and sliders and knobs for adjusting setpoints and other control parameters.

Dashboards provide a means for health care facilities to improve the productivity of scarce maintenance resources by using new technology to automatically and proactively detect potential problems. The concept of the dashboard is that the energy management system can generate displays that continuously monitor and control real-time equipment and system performance using a series of gauges, dials, lights, and buttons configured in a manner similar to the indicators on the dashboard in an automobile. The dashboard simplifies the operation of increasingly complex systems and control programming to a level readily understood by a trained operator.

It should be noted, however, that these dashboards supplement rather than replace energy management system graphic displays. A recommended practice is to use an energy management system workstation with multiple monitors to simultaneously display both the dashboard and the associated graphic display for key systems (e.g., chilled water, domestic hot water, heating water, etc.).

4.1.1 Development of Dashboards

Typically, the HFCxA initiates and facilitates the dashboard development process by working with the design team and the O&M staff to identify the dashboards needed for the project. The HFCxA verifies that the desired dashboards are included in the owner's project requirements (OPR).

The design team then develops the content and format of each dashboard and includes this information in the automatic temperature control section of the project specifications (dashboards are typically extensions of the automatic temperature control system).

As a part of the design review process, the HFCxA reviews the dashboard specifications with the O&M staff and submits comments to the design team and the owner. The HFCxA makes certain the O&M staff understand the purpose and use of the dashboards and the design team has incorporated their input into the dashboard specifications.

Once the dashboard specifications have been agreed upon, the automatic temperature control contractor designs the specific configuration of hardware and software needed. The dashboard hardware is typically the same network of control panels, sensors, and operator workstations used by the automatic temperature control system. The preferred control system network arrangement is Ethernet/IP with standard password-controlled Web browser access. A communication port outside the health facility firewall allowing remote access via the Internet is recommended. The dashboard software must include data archival, data query, and custom-reporting features. The automatic temperature control contractor incorporates the proposed dashboard configuration into the control diagrams submitted to the contractor, design team, HFCxA, and owner for review.

As a part of the submittal review process, the HFCxA reviews the control diagrams (including the proposed dashboard configuration) with the O&M staff and submits comments to the design team and owner. The HFCxA documents that the O&M staff understand how the dashboards are intended to function and that the automatic temperature control contractor has incorporated their input into the dashboard configuration.

The automatic temperature control contractor then implements the dashboards. The HFCxA and the design team review the work and verify that it is ready for functional performance testing.

When the dashboards are fully operational, the HFCxA executes functional performance tests to assure they are working properly.

Finally, the HFCxA documents O&M staff training in the proper use of the dashboards. The training includes pretesting of existing knowledge, simulating real problems (e.g., disconnecting the sensing tubes of an air terminal airflow-measuring device), identifying problems using the dashboards, troubleshooting and resolving problems using the dashboards, and post-testing to assure proficiency.

4.1.2 Systems Requiring Dashboards

Dashboards should be included for the systems and equipment described in this section. Dashboards may also be implemented for medical gas, fire alarm, and fire protection systems.

The dashboards should begin with an overall building dashboard that indicates the current status (red, yellow, or green light) of the other system and equipment dashboards, including those for energy demands and costs; air terminals; air-handling units; exhaust fans; and domestic hot water, heating water, chilled water, steam, medical gas, electrical, and other systems.

(1) **Building energy demands and costs.** The energy dashboard should indicate actual building electricity, heating fuel, and water demands and costs as well as the current cost of building operations in dollars per hour.

The energy dashboard is perhaps the most important dashboard. Its purpose is to maintain energy efficiency awareness and vigilance. The energy dashboard provides the O&M staff with instantaneous, real-time feedback regarding energy consumption and costs. O&M staff use this information to determine the immediate impact of changes they make in sequences of operation and setpoints.

The energy dashboard should display the following information:

(a) Electricity demand: A dial should indicate the instantaneous electrical demand in kW with appropriate red, yellow, and green areas.

(b) Fuel demand: A dial should indicate the instantaneous fuel consumption in MBH with appropriate red, yellow, and green areas.

(c) Energy cost: A dial should indicate the instantaneous energy cost expressed in $ and $/hour/SF with appropriate red, yellow, and green areas.

(d) Energy use intensity: A dial should indicate the instantaneous energy use intensity expressed in Btu/hour/SF with appropriate red, yellow, and green areas.

(e) Carbon footprint: A dial should indicate the instantaneous carbon footprint expressed as metric tons of CO_2 equivalent.

(2) **Air terminals.** Each air-handling unit (AHU) should have an air terminal dashboard that covers the air terminals it serves. This dashboard should indicate the terminal damper position, space temperature, temperature setpoint, discharge air temperature, heating valve position, airflow setpoint, and actual airflow for each air terminal. It should also indicate the total airflow for all air terminals served by the AHU. In addition, the dashboard should identify all terminals with no airflow and open terminal dampers (indicating a failed airflow-measuring device), terminals with closed heating water valves and high discharge air temperatures (indicating failed heating water valves), fully open terminal dampers, and fully open heating water valves.

The air terminal dashboard for each AHU should display the following information:

(a) Total airflow: Sum of the individual terminal airflows as compared to the system design airflow. The dashboard should link to a list of air terminals that indicates the supply airflow associated with each.

(b) Terminal damper positions

- Percentage of air terminal dampers open more than 90 percent (indicating air terminals are struggling to maintain airflow at setpoint). The dashboard should link to a list of these air terminals.

- Percentage of air terminal dampers open less than 50 percent (indicating the duct static pressure may be too high). The dashboard should link to a list of these air terminals.

(c) Failed airflow-measuring devices: The dashboard should indicate the number of air terminals with airflow less than 50 CFM and terminal damper position greater than 95 percent (indicating a failed airflow-measuring device). The dashboard should also link to a list of these air terminals.

(d) Failed heating water control valves: The dashboard should indicate the number of air terminals with a discharge air temperature of more than 5° F above the AHU supply air temperature and a heating water control valve less than 5 percent open (indicating a heating water valve that may have failed open or partially open). The dashboard should link to a list of these air terminals.

(e) Control temperature setpoints

- Number of air terminals with control temperature setpoints greater than 75° F. The dashboard should link to a list of these air terminals.

- Number of air terminals with control temperature setpoints less than 68° F. The dashboard should link to a list of these air terminals.

(f) Space temperatures

- The dashboard should indicate the number of air terminals with space temperature more than 2° F above their associated control temperature setpoint (indicating a possible cooling problem). The dashboard should link to a list of these air terminals that indicates the space temperature, control setpoint, and cooling bias (deadband) of each.

- The dashboard should indicate the number of air terminals with space temperature more than 2° F less than their associated control temperature setpoint (indicating a possible heating problem). The dashboard should link to a list of these air terminals that indicates the space temperature, control setpoint, and heating bias (deadband) of each.

(g) Temperature sensors: The dashboard should indicate the number of air terminals with discharge air temperature sensors that are more than 2° F below the AHU supply air temperature (indicating the discharge air temperature sensor is not accurate). The dashboard should link to a list of these air terminals.

(h) Heating and cooling loopout: The dashboard should link to a list of all air terminals that indicates the heating loopout and cooling loopout commands for each.

(i) Unoccupied mode: The dashboard should indicate the number of air terminals in unoccupied mode. Operating rooms, trauma rooms, C-section rooms, and similar occupancies have high occupied air change rate requirements and should have a reduced occupied airflow setting to save energy when the rooms are not in use. The dashboard should link to a list of air terminals in these areas.

(j) Failed points: The dashboard should indicate the number of air terminals with failed points (indicating a network or other communication problem). The dashboard should link to a list of these air terminals.

(k) Overridden points: The dashboard should indicate the number of air terminals with overridden points and link to a list of these air terminals that indicates which points have been overridden and the amount of time elapsed since the override occurred.

(l) Alarms: The dashboard should indicate the number of air terminals with parameters in alarm (analog limit or change of state) and link to a list of these air terminals.

(3) **Air-handling units.** AHU dashboards should provide key troubleshooting and diagnostic information regarding operation of air-handling units, including status, safeties, outside air conditions, supply fan speeds, valve positions, economizer cycle operation, and so on.

(a) The main air-handling unit dashboard should display the following information:

(i) Outside air conditions: Dials should display the outside air temperature, outside air relative humidity, outside air enthalpy (in Btu/lb of dry air), and outside air specific humidity (in grains).

(ii) Safeties: The dashboard should indicate the number of air-handling units with failed safeties (low limit thermostat, fire alarm, high duct static pressure, etc.) and link to a list of AHUs with failed safeties.

(iii) Building pressure: A dial should show the building pressure, using red (more negative than 0.02 inches w.g. negative or more positive than 0.03 inches w.g.), yellow (from negative 0.02 inches w.g. to neutral 0.00 inches w.g.), and green (0.0 inches w.g. to positive 0.03 inches w.g.) zones.

(iv) Air-handling unit status: The dashboard should indicate the number of air-handling units not in operation and link to a list of these AHUs.

(v) Supply airflow. The dashboard should indicate the following:

♦ Sum of the individual AHU supply airflows measured using AHU airflow-measuring stations.

♦ Sum of the individual AHU supply airflows measured using air terminal airflow-measuring stations

♦ Number of AHUs with large (more than 10 percent) discrepancies between the measured supply airflows. The dashboard should link to a list of these AHUs.

(vi) Ventilation (outside) airflow. The dashboard should indicate the following:

- Sum of the individual AHU ventilation airflows. The dashboard should contain a link to a list of the AHUs that indicates the supply and ventilation airflows associated with each.

- Number of AHUs with large (more than 10 percent) discrepancies between actual outside airflow and design ventilation airflow. The dashboard should contain a link to a list of these AHUs that indicates the measured ventilation airflow, design ventilation airflow, and economizer cycle status (a possible reason for discrepancy between actual ventilation airflow and design ventilation airflow).

(vii) Outside air damper positions: The dashboard should indicate the number of AHUs with outside air dampers open more than 95 percent and actual ventilation airflow less than 500 CFM (indicating a failed airflow measuring station). The dashboard should link to a list of these units.

(viii) Preheat coil valve positions: The dashboard should indicate the number of AHUs with preheat valve positions open more than 95 percent (indicating a possible heating problem). The dashboard should link to a list of these units.

(ix) Preheat coil valves not operating correctly: The dashboard should indicate the number of AHUs with preheat valve positions less than 5 percent open and preheat air temperatures more than 5° F above the mixed air temperature. The dashboard should link to a list of these AHUs.

(x) Humidifier valve positions: The dashboard should indicate the number of AHUs with humidifier valves more than 95 percent open (indicating a possible humidifier problem). The dashboard should link to a list of these AHUs.

(xi) Chilled water valve positions: The dashboard should indicate the number of AHUs with chilled water valve positions more than 95 percent open (indicating a possible cooling problem). The dashboard should link to a list of these AHUs.

(xii) Chilled water valves not operating correctly: The dashboard should indicate the number of AHUs with chilled water valves less than 5 percent open with cooling coil discharge air temperatures more than 2° F below the preheat air temperature. The dashboard should link to a list of these AHUs.

(xiii)   Chilled water delta T: The dashboard should indicate the number of AHUs with chilled water delta T of less than 12° F (indicating a possible valve or setpoint problem). The dashboard should link to a list of all AHUs indicating their chilled water delta T and displaying the units in ascending order from lowest delta T to highest delta T.

(xiv)   Simultaneous heating and cooling: The dashboard should indicate the number of AHUs with partially open heating and cooling valves and link to a list of these AHUs.

(xv)   Economizer cycle: The dashboard should indicate the number of AHUs operating in the economizer mode and link to a list of all AHUs that indicates the air-side economizer cycle status (enabled, disabled, or not applicable) of each.

(xvi)   Simultaneous air-side economizer cycle, cooling, and humidification: The dashboard should indicate the following:

- Number of AHUs operating in the air-side economizer mode with a partially open chilled water control valve. The dashboard should also link to a list of these AHUs indicating economizer cycle status and chilled water valve position.

- Number of AHUs operating in the air-side economizer mode with partially open humidifier valves. The dashboard should also link to a list of these units that indicates economizer cycle status and humidifier valve position.

- Number of AHUs that have partially open humidifier and chilled water control valves. The dashboard should also link to a list of these AHUs that indicates humidifier and chilled water valve positions.

(xvii)   Supply air static pressure: The dashboard should indicate the number of AHUs with supply fan or return fan speed greater than 95 percent (indicating a potential airflow problem). The dashboard should link to a list of these AHUs that indicates fan speed, static pressure, and static pressure setpoint.

(xviii)   Filter status: The dashboard should indicate the number of AHUs with a filter pressure drop of more than 0.10 inches w.g. greater than their associated loaded filter pressure drop.

The dashboard should link to a list of all AHUs that indicates their fan speed, static pressure, static pressure setpoint, pre-filter pressure drop, and final filter pressure drop.

(xix) Supply air temperature setpoints: The dashboard should indicate the number of AHUs with supply air temperature setpoints less than 55° F. The dashboard should link to a list of AHUs that shows their operating status, supply air temperature setpoint, and actual supply air temperature. The AHUs should be listed in ascending order, from lowest supply air temperature to highest supply air temperature.

(xx) Supply air temperature: The dashboard should indicate the number of AHUs with supply air temperature of more than 1° F different from setpoint. The dashboard should link to a list of these AHUs that indicates supply air temperature setpoint, supply air temperature, supply fan speed, chilled water valve position, and heating valve position.

(xxi) Return air humidity. The dashboard should indicate the following:

   • Number of AHUs with humidifiers with return air humidity greater than 5 percent less than the minimum relative humidity (RH) setpoint. The dashboard should link to a list of AHUs that indicates return air relative humidity, humidifier valve position, and return air relative humidity.

   • Number of AHUs with return air humidity greater than 55 percent RH. The dashboard should link to a list of AHUs that indicates return air RH, supply air temperature, supply air temperature setpoint, and chilled water valve position for each AHU.

(xxii) Failed points: The dashboard should indicate the number of AHUs with failed points (indicating a network or other communication problem). The dashboard should link to a list of these AHUs.

   • Overridden points: The dashboard should indicate the number of AHUs with overridden points and link to a list of these AHUs.

   • Alarms: The dashboard should indicate the number of AHUs with parameters in alarm (analog limit or change of state) and link to a list of these AHUs.

(b) Each AHU should also have its own dashboard displaying the following information:

(i) A connection to the main air-handling unit dashboard: Each individual AHU dashboard should have a link to the main AHU dashboard.

(ii) Outside air conditions: Dials should indicate the outside air temperature, outside air relative humidity, outside air enthalpy (in Btu/lb of dry air), and outside air specific humidity (in grains).

(iii) Status of safeties: Red and green lights should indicate the status of the AHU's safeties (low limit, high static, fire alarm, etc.).

(iv) AHU floor plans: The dashboard should link to a color-coded set of facility floor plans that shows the areas and air terminals served by the air-handling unit.

(v) Building pressure: A dial indicating the building pressure should be included, with red (more negative than 0.02 inches w.g. negative or more positive than 0.03 inches w.g.), yellow (from negative 0.02 inches w.g. to neutral 0.00 inches w.g.), and green (0.0 inches w.g to positive 0.03 inches w.g.) zones.

(vi) Fan status: Red and green lights should indicate the status of each supply, return, and associated exhaust fan.

(vii) Supply airflow: A dial should indicate the sum of the supply airflows measured by the air terminal airflow-measuring stations served by the AHU as well as the total airflow measured at the air-handling unit.

(viii) Ventilation (outside) airflow: A dial should indicate the ventilation airflow measured at the air-handling unit.

(ix) Damper positions: A dial should indicate the positions of the return air, relief air, and outside air dampers.

(x) Preheat coil valve position: A dial should indicate the preheat coil valve position with appropriate red, yellow, and green areas.

(xi) Preheat coil temperature: A dial should indicate the preheat coil discharge air temperature with appropriate red, yellow, and green areas.

(xii) Humidifier valve position: A dial should indicate the humidifier valve position with appropriate red, yellow, and green areas.

(xiii) Chilled water valve position: A dial should indicate the chilled water valve position with appropriate red, yellow, and green areas.

(xiv) Chilled water delta T: A dial should indicate the chilled water delta T with appropriate red, yellow, and green areas.

(xv) Simultaneous heating and cooling: A red light should indicate when both heating and cooling valves are open at the same time or the heating water valve is open during economizer operation; a green light indicates simultaneous heating and cooling is not occurring.

(xvi) Economizer cycle: Red and green lights should indicate the status of the economizer cycle.

(xvii) Simultaneous air-side economizer cycle and humidification: A red light should indicate if a humidifier valve is open during economizer operation; a green light indicates this is not occurring.

(xviii) Supply air static pressure: A dial should indicate the status of the supply air static pressure and setpoint with appropriate red, yellow, and green areas.

(xix) Filter status: Dials should indicate pre-filter and final filter pressure drops with appropriate red, yellow, and green areas.

(xx) Return air humidity: A dial should indicate the return air relative humidity and setpoints with appropriate red, yellow, and green areas.

(xxi) Failed points: The dashboard should indicate the number of AHU failed points, which indicate a network or other communication problem.

(xxii) Overridden points: The dashboard should indicate the number of AHU overridden points.

(xxiii) Alarms: The dashboard should indicate the number of AHU parameters in alarm (analog limit or change of state).

(4) **Exhaust fans.** The exhaust fan dashboard should indicate the operating status of each exhaust fan. It should also provide separate lists of exhaust fans that are not operating when their associated AHU is operating and, conversely, of exhaust fans that are operating when their associated AHU is not.

The exhaust fan dashboard should display the following information:

(a) Associated air-handling units: The dashboard should link to a list of all AHUs that identifies the exhaust fans associated with each.

(b) Exhaust fan floor plans: The dashboard should link to a color-coded set of facility floor plans that shows the areas served by each exhaust fan.

(c) Exhaust airflow: The dashboard should indicate the following:

    (i) Sum of the individual exhaust unit airflows (as measured using a piezoelectric ring at the fan inlet). The dashboard should link to a list of the exhaust fans that identifies the actual airflow and design airflow of each fan.

    (ii) Number of exhaust fans with large (more than 10 percent) discrepancies between actual exhaust airflow and design exhaust airflow. The dashboard should link to a list of these exhaust fans.

(c) Building pressure: A dial should indicate the building pressure with red (more negative than 0.02 inches w.g. negative or more positive than 0.03 inches w.g.), yellow (from negative 0.02 inches w.g. to neutral 0.00 inches w.g.), and green (0.0 inches w.g to positive 0.03 inches w.g.) zones.

(d) Exhaust fan status: The dashboard should indicate the number of exhaust fans not in operation as indicated by either a current sensor or the measured airflow. The dashboard should link to a list of these exhaust fans that indicates the status of each fan and of its associated AHU.

(e) Failed points: The dashboard should indicate the number of exhaust fans with failed points (indicating a network or other communication problem) and link to a list of these exhaust fans.

(f) Overridden points: The dashboard should indicate the number of exhaust fans with overridden points and link to a list of these exhaust fans.

(g) Alarms: The dashboard should indicate the number of exhaust fans with parameters in alarm (analog limit or change of state) and link to a list of these exhaust fans.

(5) **Domestic hot water system.** The domestic hot water system dashboard should provide key troubleshooting and diagnostic information regarding operation of the domestic hot water system, including recirculation pump operation, domestic hot water temperatures, and so on.

The domestic hot water system dashboard should display the following information:

(a) Status of domestic hot water return pumps: The dashboard should indicate the number of domestic hot water pumps not in operation as identified by current sensors.

(b) Domestic hot water supply temperature: A dial should indicate the domestic hot water supply temperature with red, yellow, and green areas.

(c) Domestic hot water consumption: A dial should indicate domestic hot water consumption in GPM (measured using a meter in the cold water supply piping).

(d) Domestic hot water return temperatures: The dashboard should include a dial indicating the lowest domestic hot water return temperature in the system as well as a link to a floor plan identifying the domestic hot water supply and return piping and the domestic hot water return temperatures at each domestic hot water return balancing valve.

(e) Failed points: The dashboard should indicate the number of domestic hot water system failed points (indicating a network or other communication problem) and link to a list of these points.

(f) Overridden points: The dashboard should indicate the number of domestic hot water system overridden points and link to a list of these points.

(g) Alarms: The dashboard should indicate the number of domestic hot water system parameters in alarm (analog limit or change of state) and link to a list of these parameters.

(6) **Heating water system.** The heating water system dashboard should provide key troubleshooting and diagnostic information regarding operation of the heating water system, including heating water supply temperature, heating water return temperature, boiler status, pump operation, etc.

The heating water system dashboard should display the following information:

(a) Links to equipment dashboards: The heating water system dashboard should contain links to individual equipment (heating water boilers) dashboards.

(b) Outside air temperature: A dial should indicate the outside air temperature.

(c) Heating water supply temperature: A dial should indicate the heating water supply temperature with red (more than 5° F from setpoint), yellow (more than 2° F from setpoint), and green (less than 2° F from setpoint) areas.

(d) Heating water supply temperature setpoint: A dial should indicate the heating water supply temperature setpoint.

(e) Heating water consumption: A dial should indicate the heating water system flow in GPM.

(f) Heating water system delta T: A dial should indicate the heating water system delta T expressed in both °F and percentage of design delta T with appropriate red, yellow, and green areas.

(g) Heating water system differential pressure: A dial should indicate the heating water system differential pressure with red (more than 2 psig from setpoint), yellow (more than 1 psig from setpoint), and green areas (less than 1 psig from setpoint).

(h) Heating water system differential pressure setpoint: A dial should indicate the heating water system differential pressure setpoint.

(i) Heating water valve positions: A dial should indicate the position of the most open air-handling unit heating water valve with red (more than 95 percent or less than 80 percent open), yellow (90–95 percent open), and green (80–90 percent open) areas. This dial should be labeled to indicate which AHU has the most open heating water control valve and should link to the dashboard for this AHU.

(j) Lowest heating water temperature difference: A dial should indicate the lowest temperature difference of the AHU water coils expressed in both° F and percentage of design delta T with red (less than 15° F), yellow (15 to 20° F), and green (more than 20° F) areas. The dial should be labeled to indicate which AHU has the lowest temperature difference and should link to the dashboard for this AHU.

(k) Heating water system load: A dial should indicate the instantaneous load on the heating water system expressed in both MBH and as a percentage of the system design capacity with red (more than 95 percent), yellow (90 to 95 percent), and green (less than 90 percent) areas.

(l) Heating water system energy consumption: A dial should indicate the instantaneous fuel consumption of the heating water boilers expressed in MBH.

(m) Heating water system efficiency: A dial should indicate the efficiency of the heating water system (ratio of instantaneous heating water system load to energy consumption) expressed as a percentage with red (less than 75 percent or more than 88 percent), yellow (75 to 80 percent), and green (80 to 88 percent) areas.

(n) Failed points: The dashboard should indicate the number of heating water system failed points (indicating a network or other communication problem) and link to a list of these points.

(o) Overridden points: The dashboard should indicate the number of heating water system overridden points and link to a list of these points.

(p) Alarms: The dashboard should indicate the number of heating water system parameters in alarm (analog limit or change of state) and link to a list of these parameters.

(7) **Chilled water system.** The chilled water dashboard should indicate which water chillers are operating, the chilled water flow rate, supply water temperature, return water temperature, temperature difference, total power requirement, average efficiency (kW/ton), pump operating status, pump speed, and differential pressure.

The chilled water system dashboard should display the following information:

(a) Links to equipment dashboards: The chilled water system dashboard should contain links to individual equipment (water chillers and cooling towers) dashboards.

(b) Chilled water valve positions: A dial should indicate the position of the most open AHU chilled water valve with red (more than 95 percent or less than 80 percent), yellow (90–95 percent), and green (80–90 percent) areas. The dial should be labeled to identify the AHU with the most open chilled water control valve and link to the dashboard for this AHU.

(c) Lowest chilled water temperature difference: A dial should indicate the lowest temperature difference of the AHU chilled water coils expressed in both °F and percentage of design delta T with appropriate red, yellow, and green areas. The dial should be labeled to indicate the AHU with the lowest temperature difference and should link to the dashboard for this unit.

(d) Chilled water system temperature difference: A dial should indicate the chilled water system temperature difference expressed in both °F and percentage of design delta T with appropriate green, yellow, and red areas.

(e) Chilled water system load: A dial should indicate the instantaneous load on the chilled water system expressed in both tons and as a percentage of the system design capacity with red (more than 95 percent), yellow (90 to 95 percent), and green (less than 90 percent) areas.

(f) Chilled water system energy consumption: A dial should indicate the instantaneous electricity consumption of the chilled water system (sum of the pumps, towers, and chillers) expressed in kW.

(g) Chilled water system efficiency: A dial should indicate the efficiency of the chilled water system (ratio of instantaneous electricity consumption to instantaneous load) expressed in kW per ton with red (less than 0.3 and more than 0.8), yellow (0.7 to 0.8), and green (0.3 to 0.7) areas.

(h) Chilled water supply temperature: A dial should indicate the chilled water supply temperature with red (more than 46° F or less than 40° F), yellow (44 to 46° F and 40 to 42° F), and green (42 to 44° F) areas.

(i) Chilled water system supply temperature setpoint: A dial should indicate the chilled water system supply temperature setpoint.

(j) Condenser water supply temperature setpoint: A dial should indicate the condenser water supply temperature setpoint.

(k) Failed points: The dashboard should indicate the number of chilled water system failed points (indicating a network or other communication problem) and link to a list of these points.

(l) Overridden points: The dashboard should indicate the number of chilled water system overridden points and link to a list of these points.

(m) Alarms: The dashboard should indicate the number of chilled water system parameters in alarm (analog limit or change of state) and link to a list of these parameters.

(8) **Water chillers and cooling towers.** The dashboards for this equipment should indicate equipment operating status, flow, entering and leaving water temperatures, and power consumption.

(a) A water chiller dashboard should display the following information:

(i) A link to the chilled water system dashboard: Each water chiller dashboard should link to the chilled water system dashboard.

(ii) Water chiller load: A dial should indicate the instantaneous load on the water chiller expressed in both tons and as a percentage of the system design capacity with red (more than 95 percent), yellow (90 to 95 percent), and green (less than 90 percent) areas.

(iii) Water chiller energy consumption: A dial should indicate the instantaneous electricity consumption of the water chiller expressed in kW.

(iv) Water chiller efficiency: A dial should indicate the efficiency of the water chiller (ratio of instantaneous electricity consumption to instantaneous load) expressed in kW per ton with red (less than 0.3 and more than 0.6), yellow (0.55 to 0.6), and green (0.3 to 0.55) areas.

(v) Water chiller leaving chilled water temperature: A dial should indicate the leaving chilled water temperature with red (more than 46° F or less than 40° F), yellow (44 to 46° F and 40 to 42° F), and green (42 to 44° F) areas.

(vi) Water chiller entering condenser water temperature: A dial should indicate the entering condenser water temperature with red (more than 87° F or less than 60° F), yellow (84 to 86° F and 60 to 65° F), and green (65 to 85° F) areas.

(vii) Evaporator approach: A dial should indicate the evaporator approach temperature difference (the difference between the leaving chilled water temperature and the evaporator refrigerant temperature) using red (more than 2° F), yellow (1.5 to 2° F), and green (less than 1.5° F) areas.

(viii) Condenser approach: A dial should indicate the condenser approach temperature difference (the difference between the condenser refrigerant temperature and the leaving condenser water temperature) using red (more than 2° F), yellow (1.5 to 2° F), and green (less than 1.5° F) areas.

(ix) Failed points: The dashboard should indicate the number of water chiller failed points (indicating a network or other communication problem) and link to a list of these points.

(x) Overridden points: The dashboard should indicate the number of water chiller overridden points and link to a list of these points.

(xi) Alarms: The dashboard should indicate the number of water chiller parameters in alarm (analog limit or change of state) and link to a list of these parameters.

(b) A cooling tower dashboard should display the following information:

    (i) A link to the chilled water system dashboard: Each cooling tower dashboard should link to the chilled water system dashboard.

    (ii) Failed points: The dashboard should indicate the number of cooling tower system failed points (indicating a network or other communication problem) and link to a list of these points.

    (iii) Condenser water supply temperature setpoint: A dial should indicate the condenser water supply temperature setpoint with appropriate red, yellow, and green areas.

    (iv) Cold water basin temperature: A dial should indicate the cooling tower cold water basin temperature with appropriate red, yellow, and green areas.

    (v) Makeup water rate: A dial should indicate the average makeup water rate expressed in gallons per hour and the percentage of total water flow for the prior 6-hour period with appropriate red, yellow, and green areas.

    (vi) Fan speed: A dial should indicate the cooling tower fan speed with appropriate red, yellow, and green areas.

    (vii) Basin water level: A dial should indicate the cooling tower basin water level with appropriate red, yellow, and green areas.

    (viii) Overridden points: The dashboard should indicate the number of cooling tower overridden points and link to a list of these points.

    (ix) Alarms: The dashboard should indicate the number of cooling tower parameters in alarm (analog limit or change of state) and link to a list of these parameters.

(9) **Steam system.** The steam dashboard should indicate which boilers are operating, the steam flow rate, makeup water flow rate, makeup water temperature, feedwater temperature, deaerator steam flow rate, fuel consumption, power consumption, and average fuel-to-steam efficiency.

The steam system dashboard should display the following information:

(a) Links to equipment dashboards: The steam system dashboard should contain links to individual equipment (steam boilers) dashboards.

(b) Steam flow: A dial should indicate the instantaneous steam flow expressed in both lbs/hour and as a percentage of the system design capacity using red (more than 95 percent), yellow (90 to 95 percent), and green (less than 90 percent) areas.

(c) Steam system energy consumption: A dial should indicate the instantaneous fuel consumption of the steam system (sum of the individual boilers) expressed in MBH.

(d) Fuel to steam efficiency: A dial should indicate the efficiency of the steam system (ratio of instantaneous useful heat output to the steam system energy consumption) expressed as a percentage using red (less than 70 and more than 90), yellow (70 to 75 and 86 to 90), and green (80 to 86) areas.

(e) Feedwater flow: A dial should indicate the total boiler feedwater flow rate with appropriate red, yellow, and green areas.

(f) Deaerator steam flow: A dial should indicate the deaerator steam flow rate with appropriate red, yellow, and green areas.

(g) Chemical residuals: A dial should indicate instantaneous oxygen scavenger and corrosion inhibitor residuals with appropriate red, yellow, and green areas.

(h) Makeup water rate: A dial should indicate the average makeup water rate for the previous 6 hours with appropriate red, yellow, and green areas.

(i) Feedwater temperature: A dial should indicate the feedwater temperature with appropriate red, yellow, and green areas.

(j) Makeup water hardness: A dial should indicate the makeup water hardness with appropriate red, yellow, and green areas.

(k) Condensate pH: A dial should indicate the steam condensate pH with appropriate red, yellow, and green areas.

(l) Steam pressure: A dial should indicate the steam pressure using appropriate red, yellow, and green areas.

(m) Failed points: The dashboard should indicate the number of steam system failed points (indicating a network or other communication problem) and link to a list of these points.

(n) Overridden points: The dashboard should indicate the number of steam system overridden points and link to a list of these points.

(o) Alarms: The dashboard should indicate the number of steam system parameters in alarm (analog limit or change of state) and link to a list of these parameters.

(10) **Boilers.** Boiler dashboards should indicate equipment operating status, feedwater flow, feedwater temperature, steam flow, fuel flow, stack temperature, combustion efficiency, and power consumption.

(a) A heating water boiler dashboard should display the following information:

(i) A link to the heating water system dashboard: Each heating water boiler dashboard should link to the heating water system dashboard.

(ii) Boiler load: A dial should indicate the instantaneous load on the heating water boiler expressed in both MBH and as a percentage of the system design capacity with red (more than 95 percent), yellow (90 to 95 percent), and green (less than 90 percent) areas.

(iii) Boiler energy consumption: A dial should indicate the instantaneous fuel consumption of the boiler expressed in MBH.

(iv) Boiler efficiency: A dial should indicate the efficiency of the boiler (ratio of instantaneous load to energy consumption) expressed as a percentage with appropriate red, yellow, and green areas.

(v) Boiler leaving water temperature setpoint: A dial should indicate the boiler leaving water temperature setpoint.

(vi) Boiler leaving heating water temperature: A dial should indicate the leaving heating water temperature with appropriate red, yellow, and green areas.

(vii) Overridden points: The dashboard should indicate the number of boiler overridden points and link to a list of these points.

(viii) Alarms: The dashboard should indicate the number of boiler parameters in alarm (analog limit or change of state) and link to a list of these parameters.

(ix) Failed points: The dashboard should indicate the number of heating water boiler failed points (indicating a network or other communication problem) and link to list of these points.

(b) A steam boiler dashboard should display the following information:

(i) A link to the steam system dashboard: Each steam boiler dashboard should link to the steam system dashboard.

(ii) Boiler steam flow: A dial should indicate the instantaneous load on the steam boiler expressed in both lbs/hour and as a percentage of the system design capacity using red (more than 95 percent), yellow (90 to 95 percent), and green (less than 90 percent) areas.

(iii) Boiler feedwater flow: A dial should indicate the instantaneous boiler steam flow with appropriate red, yellow, and green areas.

(iv) Chemical residuals: Dials should indicate corrosion inhibitor, sulfite, and other chemical residuals with appropriate red, yellow, and green areas.

(v) Boiler stack temperature: A dial should indicate the boiler stack temperature using appropriate red, yellow, and green areas.

(vi) Oxygen content: A dial should indicate the boiler stack oxygen content with appropriate red, yellow, and green areas.

(vii) Combustion efficiency: A dial should indicate the boiler's combustion efficiency (calculated using the boiler stack temperature and oxygen content) with appropriate red, yellow, and green areas.

(viii) Boiler energy consumption: A dial should indicate the instantaneous fuel consumption of the boiler expressed in MBH.

(ix) Boiler fuel-to-steam efficiency: A dial should indicate the efficiency of the boiler (ratio of instantaneous load to energy consumption) expressed in a percentage with appropriate red, yellow, and green areas.

(x) Boiler steam pressure setpoint: A dial should indicate the boiler steam pressure setpoint.

(xi) Boiler steam pressure: A dial should indicate the boiler steam pressure using appropriate red, yellow, and green areas.

(xii) Overridden points: The dashboard should indicate the number of boiler overridden points and link to a list of these points.

(xiii) Alarms: The dashboard should indicate the number of boiler parameters in alarm (analog limit or change of state) and link to a list of these parameters.

(xiv) Failed points: The dashboard should indicate the number of steam boiler failed points (indicating a network or other communication problem) and a link to a list of these points.

(11) **Fuel oil system.** The fuel oil dashboard should indicate the operating status of the fuel oil pump and the fuel oil storage level.

A fuel oil system dashboard should display the following information:

(a) Links to the essential power and the steam system dashboards: The fuel oil system dashboard should contain links to the essential power and steam system dashboards.

(b) Fuel oil use: A dial should indicate the total instantaneous fuel oil consumption of boilers and generators in GPH.

(c) Fuel oil storage: A dial should indicate the fuel oil storage level in gallons.

(d) Fuel oil inventory: Dials should indicate the available fuel oil supply in hours at the current instantaneous fuel oil consumption rate and the design fuel oil consumption rate.

(e) Tank monitoring system: Red and green lights should indicate the operating status of the fuel oil tank monitoring system.

(f) Fuel oil pump status: Red and green lights should indicate the status of the fuel oil pumps.

(g) Overridden points: The dashboard should indicate the number of fuel oil system overridden points and link to a list of these points.

(h) Alarms: The dashboard should indicate the number of fuel oil system parameters in alarm (analog limit or change of state) and link to a list of these parameters.

(12) **Normal power system.** The normal power system dashboard should indicate voltage, amps, apparent power, real power, power factor, and main breaker status.

A normal power system dashboard should display the following information:

(a) A link to the essential power system dashboard: The normal power system dashboard should link to the essential power system dashboard.

(b) Electricity demand: A dial should indicate the instantaneous electrical demand in kW.

(c) Power factor: A dial should indicate the instantaneous power factor as a percentage (leading or lagging).

(d) Voltage: A dial should indicate the electrical service voltage.

(e) Amperes: Dials should indicate the electrical system current in amperes.

(f) Breaker status: Red and green lights should indicate the status of main circuit breakers.

(g) Overridden points: The dashboard should indicate the number of normal power system overridden points should link to a list of these points.

(h) Alarms: Number of normal power system parameters in alarm (analog limit or change of state). The dashboard should link to a list of these parameters.

(13) **Essential power system.** The essential power system dashboard should indicate which generators are operating and the position of the automatic transfer switches.

An essential power system dashboard should display the following information:

(a) Link to normal power system dashboard: The essential power system dashboard should link to the normal power system dashboard.

(b) Generator status: Red and green lights should indicate the status of generators.

(c) Generator load: Dials should indicate instantaneous generator loads expressed in both kW and percent capacity with appropriate red, yellow, and green areas.

(d) Generator fuel consumption: Dials should indicate instantaneous generator fuel consumption in gallons per hour.

(e) Breaker status: Red and green lights should indicate the status of main circuit breakers.

(f) Automatic transfer switch status: Red and green lights should indicate the status of automatic transfer switches.

(g) Overridden points: The dashboard should indicate the number of essential power system overridden points and should link to a list of these points.

(h) Alarms: The dashboard should indicate the number of essential power system parameters in alarm (analog limit or change of state) and link to a list of these parameters.

4.2 FACILITATE MAINTENANCE STAFF TRAINING

4.2.1 Planning O&M Staff Training

Training requirements should be coordinated with the facility staff to assure the planned level of training, schedule, and delivery will meet the needs of the staff. Training goals and criteria should be developed early in the project and documented in the OPR, and the training specifications should accommodate these.

(1) **Training goals and criteria.** Planning for O&M staff training should be initiated at the onset of the commissioning process during development of the OPR document. System selections and designs must consider existing maintenance resources (e.g., staffing level, staff knowledge and expertise, etc.) and the training needed to achieve sustainable high performance of building systems. Highly complex and sophisticated systems with the potential to improve energy efficiency will not be successful if the O&M staff do not have the knowledge and expertise to maintain them.

The OPR training goals and criteria should include the following:

(a) A clear description of the purpose for training

(b) A list of equipment and systems for which training should be provided

(c) Defined training levels to be provided for different owner personnel

(d) A list of personnel to be included in the training process

(e) Milestone scheduling for when training will be provided during each phase of the project

(f) A plan for documenting training effectiveness

(g) A list of training deliverables

(h) A description of how training documentation will be archived for future reference.

(2) **Training components.** A more detailed outline of the OPR training components is provided below:

(a) A clear statement of the purpose of the training program. Following is a sample purpose statement:

"The purpose of training for this project is to assure the building occupants and O&M staff have the knowledge and expertise required to cost-effectively operate and maintain the building and its associated systems after initial occupancy. The training program will provide building occupants and O&M staff with the functional knowledge necessary to sustain comfort, productivity, air quality, environmental quality, reliable operation, equipment longevity, optimal energy performance, code compliance, and warranty compliance."

(b) The equipment and systems for which training will be provided. Refer to Section 1.1.1 of the *HFCx Guidelines* for a list of equipment and systems that might be included. In addition to the listed equipment and systems, consider providing training on design intent, sustainability initiatives (e.g., LEED, *Green Guide for Healthcare*, EPA Energy Star, etc.), and the project energy performance goals.

(c) The specific O&M staff for whom training should be provided, including those listed below:

   (i) Facility manager and supervisors

   (ii) O&M personnel (including boiler operators, electricians, control technicians, HVAC technicians, and information technology technicians)

   (iii) Future building occupants or user group personnel

   (iv) Safety and security personnel

   (v) Night and weekend shift personnel

   (vi) Environmental services personnel

   (vi) Local emergency response personnel

   (vii) Local utility personnel

   (viii) Outsource or contract personnel including vendors and suppliers

(d) Training the owner will provide

(e) Any follow-up training the owner will require after project occupancy

(f) The training venues desired by the owner. Some examples include:

   (i) On-site training with a group of staff

   (ii) On-site one-on-one training with staff

   (iii) Classroom style training

   (iv) On-site vendor training

   (v) Off-site vendor training

(g) The level of training to be provided for different personnel at different stages of the project. A training schedule matrix can be used for clarity. The level of training and relevant personnel should be identified for the following project phases:

    (i) Predesign phase

    (ii) Design phase

    (iii) Construction phase

    (iv) Pre-occupancy phase

    (v) Warranty phase

    (vi) Ongoing/follow-up training

(h) A clear definition of the owner's intent to quantify the effectiveness of training programs. Multiple options are available for documenting training effectiveness, including these:

    (i) Conducting pre-testing and post-testing of the owner's staff to quantify how much knowledge was acquired as part of the training effort. See Section 4.2.2 below for more details regarding testing staff knowledge.

    (ii) Conducting training surveys. The staff can state their impression of the training through surveys, and provide comments on how to improve the training. Surveys are typically distributed at the end of a training class and completed by those who attended the training.

    (iii) Conducting verbal testing at the end of the training session. This can identify subjects needing additional training.

    (iv) Conduct warranty period training to follow up with operational staff after they have "lived" with the new systems and equipment. Warranty period training is typically much more effective than construction period training.

(i) The deliverables for a successful training program. It is the responsibility of the contractor to provide the necessary training deliverables to be verified by the HFCxA. Potential training deliverables might include the following:

    (i) Access to various online or Internet resources for training support

    (ii) Access to phone numbers or help desks for training support

    (iii) Training materials, including books, papers, presentations, DVDs, CDs, etc.

(iv) Audio recordings of training sessions for future reference and training programs

(v) Video recordings of training sessions for future reference and training programs

(vi) Samples or spare parts to be used for future training programs

(j) Clear documentation of the owner's desire to obtain training information and deliverables in a hard copy or electronic copy format. The OPR should also specify the number of copies of different materials the owner would like to receive, if necessary.

(3) **Training specifications.** The HFCxA should work with the design team to assure comprehensive training specifications are included in the design documents. At minimum, it is recommended the training specifications cover the following:

(a) A clear definition of the role of the HFCxA in training for the O&M staff

(i) The HFCxA will review the training syllabus.

(ii) The HFCxA will review the proposed staff or faculty qualifications.

(iii) Is the HFCxA responsible for scheduling training?

(iv) Who is responsible for assuring the training will be recorded?

(b) Identification of training venues

(c) The role of the contractor, the design team, the owner, and vendors in meeting training requirements

(d) A recommended training schedule for each phase of the project.

(e) he training deliverables required from the contractor

(4) **The training program.** The project construction team should develop a training program with support from manufacturers and vendors that addresses the specific needs of the owner as outlined above. A detailed program should be documented and submitted—as part of the submittal review process—to the design team, the owner, and the HFCxA for review and approval well before the training will be executed. The contractor team and the HFCxA then use the training program as a guideline for scheduling and monitoring the training process.

(5) **The training plan.** The contractor should develop a training plan for review by the owner and the HFCxA once equipment submittal reviews

for the project have been completed. In addition to training provided by the contractor, it is recommended the HFCxA provide ongoing training for the owner's staff during construction. This level of effort may or may not be documented in the contractor's training plan.

(a) It is recommended that the training plan provide the following information:

  (i)   A detailed list of training sessions, including a description of the equipment or systems for which training is being provided

  (ii) A list of personnel to attend each training session

  (iii) A schedule showing dates, venues, and the party responsible for each training session. The schedule should also show when all preparation materials will be delivered for review.

  (iv) A list of faculty or personnel who will be responsible for conducting each training session. The faculty's experience and qualifications should be documented.

  (v)   A list of all training deliverables to be provided by the contractor

(b) Training syllabus. The contractor should provide a detailed syllabus for each training session to the owner and HFCxA for review and approval.

(c) Training materials. It is recommended that the contractor submit training materials to the owner's personnel at least one week in advance of the training session for review. This will enhance the effectiveness of the training sessions.

(d) Training results. Depending on the requirements of the OPR, the contractor shall quantify the results of the training programs to demonstrate that all owner personnel and staff have been trained effectively. The quantified results shall be provided to the owner and HFCxA for review and approval.

(e) Training library documents. Depending on the requirements of the OPR, the contractor shall provide all required training documents (extra copies of training materials, sample parts, CDs, DVDs, drawings, etc.) to the owner for inclusion in training libraries.

4.2.2 Testing Staff Knowledge

The HFCxA should also develop testing to assess the O&M staff's knowledge, first to assess what level of training is needed and then to assess how successful the training was. The testing procedures can be developed so they also satisfy the documentation requirements of accrediting agencies.

(1) Suggested means of testing include these:

 (a) Written tests to determine how much specific knowledge has been retained by the staff members

 (b) Practical performance testing to evaluate whether staff members have retained the skills that enable them to perform required functions. Plan to continue conducting skills testing throughout the warranty period.

(2) Recommendations for testing approaches include these:

 (a) Focus testing on integrated system operation rather than individual system components. This focus will help ensure the operational staff has a complete understanding of system operations and design intent.

 (b) Focus testing on specific system set points, alarms, and monitored points.

  (i) Testing on system set points helps ensure operational staff have a firm understanding of the recommended systems operational parameters and can query system set points to check for anomalies.

  (ii) Testing on specific system alarms assesses appropriate operational response to various system alarms. This level of testing helps insure that operational staff understand the specific meanings of various alarms and may result in minimal system overrides over the long term.

  (iii) Testing on monitored points includes setting up and reviewing various system trend reports. Regularly reviewing system trend logs helps staff diagnose potential system operational problems and maintain optimum system performance.

(3) Testing results can be improved in several ways:

 (a) Management review of lessons learned from skills testing can be used to identify opportunities to improve subsequent training sessions.

 (b) If testing results do not show sufficient knowledge gain from the training programs, additional training is recommended. This should be structured to address the specific areas of concern identified by the testing results.

(c) Though initial testing may be conducted anonymously, it may become necessary to conduct individual assessments for the purpose of determining the level of retraining required. If additional training is required to obtain the necessary system knowledge and skill, it is best to conduct this type of training in a one-on-one environment and to schedule appropriate follow-up sessions to reinforce knowledge retention.

4.2.3 Training Program Components

(1) Instructor resumes

(2) Description of the general purpose of the equipment or system the training is intended to cover

(3) Simplified system schematics showing different modes of operations such as heating, cooling, occupied, unoccupied, and so on.

(4) List of O&M manuals to be used during training

(5) Material addressing these operational modes:

   (a) Start-up

   (b) Normal operation

   (c) Shutdown

   (d) Unoccupied operation

   (e) Seasonal changeover

   (f) Manual operation

   (g) Controls setup and programming

   (h) Troubleshooting

   (i) Alarms

(6) Description of how the equipment and/or system interacts with other building systems and how it is included in operations dashboards

(7) Adjustments and optimizing methods for energy conservation

(8) Relevant health and safety issues

(9) Special maintenance and replacement sources

4.3 FACILITATE IMPLEMENTATION OF HVAC CONTROL SYSTEM TRENDS

The contract design scope should require creation of various trends to help the O&M staff monitor the operation of key equipment and systems in the facility. Often, the design documents require the HVAC control system to be capable of trending the systems but do not define these trends. In such cases, the HFCxA should assist the O&M staff in implementing key trends.

4.3.1 Purposes of Trending

Trends provide critical feedback on space conditions and energy use that help O&M personnel manage the facility building systems and minimize energy costs. Trends can be implemented for various systems, but the focus should be on systems that have the most impact on energy use and space conditions. Trends make it easier to diagnose control problems and identify system operations that waste energy or negatively affect space conditions and/or critical pressure relationships. Trends also identify how well control loops are tuned.

Review of trends after a building has been occupied is discussed in Section 5.1 (Review Trend Data).

4.3.2 Trends to Consider for Development

Several examples of trends that should be considered are listed in this section. Additional trends may be relevant depending on the specific needs of a facility.

(1) **Terminal boxes and other zone control devices.** Terminal boxes are either variable air volume (VAV) or constant volume (CAV) boxes. Trending terminal boxes can identify boxes that are performing incorrectly or wasting energy. Trends for similar criteria for other zone control devices (e.g., fan coil units, fan-powered boxes, etc.) should also be defined. Trends for these types of equipment should monitor the following:

   (a) Discharge air temperature

   (b) Airflow

   (c) Box damper position

   (d) Thermostat setpoint

   (e) Space temperature

   (f) Reheat hot water valve position

(2) **Heating hot water systems.** Heating hot water systems should be controlled to minimize energy use for pump horsepower and water temperature. The supply water temperature should be reset based on load requirements and/or outside air temperature. The pumping system should be controlled based on demand (static pressure). Points that should be trended include:

   (a) Outside air temperature

   (b) Supply and return water temperature

   (c) Steam valve(s) position

   (d) Differential pressure setpoint

(e) Actual static pressure at controlling sensor

(f) Pump speed and status

(g) System flow

(3) **Air-handling units.** Like terminal boxes, AHUs are either VAV or CAV. They can serve one zone or multiple zones; be low-, medium-, or high-pressure; and have chilled water coils, DX coils, or steam or hot water preheat or reheat coils (also, some coils may have loop pumps). AHUs can have unit-mounted humidifiers and other associated equipment. Setpoints for supply air temperature and static pressure control should be reset based on load or outside air conditions. Points that should be trended include these:

(a) Supply air temperature and setpoint

(b) Airflows for supply, return, and outside air

(c) Static pressure setpoint and actual reading (may be multiple readings)

(d) Outside, return, and mixed air temperatures

(e) Control valve positions on the chilled water coils, preheat and reheat coils, and humidifier. The steam line to the humidifier should also have an automatic isolation valve that is monitored.

(f) Relative humidity reading in AHU supply air and at the space sensor

(g) Coil pump status (if applicable)

(h) Fan speed

(4) **Chilled water system.** The chilled water system (CHW) is usually the greatest energy load in the facility as well as the one most likely to operate inefficiently. This is due to the criticality of the chilled water temperature and how it affects the supply air temperature in surgery and other mission-critical areas. The two chilled water designs most frequently used today are variable flow primary and primary/secondary systems. Many designs also include a water-side economizer that makes use of various elements of the chilled water system to provide "free cooling." Each system contains numerous elements that must be monitored. Points that should be trended include these:

(a) Pump speeds for primary and secondary chilled water, condenser water pumps, plate and frame pumps

(b) Differential pressure setpoints and actual readings

 (c) Water flows for primary and secondary chilled water, condenser water

 (d) Chiller start/stops, chiller run time

 (e) Outside air and water temperature setpoints and actual readings

 (f) Isolation valves for chillers and cooling towers

 (g) Cooling tower start/stops, fan speeds

4.4. PREPARE THE COMMISSIONING REPORT AND SYSTEMS MANUAL

4.4.1 Commissioning Report

The HFCxA completes the commissioning report and systems manual at the completion of the construction phase. The commissioning report summarizes and documents the methodology and results of the commissioning process and includes documentation of all commissioning activities. The report generally includes:

 (1) An executive summary (This should summarize the process and the results of the commissioning process.)

 (2) A history of the action items and deficiencies noted and how they were resolved

 (3) System performance tests and evaluations

 (4) A summary of the design review and submittal processes

 (5) A summary of the O&M documentation and training processes

 (6) Commissioning documentation from throughout the process, including:

  (a) Meeting minutes

  (b) Completed documents such as start-up documents, completed pre-functional checklists, functional performance test results, training data, and so on.

4.4.2 Systems Manual

The HFCxA also compiles the systems manual, which focuses on operating systems and serves as a condensed system-level troubleshooting guide for O&M personnel. At minimum, the systems manual should include the following:

 (1) Final version of the OPR and BOD

(2) System single-line drawings

(3) As-built sequences of operation

(4) Control shop drawings

(5) Original control setpoints

(6) Operating instructions for integrated systems

(7) Recommended retesting schedule and blank test forms

(8) Sensor and actuator recalibration schedules

4.5 FACILITATE DEVELOPMENT OF THE MAINTENANCE BUDGET

The HFCxA should assure that the health care administrative staff and facility manager have an accurate and thorough understanding of the resources needed to maintain and operate the health care facility in a cost-effective manner (e.g., staffing, materials, service contracts, etc.). Facility managers can predict maintenance and operating staffing levels using either the more comprehensive and time-consuming ASHE benchmarking tool or a tool developed in 2011 by one of the authors of this handbook using the raw data collected during an ASHE-IFMA (International Facility Management Association) survey of health care facilities.

ASHE created its original benchmarking tool from data collected directly from hospitals. Unlike more generic benchmarking methods, the ASHE tool considers site-specific information. Figure 4-1 shows staffing levels and maintenance and operating costs for four different sizes and types of hospitals; this data is the average of input from facilities that participated in development of the ASHE benchmarking tool.

The costs and staffing levels indicated in Figure 4-1 include grounds, but not data management, compliance, housekeeping, biomedical equipment maintenance, or security. The staffing levels vary from 12,000 square feet per full-time employee (FTE) for a small 100,000-square-foot facility up to 42,000 square feet per FTE for a massive 4 million-square-foot facility. The maintenance and operating costs (including energy costs) vary inversely from $11 per square foot for the smaller facility down to $7 per square foot for the larger facility. The vast difference between the smaller and larger facilities suggests that more simplified benchmarking approaches that do not consider the impact of the floor area on the floor area per FTE ratio may not yield useful or actionable results.

The new tool developed from the ASHE-IFMA data can be used to predict staffing levels for each trade based on floor area only (it does consider floor area impact on the floor area per FTE ratio). A sample output is provided in Figure 4-2.

For a sample display of data from the ASHE-IFMA hospital staffing tool, see Appendix 4.

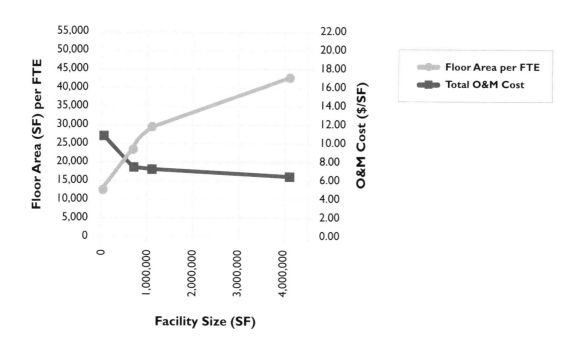

Figure 4-1: Staffing Level Output from ASHE Benchmarking Tool

Input Floor Area (GSF)	650,000

CATEGORY	GSF/FTE	Recommended FTEs
Electricians	151,982	4.3
Plumbers	414,535	1.6
Low Voltage	494,075	1.3
HVAC	230,762	2.8
Stationary Engineers	117,320	5.5
Carpenters	335,282	1.9
General Mechanics	104,658	6.2
Locksmiths	800,658	0.8
Painters	335,654	1.9
Supervisors	378,922	1.7
Managers	479,409	1.4
Help Desk	335,654	1.9
Administrative Assistant	519,939	1.3
Total	21,147	32.7

Figure 4-2: Sample Staffing Level Output from New Tool Based on ASHE-IFMA Data

A comparison of staffing levels predicted using the original ASHE bench-marking tool and the new tool can be found in Figure 4-3.

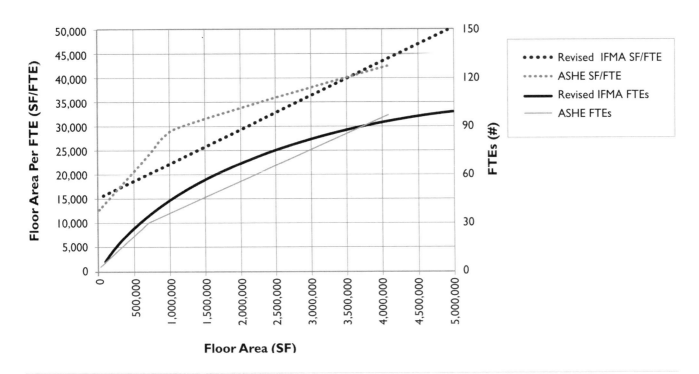

Figure 4-3: Comparison of Predicted Staffing Levels

A facility's annual utility budget can be developed using the EPA Target Finder and the applicable utility unit costs. Target Finder predicts annual energy consumption as a function of the Energy Star rating. If the health care facility is designed to earn the Energy Star as confirmed by an energy model, the HFCxA can enter 75 into Target Finder and it will automatically predict annual energy consumption.

The prediction of annual energy consumption and costs should initiate the process of developing and continuously updating the facility's strategic energy plan.

4.6 FACILITATE FIRE AND SMOKE DAMPER INSPECTIONS AND TESTING

4.6.1 Code Requirements

National codes require health care facilities to inspect and test their fire and smoke dampers within 12 months of installation and every six years there-after. To reduce costs and minimize disruption, the HFCxA works with the contractor to complete the initial damper inspection and testing at the completion of the construction phase, immediately before the building is occupied.

The HFCxA prepares a written report of specific information on each fire and smoke damper, listing the damper number, damper location, date of inspection, damper inspection results, and associated corrective work, if required. The facility manager uses this report as the basis for conducting regular required inspections.

Fire and smoke damper testing is required by NFPA 90A: *Standard for the Installation of Air-Conditioning and Ventilating Systems*. Smoke damper testing should be conducted in concert with smoke detector and fire alarm testing as required by NFPA 72: *National Fire Alarm and Signaling Code*. In all applications other than hospitals, the testing interval is every four years. In hospitals, the testing interval is every six years.

4.6.2 Scope for Damper Inspection and Testing

The fire and smoke damper testing must be completed after the HVAC system has been fully installed and balanced. All tests need to be completed safely by personnel wearing appropriate protective equipment, including safety glasses. The testing should verify that full and unobstructed access to all dampers and related components is available.

Testing must be documented, indicating the location of the damper, the date of testing, the name of the inspector, and any deficiencies discovered. This documentation should also have a space to indicate when and how deficiencies are corrected.

Inspection and testing work items include the following activities:

(1) Verify that the record drawings accurately indicate the location of all fire and smoke dampers and that the dampers are properly labeled.

(2) Locate all fire and smoke dampers. Verify that the dampers are properly tagged.

(3) Remove and reset fusible links on fire dampers to verify each damper fully closes. Replace fusible links as required.

(4) Lubricate all moving parts on each damper.

(5) Clear each damper of any obstruction impeding its normal operation.

(6) Manually activate each smoke damper and combination fire-and smoke-damper actuator to verify proper operation.

4.7 FACILITATE COMPLETION OF THE STATEMENT OF CONDITIONS (SOC)

When a Joint Commission Statement of Conditions is required for a facility, the HFCxA works with the owner and the design team to see that it is completed.

The Joint Commission developed the SOC document to help health care facilities create and maintain a safe environment and demonstrate compliance with the *Life Safety Code*. The SOC has four parts:

+ Part 1: Introduction and Instructions. This contains instructions for completing Parts 2 through 4.

+ Part 2: Basic Building Information. This section collects general information regarding the building, including address, Joint Commission organization identification number, occupancy, and number of stories.

+ Part 3: Life Safety Assessment. This sectionis used to verify compliance with *Life Safety Code* requirements, including fire and smoke barriers and exits.

+ Part 4: Plan for Improvement (PFI). In this section, plans to resolve life safety deficiencies are described.

The Joint Commission generally requires an SOC for buildings occupied by patients. An SOC is not required for Business Occupancies that are either freestanding or separated from other areas of the health care facility by a 2-hour fire barrier as long as they do not serve as a required exit from the health care facility.

The HFCxA should assure that the SOC is completed prior to occupancy. The person completing the SOC should have extensive knowledge of the building and the *Life Safety Code*.

Any deficiencies noted during development of the SOC should be added to the project issues log for immediate resolution by the project team. Developing a PFI and deferring resolution of the deficiency to the postoccupancy period should not be an option for new construction or renovation projects.

The SOC is continuously maintained by the facility within the Joint Commission database. This electronic version of the SOC is referred to as the eSOC.

4.8 FACILITATE DEVELOPMENT AND IMPLEMENTATION OF THE BUILDING MAINTENANCE PROGRAM

4.8.1 Timing and Software Requirement

Once the project design has been completed but well before the building is ready for occupancy, the HFCxA should work with the facility manager, design team, and contractor to develop and implement a building maintenance program (BMP) for new facilities or to update the existing BMP for renovations and additions.

A computerized maintenance management system (CMMS) software program should be used to develop the BMP. The specific program to be used should be selected by the health facility maintenance staff based on their specific needs and preferences. At a minimum, the software should provide a means to maintain a complete equipment and system inventory, automatically generate and track scheduled maintenance work orders, track unscheduled maintenance work orders, and monitor maintenance staff productivity (percentage of available work hours actually spent maintaining equipment and systems).

The HFCxA should assist the health facility manager in selecting the CMMS program for new facilities by documenting needs and preferences and identifying alternatives. For renovation projects, the HFCxA should assist the health facility manager by assessing the existing CMMS program and determining if it should be replaced or upgraded within the project scope.

4.8.2 HFCxA Scope for BMP Effort

The scope of the HFCxA's involvement in the development and implementation of the maintenance management program should include the following items of work:

(1) Assure that all equipment is numbered and labeled in a manner consistent with facility standards. (For renovation and addition projects, the equipment numbers should begin with the next available number rather than starting over again at 1.)

Proper equipment numbering and labeling is often overlooked and is a common problem in many health care facilities. Assuring proper numbering and labeling begins with the HFCxA's drawing review. The equipment labels indicated on the drawings must be consistent with the actual labels affixed to the equipment, point names used by the building automation system, and the CMMS inventory.

(2) Assure that room numbers indicated on the construction drawings are consistent with facility standards and actual room numbers. Use of incorrect room numbers prevents an easy transition from construction completion to sustainable operation.

Room numbers are frequently assigned by the architect early in the design process. Many health care facilities, however, have organized room-numbering systems. The HFCxA must facilitate a conversation at the onset of the project to assure the room numbers indicated on the drawings match the room numbers assigned by the health care facility and the actual room numbers indicated by the wayfinding (signage) system.

Building names can be equally problematic in that these often change postoccupancy due to philanthropic gifts. The HFCxA should facilitate a conversation at the onset of the project to assure the building name used to identify building equipment, systems, and spaces is sufficiently generic to be consistent with potential naming conventions.

(3) Assure the owner receives an electronic archive of all information required to operate and maintain the facility. This archive can be inserted into a three-dimensional electronic model of the building, called a building information model, or BIM.

Comprehensive and accurate maintenance and operating information is absolutely essential for a successful transition to sustainable high-performance operation. This information is the cornerstone of the maintenance staff training program. The HFCxA must assure that all members of the team understand the importance of this task and that it is properly completed. If a building information model is used, the HFCxA must also assure the maintenance staff have the computer hardware and software needed to access the stored have information and are fully trained in its use.

The operations and maintenance archive should include the following:

(a) Design calculations

(b) Record drawings

(c) Project manual

(d) Submittals

(e) Shop drawings

(f) Coordination drawing

(g) Factory test reports

(h) Pre-functional checklists

(i) Equipment start-up reports

(j) TAB reports

(k) Functional performance test results

(l) Other test results

(m) Installation requirements

(n) Operations and maintenance manuals

(o) Spare parts inventory

(p) Recommended schedule and frequency for maintenance procedures

(q) Parts lists

(r) Warranties

(s) Service contracts

(t) Service provider contact information

(4) Assure each item of equipment and its associated maintenance and operating information is identified in the CMMS.

It is not uncommon for CMMS programs to be set up with groups of similar equipment (air terminals, fan coil units, etc.) or an entire system (e.g., a fire alarm system) covered by a single equipment identifier instead of a separate and unique identifier for each component. Although this arrangement expedites the CMMS setup process, it is not appropriate for health care facilities and should not be used. The CMMS system must maintain an individual service history for each piece of equipment, and this is not possible unless each item is uniquely identified. The HFCxA should assure the CMMS setup meets this requirement.

CMMS programs that can link directly to a building information model are currently under development. Linking the CMMS to a BIM model has the potential to significantly expedite the CMMS setup process.

(5) Assure the CMMS automatically generates work orders for recommended maintenance procedures at the recommended frequency.

The HFCxA and the health facility manager should review equipment maintenance manuals to determine the proper frequency for these procedures.

(6) Assure a complete service history for each item of equipment (scheduled maintenance, unscheduled maintenance, etc.) is maintained in the CMMS.

The HFCxA and the health facility manager should assure the CMMS includes records for all service-related events for each item of equipment, including service calls, unscheduled maintenance, and preventive maintenance. The health facility manager should assure that service histories are readily available and continuously updated.

(7) Assure the CMMS provides for regular (annual or more frequent) calibration of temperature, pressure, and other sensors critical to efficient system performance.

The HFCxA and the health facility manager should identify the control equipment and components that are most critical to efficient system performance (e.g., AHU supply air temperatures). The frequency of the preventive maintenance procedures for these devices should be adjusted accordingly.

Postoccupancy and Warranty Phase

5.1 REVIEW TREND DATA

When a facility is occupied and its building systems are being subjected to actual load conditions, automatically recorded trend data can help the facility manager optimize system operations for both building comfort and energy management. Integrating trend data into the operations and maintenance (O&M) dashboards can provide vital real-time feedback. (See Section 4.3, Facilitate Implementation of HVAC Control System Trends, in both the *Health Facility Commissioning Guidelines* and this handbook for more information on collecting trend data.)

Ideally, the facility staff's involvement in the functional performance testing process and during training sessions has equipped them with the knowledge needed to review trends and modify the HVAC controls to optimize performance. Their everyday presence at the facility and access to the systems make these staff members the most logical choice to observe the trends, evaluate the data, and make the necessary adjustments. Where additional technical support is needed, the HFCxA can assist facility staff in interpreting trend data and adjusting control system setpoints to improve system performance.

5.1.1 Terminal Boxes

The facility staff should regularly review trend data for the operation of terminal boxes to look for problems such as these:

(1) **Simultaneous heating and cooling.** Unchecked, terminal boxes often waste energy by cooling and heating simultaneously. For variable volume boxes, the box damper should modulate airflow to satisfy setpoint before the reheat valve opens, but often this does not occur. Therefore, the trend should compare the performance of the damper and the reheat valve to assure that on a call for heating the damper closes to the

minimum position before the reheat control valve begins to modulate open. Conversely, on a call for cooling, the trend should indicate the reheat control valve remains closed as the damper modulates open to satisfy setpoint.

(2) **Malfunctioning box dampers and reheat hot water control valves.** The trending of the damper position, reheat control valve position, and thermostat call for heating or cooling will reveal if the terminal box elements are programmed correctly. If the reheat control valve is open when the thermostat is calling for cooling or the damper is closing, then these components are programmed incorrectly. The opposite would be true on a call for heating. These conditions are readily apparent from the readings in the trend data.

(3) **Blockages in the heating water piping system.** If the trend data show a problem with the heating hot water system but it has been confirmed that the box damper and reheat control valve are operating and sequencing correctly, the piping system may be partially or completely blocked. Trending the discharge air temperature readings and the reheat control valve position will reveal whether this is the case. This trend should concurrently review the supply heating hot water temperature. If the reheat valve is shown to be 100 percent open and the discharge air temperature is below the design heating discharge air temperature, there is a blockage in the heating hot water system. The blockage may be at the strainer if one is provided in the box coil supply, or it may be in the coil itself. At times, piping serving boxes located at the lowest point in a heating hot water distribution system can be clogged with dirt that migrates to the bottom of the system.

(4) **Capability of the boxes to satisfy space temperature.** Assess whether the terminal box is maintaining the space temperature setpoint at all times. Trending the actual space temperature against the setpoint called for at the thermostat will identify a system's ability to maintain setpoint.

(5) **Excessive energy use from "over-airing" the space.** Monitor airflows against the sequence of operation to determine if the box resets to the specified airflows as conditions change in the space. The HVAC control system or building automation system should provide data on the actual airflow and the setpoints for minimum and maximum flow. The minimum flow should be reported when the system is in the heating mode, and the maximum flow would only occur when the system is modulating to cool to setpoint. Trending the actual airflow against the damper position and the call for heating and cooling would reveal "over-airing."

5.1.2 Heating Hot Water System

Trend data for the heating hot water system are regularly reviewed to identify problems such as these:

(1) **Outside air and supply water temperature.** Often the heating hot water supply temperature setpoint is designed to reset based on actual outside air temperature. The supply water setpoint decreases as the outside air temperature rises and increases as the outside temperature drops. These automatic resets should be limited by programming in maximum and minimum allowable setpoints. Trending the actual outside air temperature, the sliding scale setpoint, and the actual supply water temperature will reveal whether the supply temperature setpoint is responding to changes in the outside air temperature as required.

(2) **Supply and return water temperatures.** The heating hot water system is designed for a temperature drop across the system, and trending these temperatures can reveal if flow in the system is adequate. Comparing the supply and return water temperature differential to the design temperature could show whether there is too much flow in the system: If the actual temperature differential is significantly less than design, there could be too much water flow and the static pressure setpoint may be greater than necessary. Conversely, if the temperature differential is significantly greater than design, there could be too little flow and the system static pressure setpoint could be too low.

(3) **Steam valve(s) position.** The valve position should be trended against the supply water temperature setpoint and actual water temperature. The position of the steam valve will indicate how well the control loop is tuned and the steam system's ability to serve the load. The valve position should not fluctuate and cause the actual water temperature to vary above and below setpoint. Rather, the valve should modulate to maintain setpoint. A properly tuned PID loop will control the valve so the actual water temperature tracks setpoint. If more than one steam valve serves a system, the valves should be different sizes, generally 1/3 – 2/3. Trending the position of these valves will indicate if they are sequencing properly. The smaller valve should operate during low load conditions, and the larger valve should not open until the smaller cannot maintain setpoint, at which point the larger valve picks up the load as the smaller valve closes. When the load exceeds the capacity of the larger valve, the smaller valve again opens to satisfy the load. This sequencing should be monitored against the system's ability to maintain setpoint. At no time should both valves be partially open except in transition of control from one to the other.

(4) **Differential pressure, setpoint and actual reading, and pump speed.** Review trending data to make sure the pump speed reflects variations in load demand and that the control loop is tuned. Static pressure setpoint and actual readings should be trended against the VFD (variable frequency drive) output. The VFD should modulate the speed of the pump to maintain the setpoint as the load varies. The static pressure setpoint should be determined during the TAB (testing, adjusting, and balancing) process and identified in the control system. Often the setpoint is found to be higher than necessary, thus wasting pump energy. The setpoint can be varied down to determine if the system can maintain the pressure at lower pump speeds while the terminal boxes are monitored to assure they maintain space condition setpoints.

(5) **Pump status.** Pumps are programmed to operate in series or in parallel, depending on the design. Pumps that are designed to run in series should not operate simultaneously. Pumps that are designed to operate in parallel should operate at equal speeds. Trending pump status will indicate when series pumps are being operated individually, and trending VFD output on parallel pumps will reveal whether they are modulating properly.

5.1.3 Air-Handling Units (AHUs)

Trend data for AHUs are reviewed to identify problems such as these:

(1) **Static pressure.** Similar to pump controls, the static pressure setpoint can result in consumption of unnecessary energy if it is set higher than needed. The static pressure setpoint adequate to serve the load should have been identified during the TAB process. Trending the static pressure setpoint and actual readings along with the VFD output will show if the system is maintaining adequate static pressure. The VFD should modulate the speed of the AHU supply fan to maintain the static pressure setpoint as the load varies without overshooting the setpoint. If the system is designed properly, the VFD should not be operating at 100 percent at all times.

(2) **Simultaneous heating and cooling.** There are several scenarios in which simultaneous heating and cooling could occur:

(a) The preheat coil should not operate during the cooling cycle. Comparing the trend data for the air temperature entering the preheat coil to the temperature coming off the coil will reveal whether the airflow is picking up heat from the coil during the cooling season. This could occur if the coil control valve is commanded open errantly or held slightly open due to debris in the valve.

(b) The preheat coil should not overheat the airflow in the winter season. Overheating the airstream to a temperature higher than the supply air temperature setpoint will require the chilled water coil to operate to maintain supply air temperature. The air temperature off the preheat coil should be trended against the supply air temperature setpoint to assure the preheat coil does not overheat the airstream.

(c) In all but very dry climates, the steam to the humidifier is not required and should be turned off during the cooling season. Usually an automatic shutoff valve is installed in the steam supply to the humidifier. Trending the air temperature across the humidifier will indicate if heat is being gained as the airstream crosses the humidifier.

(3) **Humidifier.** The humidifier control should modulate to maintain space relative humidity without exceeding the high-limit humidity setpoint in the supply duct. At steady state, the humidifier valve should not modulate excessively. Trend the humidifier valve position and the actual relative humidity in both the space and the duct; compare the space humidity to setpoint and review the duct humidity to assure the high limit is not exceeded.

(4) **Fan tracking.** In variable volume air-handling systems, the differential between the fans must be a constant air quantity to maintain building pressurization. Trend the supply airflow against the return flow to assure the differential setpoint is maintained. If the actual differential is greater than the design differential, the system is drawing more outside air into the building than intended by the design and thus using more energy than required. If the differential is less than design, the overall building pressure will be negative, subjecting the facility to conditions that may foster mold growth or, at least, draw in outside air through doors or other openings in the building envelope.

(5) **Coil pumps.** These pumps are designed to operate only under certain conditions; however, they can operate 24/7 without affecting temperature control but using excessive energy. Trend the status of the pump operation and compare it to that required by design.

(6) **Control valves.** Assess whether the AHU valve positions modulate with the load and if the control loops are tuned. Trend the control

valve positions against the corresponding actual coil entering and leaving conditions to assure setpoints are being maintained without overshooting.

5.1.4 Chilled Water System

The chilled water system (CHW) has the largest impact on energy consumption of any single system in the facility. Chillers should be controlled in conjunction with the condenser water system and pumping system to meet load requirements while minimizing energy usage. Generally, chillers operate more efficiently when fully loaded; thus, it is critical to load them properly and maintain the design load side water temperature differential. Chiller manufacturers offer integration panels that share chiller performance information with the building automation system. This data-sharing allows facility staff to monitor critical performance criteria in the chillers and optimize system performance.

Trend the chilled water system to identify problems such as these:

(1) **Chiller loading.** Trend the chillers to assure they operate fully loaded. The integration panel should be able to identify the connected load as a percentage of full load for each chiller, and this input should be trended. The load percentage is not the only factor that requires a chiller to operate, however. Other elements in the overall chilled water system may call for a chiller to operate while not fully loaded. For example, chillers are often started unnecessarily to satisfy water flow demands. If the water flow is not balanced on the load side of a system, operation of multiple chillers may be required to satisfy flow demands rather than tonnage demand. If the temperature differential on the load side is less than the design temperature differential of the chiller, there will be no way to fully load the chiller(s). Adjustments must be made to the load side of the system to assure the system is hydraulically balanced and to increase the differential between the supply and the return water temperatures to one greater than the chiller design differential so the chillers can be loaded properly. Thus, if multiple chillers are operating at partial loading, the controls and load side conditions should be investigated.

(2) **Chiller stops and starts.** The sequencing of chillers on and off should be defined by the building automation system to assure chillers are not started and stopped unnecessarily. The starts and stops for each chiller should be trended/monitored and compared to total hours of operation. The base load of a facility should require a set number of chillers to operate with an additional chiller to satisfy the day's peak demands. During the course of a normal day and evening, the load in the facility may vary, requiring one lag chiller to start once each day to

satisfy demand. The lead chiller(s) should have relatively few starts as compared to the lag chiller, but the lag chiller generally should have no more than one start per day as needed. If trending indicates multiple starts for the lead chiller(s) or more than one start per day for the lag chiller, the system lead/lag controls should be investigated.

(3) **Chiller run time.** Operating times for chillers in a system should be equally divided to maximize the useful life of the equipment. However, this assumes all chillers in the system are equally sized and equally efficient, and chillers frequently have differing efficiencies due to their age or variations in their tonnage. Because chillers operate most efficiently fully loaded, the capacity of different combinations of chillers may need to be matched to the anticipated building loads according to the time of year. Chiller run time can be trended or monitored using the building automation system.

(4) **Primary CHW flow vs. secondary CHW flow.** In primary/secondary systems, it is critical to assure the total flow in the primary loop is greater than that in the secondary loop so the chilled water supply temperature serving the facility is maintained at setpoint. The primary supply and the secondary supply water temperatures should be the same. Warmer secondary return water is mixed with supply water from the primary loop when the flow in the secondary loop exceeds the primary flow. This results in warmer than design secondary supply water. Trending the secondary water supply temperature against the primary loop supply temperature will indicate if the secondary loop flow is greater than the primary loop flow. Some systems have a flow sensor in the decoupler line between the primary and secondary loops. This flow reading should also be trended because a negative reading here also indicates flow in the secondary system is greater than that in the primary system.

(5) **Primary CHW temperature vs. secondary CHW temperature.** Chillers are designed to operate to a set differential between supply and return water temperatures. As long as the differential between the supply and return temperatures equals or exceeds this chiller design differential, the chiller can be fully loaded. However, the load side differential is often found to be less than the chiller design differential. Usually, this is a result of inadequate heat transfer at the air-handling units. In primary/secondary systems, the design primary loop temperature differential should be less than or equal to the secondary loop temperature differential. If the primary differential design temperature is greater than that in the secondary system, it will not allow the chillers to load properly. The primary supply and return water

temperatures should be trended to calculate their actual differential. This should also be done for the secondary supply and return water temperatures.

(6) **Differential pressure, setpoint and actual reading, and pump speed.** The secondary pumps are controlled by VFDs to deliver adequate flow to the loads. Review trend data to make sure the control loop is tuned and the pump speed reflects variations in load. Static pressure setpoint and actual readings should be trended against the VFD (variable frequency drive) output. The VFD should modulate the speed of the pump to maintain the setpoint as the load varies without overshooting the setpoint. The static pressure setpoint should have been determined during the TAB process and identified in the control system, but the setpoint is often found to be higher than necessary, wasting pump energy. The setpoint can be varied down to determine if the system can maintain the pressure at lower pump speeds while the AHU boxes are monitored to assure they maintain discharge air temperature setpoints.

5.1.5 Cooling Towers and Condenser Water Systems

Cooling towers and condenser water systems are operated to reject heat from the chillers. Many systems with multiple cooling towers are piped in a common piping arrangement (with common supply and common return water headers). In a "common system," isolation valves are installed to direct the condenser waterflow to the appropriate cooling tower(s). A less frequently used system utilizes dedicated piping between the cooling tower, condenser water pump, and associated chiller. For this discussion, it is assumed the "common header" system is being utilized. It is industry standard to design a multiple cooling tower system with at least some of the cooling tower fans driven by VFDs. Some systems may also have plate and frame heat exchangers to allow for "free" hydronic cooling in the winter months.

(1) **Staging cooling towers and cooling tower fans.** At some times of the year, cooling towers can maintain the condenser water supply (CWS) temperature without operating the cooling tower fans. In addition, depending on outside conditions, the flow of one or more cooling towers can be distributed across multiple cells to maintain the heat transfer needed to serve the operating chiller(s). The fans are only operated as needed to maintain condenser water supply temperature. To assure the cooling tower fan is not started until the differential between the CWS and the condenser water return (CWR) cannot be maintained by distributing the water over multiple cells, the condenser water supply and return temperatures should be trended against the operation of the cooling tower fan and the VFD output. As well, the VFD output should

be trended to assure the fan speed modulates as needed to maintain CWS setpoint. The fan speed should be limited to that needed to maintain the condenser water supply temperature at setpoint.

(2) **Run time.** The common header system allows any cooling tower cell and associated fan, or any condenser water pump, to serve any chiller in the system (assuming the cooling towers and chillers are equally sized). Cooling tower fan run time and condenser pump run times should be equally divided among the various cells and pumps. These run times should be trended to assure the various pieces of equipment are being operated equally.

(3) **Optimal CWS temperature.** Some chillers operate more efficiently at a CWS temperature that is lower than the design CWS temperature setpoint. The CWS temperature can be varied below the design setpoint to determine optimal chiller performance. The efficiency of the chillers can be trended against the varying CWS temperatures to determine the CWS temperatures at which the chillers operate most efficiently.

(4) **Plate-and-frame approach.** When a plate-and-frame system is used to create chilled water directly from the condenser water, there is a design-defined CWS temperature that will be required to maintain the desired chilled water supply (CHS) temperature. When a plate-and-frame heat exchanger becomes fouled, the heat transfer is reduced and the CHS supply temperature rises above setpoint. Trends of the CHS temperature and the CWS temperature should be taken to monitor the efficiency of the heat exchanger and identify when the equipment should be serviced.

5.2 MEASURE AND VERIFY ACTUAL ENERGY PERFORMANCE

To measure energy performance, the HFCxA and the facility manager can collaborate to establish a Portfolio Manager account on the EPA Energy Star website. Once the required building information has been entered into the Portfolio Manager account, the facility manager should enter actual electricity and heating fuel costs as well as water consumption and costs. After 12 months of data have been entered into the Portfolio Manager account, the facility receives a baseline Energy Star rating. Because the Energy Star rating is normalized to weather and other parameters entered into Portfolio Manager, it can be used to compare year-by-year performance for the life of the facility. An energy efficiency scorecard can be established using the Portfolio Manager data, and the facility manager should publish this each month to help staff manage energy use.

When the baseline Energy Star rating is lower than that projected during project design, the HFCxA can help the facility make adjustments to improve energy efficiency. However, caution should be taken when comparing monthly actual figures from the first 12 months of operation to the consumption and costs predicted by the design phase energy model (see Section 2.2, Set Project Energy Efficiency Goals). The design phase energy model makes many assumptions concerning actual weather and operation of the building that may not be realized, sometimes resulting in inaccurate predictions of energy consumption, demand, or costs. Consequently, the design phase energy model should be recalibrated using actual monthly utility bills, weather data, operational data, and system-level trend data (as well as ASHRAE 90.1 baseline building energy consumption levels, if applicable), as described below. If actual consumption and costs exceed predicted levels, the HFCxA works with the facility manager, design team, and contractor to identify the cause of the discrepancy and implement corrective action. An energy model recalibrated using actual data reflects the performance of the building and can be used to identify building systems that are not performing as intended.

5.2.1 Measurement and Verification

Energy, water, or demand savings cannot be directly measured since this type of saving represents an absence of use or demand. Instead, savings are determined by comparing measurements of use or demand before and after implementation of an energy management program, making suitable allowances for differences in environmental conditions. In a new construction project, where no previous measurements exist, a baseline building defined by an energy code or standard (e.g., ASHRAE 90.1) is typically used for comparison.

(1) **The process.** Measurement and verification (M&V) is the process of using measurements to reliably determine the actual savings a facility achieves once it has implemented an energy management program. M&V activities include some or all of the following:

   (a) Meter installation, calibration, and maintenance

   (b) Data gathering and screening

   (c) Development of a method for computing calibrated savings and acceptable calibration accuracy. (Criteria are provided in the International Performance Measurement & Verification Protocol (IPMVP), Volume III: *Concepts and Options for Determining Energy Savings in New Construction*; ASHRAE Guideline 14: *Measurement of Energy Savings*; and/or the Federal Energy Management Program (FEMP)'s *M&V Guidelines: Measurement and Verification for Federal Energy Projects Version*.)

(d) Computations using data collected. (The IPMVP offers four different computation options; Option D, "Whole Building Calibrated Simulation," is the most commonly used when a design phase energy model has been generated.)

(e) Reporting, quality assurance, and third-party verification of reports

(2) **Recommended practices.** Good M&V practices yield results that are:

(a) Accurate—M&V reports should be as accurate as the M&V budget will allow. M&V costs are normally small relative to the monetary value of the savings being measured.

(b) Comprehensive—Energy savings reporting should consider all effects from a project. For example, in addition to the reduction in lighting and cooling energy, a lighting retrofit should take into account any increases in heating energy.

(c) Conservative—If judgments must be made about uncertain data, M&V procedures should be designed to underestimate savings. Any assumptions or stipulations should be founded and well-documented.

(d) Consistent—All M&V procedures and reports should be consistent with an industry standard convention such as the IPMVP, ASHRAE Guideline 14, or the FEMP *M&V Guidelines*.

(e) Relevant—Direct measurements and trending from the M&V process should focus on the performance parameters of most concern, while other less critical or predictable parameters may be estimated or stipulated. The results of the M&V analysis should inform the facility manager as to the actual savings from implementation of a project, relating them to pre-implementation building performance or baseline building data and comparing them to design phase energy model predictions. The M&V analysis should also identify systems not performing as intended and provide suggestions for corrective actions.

(f) Transparent—All M&V activities should be clearly and fully disclosed.

5.2.2 EPA Energy Star Portfolio Manager

The EPA Energy Star Portfolio Manager is an interactive energy management tool that supports tracking and assessment of energy and water consumption across an entire portfolio of buildings in a secure online environment. Portfolio Manager can be used to identify underperforming buildings so they can be targeted for energy efficiency improvements and to establish baselines for setting and measuring progress for energy efficiency improvement projects. The HFCxA should work with the owner's staff to set up Portfolio Manager and to interpret the data it generates.

(1) **Data collection.** Data collection for input into Portfolio Manager should begin as soon as commissioning has been completed and the facility has been put into operation. To get an accurate Energy Star rating, it is necessary to collect data for at least 12 months so it will reflect building system performance in a way that takes into account seasonal variations and full occupancy of the facilities. If significant portions of the building are not immediately put into operation, the energy usage will not correlate well with the building energy model developed during design, which will have assumed full building operation.

(2) **Energy model calibration.** As actual building energy and water usage are measured, the data should be compared to the usage predicted by the design phase energy model. Apply actual use data to recalibrate the model so it can be used for accurate predictions of future energy and water use. Using long-term trend data for various key building systems will help assure the recalibration process results in an energy model that more closely reflects the performance of the building at system level. The HFCxA should assist the building owner and design team in recalibrating the building energy model.

(3) **Initial setup.** EPA Portfolio Manager is designed to benchmark the performance of many different types of buildings. Health care space is divided into three types:

(a) Acute care and children's hospital campuses

(b) Freestanding acute care and children's hospitals

(c) Freestanding medical office buildings

The acute care hospital, children's hospital, or medical office space must be at least 50 percent of the total health care property to use the rating system. Only one of these categories can be used to define the primary space type for a project. Specific guidance on defining your health care property type can be found on the EPA Portfolio Manager website.

(4) **Data requirements.** A data collection worksheet is available on the Portfolio Manager website.

(a) The initial data required to set up a hospital worksheet are:

      (i) Gross square footage of floor area

     (ii) Number of licensed beds

   (iii) Maximum number of floors

   (iv) Tertiary care facility (as defined by Energy Star)—yes or no

  (b) Optional data include:

      (i) Laboratory on-site—yes or no

     (ii) Laundry facilities on-site—yes or no

   (iii) Number of buildings

   (iv) Ownership status (choose from dropdown options)

  (c) The initial data required to set up a medical office worksheet in Portfolio Manager are:

      (i) Gross square footage of floor area

     (ii) Number of workers on main shift

   (iii) Weekly operating hours

   (iv) Percentage of floor area cooled in 10 percent increments

    (v) Percentage of floor area heated in 10 percent increments

(5) **Viewing and interpreting results.** Once 12 months of utility data have been entered into Portfolio Manager, the system produces a baseline rating from 1 to 100. A rating of 75 or better allows users to display the Energy Star label to create awareness that the facility has been nationally recognized for its energy efficiency. The label also demonstrates an organization's commitment to reducing environmental pollution and emissions that contribute to global warming. Achieving Energy Star status will also demonstrate to organizational leadership that the facility department is saving money and boosting the organization's bottom line.

(6) **Tracking progress over time.** Portfolio Manger comes pre-populated with nine standard summary views of facility data, which are displayed in the My Portfolio summary page. These include:

     Summary: Energy Use

     Performance: Greenhouse Gas Emissions

     Performance: Financial

     Performance: Water Use

In addition, users can create and save custom downloadable views by choosing from more than 70 different metrics. All data can be exported to Microsoft Excel®.

(7) **Verifying and documenting results.** Portfolio Manager can be used to quickly and accurately document reductions in energy use, greenhouse gas emissions, water use, and energy costs for an individual building or an entire portfolio. This information can be used to provide transparency and accountability for capital projects and to help demonstrate strategic use of funding. The HFCxA should help the building owner compare the facility's actual performance to the performance predicted by its energy model. At the end of project delivery, this comparison can help identify potential problems and items that need to be corrected by the contractor prior to the end of the warranty period.

5.3 CONDUCT POSTOCCUPANCY PERFORMANCE TESTS

The systems that serve a new construction, renovation, or mechanical/electrical/plumbing (MEP) infrastructure upgrade project are designed to operate in multiple modes depending on the season or the state of occupancy of the facility. Anticipated modes may include normal/occupied, unoccupied, and emergency for each of the cooling, heating, and shoulder seasons of operation.

At the outset of a project, the scope of work for postoccupancy performance testing of the various modes during each season in the first year of occupancy should be included in the contracts for the entire commissioning team. When construction approaches the acceptance phase of the project, the HFCxA, the construction team, the design team, and facility O&M staff should collaboratively work together to identify the performance tests required to be completed after occupancy.

An effective plan for this postoccupancy performance testing comprises the following steps:

(1) Identify the seasonal or deferred performance tests in the commissioning or turnover plan.

(2) Discuss and document open issues, and make sure they are included in the HFCxA's issues log and substantial completion minutes and that they are discussed during O&M staff walkthroughs and end user occupancy training.

(3) Inform the end users how hot and cold calls or other expected issues will be handled until the systems have been fully tested and accepted.

(4) Plan for the implementation of performance testing, including a coordination meeting to be held before testing begins and a procedure for testing that includes risk assessments for the occupied spaces and adequate resource representation.

(5) Implement performance testing with proper notification to all affected parties.

(6) Maintain a deficiency log of items discovered during testing; repair and retest as required.

(7) Complete O&M staff training related to system performance requirements unique to each season.

(8) Formally accept the completed system.

(9) Include the performance test documentation in the commissioning report and turnover plan.

5.4 PARTICIPATE IN THE END-OF-WARRANTY REVIEW

The HFCxA participates with the commissioning team (owner, contractor, and design team) in a comprehensive review of the project near the end of the warranty phase (eight to 10 months after substantial completion). This review identifies outstanding construction deficiencies and additional deficiencies discovered by the O&M staff after occupancy.

The HFCxA should assist the owner with documentation of warranty period issues. The owner and HFCxA should maintain a record of deficiencies and problems discovered during the warranty period and identify any unresolved items so they may be addressed at the end-of-warranty review meeting. Routine maintenance items should not be misrepresented as warranty items. Documentation is critical, especially for issues that are not corrected in a timely manner by the contractor.

The warranty review meeting should also address any items related to incomplete scope of work for any member of the commissioning team. Examples of such items are inadequate or incomplete O&M training, incomplete postoccupancy testing, inadequate or incomplete O&M documentation, incomplete or inaccurate record documents, and so on. Open items that remain on the commissioning master issues log should be addressed in the meeting as well.

The HFCxA coordinates with the owner to schedule the warranty review meeting with the project team. The HFCxA develops an agenda for the meeting based on input from the owner and the commissioning team and publishes the agenda at least one week prior to the meeting. The agenda should include an opportunity for team members to share lessons learned during the HFCx process. The HFCxA will chair the meeting, prepare and issue meeting minutes, and follow up on outstanding issues to facilitate resolution before the end of the warranty period. No less than one month prior to the end of the warranty, the HFCxA provides a written report to the owner defining any remaining open items, copying all other members of the commissioning team.

If several attempts and a significant amount of time are required to correct an issue, the owner may need to negotiate an extended warranty with the contractor. For example, if it takes several tries to correct a leaky roof or window, the owner should get a full 12-month warranty for the properly installed system.

5.5 BENCHMARK ONGOING ENERGY PERFORMANCE

5.5.1 Benchmarking as an Ongoing Activity

Over time, numerous events and other influences can affect a facility's energy consumption. For instance, systems degrade as they age (sensors fail, control devices fail, devices drift out of calibration, etc.), and system programming can accidentally be changed. Thus, to maintain and strive to improve a facility's energy performance over time, the owner or the HFCxA should continue the benchmarking process indefinitely after the facility's energy performance baseline has been established after a year in service.

Energy performance benchmarking is a critical first step in all measurable, documented energy or carbon reduction initiatives. An ongoing program is required to identify continued energy-related returns on investment (ROIs) such as costs per kWh saved.

Since hospitals operate around the clock every day of the year, many ongoing O&M activities (e.g., vibration analysis, TAB, staff training, and pump and fan efficiency programs) will yield an annual energy reduction impact three to five times that of similar projects in commercial buildings. Ongoing commissioning is an important component in sustaining the successful implementation of energy conservation measures and design concepts.

5.5.2 The ASHE Energy Efficiency Commitment Program

The ASHE HFCx commissioning process recognizes that facility managers and plant engineers are required to be knowledgeable about energy usage, management, and conservation. ASHE is committed to helping facility managers identify how their new facility, renovated space, or MEP infrastructure currently uses energy and what the statistical breakdown of its energy use is by source and load. This commitment is fleshed out in the ASHE Energy Commitment (E^2C) program.

Building on past successes in energy benchmarking through EPA Energy Star and the ASHE publication *Healthcare Energy Guidebook*, ASHE and the EPA collaborated to create ASHE E^2C in 2006. The program facilitates peer networking and sharing of fundamental concepts, real data, proven strategies, financial tools, and local success stories among ASHE members.

No fees or costs are associated with participation in E^2C; this is an ASHE member service. The Society's commitment is to help facility managers share their knowledge with their peers and learn from each other's experiences. This cooperation will not only help improve individual facility operations, it will also improve the state of the art of energy management.

To get started with E^2C, visit the ASHE E^2C Web page at www.ashe.org/e2c.

Retrocommissioning Activities

6.1 THE RETROCOMMISSIONING PROCESS

6.1.1 Who Leads the Effort

Retrocommissioning is generally undertaken to optimize the performance of the building systems in an existing facility. A health facility commissioning agent (HFCxA) should lead the retrocommissioning effort.

The individual who serves as retrocommissioning team leader (RTL) should have extensive health care facility design, construction, and operations experience. To sell retrocommissioning to the health facility C-suite (chief executive officer, chief operating officer, chief financial officer, and so on), the RTL must speak their language, using concepts like payors, case mix, patient days, internal rate of return, net present value, and so on. The RTL must also possess detailed knowledge of utility rate structures, HVAC systems, automatic temperature control, energy efficiency measures, and measurement and verification techniques, and be capable of reading, modifying, and writing control programs using the facility's energy management system (EMS). In short, the RTL must be equally comfortable in the health care organization's boardroom and its boiler room.

The health care facility should select the RTL based on qualifications. Since a more qualified RTL could achieve significantly higher life cycle energy cost savings than a less qualified RTL, fee should not be a significant factor in the selection process. After selecting the RTL, the health care facility should negotiate a reasonable fee for the requested services. The fee for basic retrocommissioning services typically ranges from 15 to 30 cents per square foot of floor space, with larger facilities (more than 1 million square feet) on the low end of the range and smaller facilities (less than 100,000 square feet) on the high end. Basic retrocommissioning services generally include energy benchmarking, review of current utility procurement practices (commonly referred to as a supply-side energy audit), and a review of the facility's energy-consuming systems and equipment.

It is important to note that the fee for basic retrocommissioning services does not represent the entire cost of a retrocommissioning effort. In many instances, the initial work also includes equipment testing; air and water testing, adjusting, and balancing (TAB); and automatic temperature control system repairs and programming revisions. The cost of these additional services typically ranges from 30 to 70 cents per square foot, with larger facilities on the low end of the range and smaller facilities on the high end. After the retrocommissioning team has completed their initial work, the health care facility may also implement capital-intensive energy conservation measures identified by the RTL and the retrocommissioning team (e.g., equipment replacements, system conversions, etc.). The cost of implementing these energy cost reduction measures can range from $1 to $20 per square foot.

The retrocommissioning team must include the health facility O&M staff. O&M staff members operate the systems and equipment and know the changes in sequences of operation and setpoints that have occurred since the building was constructed. They also have knowledge of maintenance challenges and energy conservation opportunities. Most importantly, the O&M staff will be responsible for implementing any changes in procedure suggested by the retrocommissioning effort. If O&M staff predict a specific action will work, they will make certain it does work. If they predict a specific action will not work, generally that is true as well. To the fullest extent possible, the O&M staff should implement the retrocommissioning work. This provides valuable training and vests staff members in a positive outcome. The likelihood of positive and sustainable retrocommissioning results is directly proportional to the level of O&M staff involvement.

The retrocommissioning effort strives for continuous progress toward optimum performance. Optimizing performance can take many forms, including improved energy efficiency, equipment and system longevity, equipment and system reliability, thermal comfort, lowered infection rates, business continuity, and patient, staff, and visitor satisfaction. Unlike most standard commissioning services, the scope of retrocommissioning work is not restricted to assuring that building systems meet the design intent. In many cases, the retrocommissioning effort actually corrects deficiencies in the original building design.

6.1.2 Items of Work for Retrocommissioning Energy-Consuming Systems

The retrocommissioning process for energy-consuming systems in health care facilities should include these items of work:

(1) Establish an Energy Star® Portfolio Manager account for the health care facility.

Energy Star is a free Internet-based service of the U.S. Environmental Protection Agency designed to track energy consumption and costs. Health care facilities can use Energy Star to benchmark their energy consumption against that of similar facilities. Energy Star uses energy consumption, floor area, and other factors to establish a weather-adjusted percentile ranking. For example, a ranking of 75 indicates a health care facility is more energy-efficient than 75 percent of its peers and less energy-efficient than 25 percent of its peers.

The first step in the Energy Star benchmarking process is to set up a Portfolio Manager account. Portfolio Manager is the program provided by Energy Star for entering data and generating reports. Once a Portfolio Manager account has been set up, it can be accessed at any time using standard Internet web browser software. Access to the facility's account is controlled by a user-defined password.

Instructions for setting up a Portfolio Manager account can be found on the ASHE website at www.ashe.org/e2c and at www.energystar.gov/benchmark.

(2) Obtain 24 months of utility bills (natural gas, fuel oil, steam, chilled water, electricity, water, sewer, etc.) and enter them into the Portfolio Manager account.

EPA Energy Star establishes a baseline rating for a facility based on its historical utility consumption and other facility-specific information. A health facility O&M staff member manually enters utility consumption and cost figures taken from monthly utility bills into Portfolio Manager. Although the RTL or other consultant can enter the data, it is best if the O&M staff accomplishes this task (involving the O&M staff to the fullest extent possible is desired for the reasons previously mentioned). Utility account representatives for the health care facility may be able to provide the consumption and cost data in a summary format. If the health care facility purchases natural gas in an "unbundled" manner [as described in Section 6.1.2 (12)(k)], all costs including commodity, transportation, local distribution, cash-in/cash-out, and transportation fuel must be included (thus accounting for the total cost of natural gas delivered to the burner tip). The costs entered into Portfolio Manager should match the health care facility's utility expenditures for the corresponding time period. To assure accuracy and consistency, the RTL should always review the data entered into Portfolio Manager.

Portfolio Manager allows the user to select any 12 consecutive months within the prior 60 months as the time period used to determine a facility's baseline Energy Star rating. Although a baseline rating can be determined from only 12 months of data, a more extensive data set (a minimum of 24 months, if possible) helps the retrocommissioning team identify performance opportunities, spot trends and anomalies, and understand how the facility reacts to weather and other factors.

(3) Enter other required facility data into the Portfolio Manager account. Obtain a baseline Energy Star rating for the facility.

An algorithm that considers a facility's source energy consumption, zip code (climate), building location, gross floor area (excluding parking facilities), number of beds, number of floors, and the presence or absence of tertiary care (specialized care such as high-risk pregnancies, oncology, neurosurgery, trauma surgery, and organ transplants) determines the Energy Star rating. To be considered a hospital, the health care facility must use at least 51 percent of its floor area for acute care services. The algorithm allows a direct comparison of the Energy Star rating for a small 25-bed hospital in a cold climate (e.g., Minnesota) to a large 1,000-bed hospital in a hot and humid climate (e.g., Florida). Thus, the O&M staff should enter site-specific information into Portfolio Manager.

Because of the dynamic nature of the health care facility business—due to changing technology, emerging competition, shifting demographics and market areas, and an aging population—most health care facilities are continuously evolving through renovations, additions, and construction of new buildings. To assure the accuracy of the Energy Star rating at any point in time, the O&M staff must promptly enter all changes in gross floor area, number of floors, and number of beds into the Portfolio Manager account.

Once the health care facility has set up the Portfolio Manager account, populated it with utility bill and site-specific facility data, and defined a baseline period, EPA Energy Star automatically establishes the facility's baseline Energy Star rating. The average baseline rating is 50. If the hospital has a baseline rating above 50, the facility operates more efficiently than its peers. If the hospital has a baseline rating below 50, the facility operates less efficiently than its peers.

The health facility O&M staff may worry that a low baseline rating casts a bad light on their job performance. On these occasions, the RTL must act quickly to alleviate their fears. The baseline represents nothing more than point A—a starting place. The

Area	Average Electricity Demand (watts/SF)	
	Minimum	Maximum
Hospital	**4.8**	**7.5**
Outpatient facility	4.6	7.2
Nursing facility	4.6	7.0
Administrative and educational areas	4.5	6.8
Laboratory and research areas	5.5	8.2
Residential facility	3.8	6.5

Table 6-1: Typical Health Facility Average Electricity Demand

retrocommissioning team should not focus on point A but on demonstrating progress toward point B—the target rating. Instead of fearing a low baseline rating, O&M staff should embrace the opportunities it represents.

The retrocommissioning team should consider other performance benchmarks in addition to the baseline Energy Star rating. Other relevant performance benchmarks include average monthly billed demand per square foot (watts/SF), annual electricity consumption per square foot (kWh/SF), annual natural gas use per square foot (kBtu/SF), and annual water consumption (gallons/SF). The figures shown in Tables 6-1 through 6-4 indicate typical ranges for these performance benchmarks for various types of health care facilities.

The retrocommissioning team should also use submeter data (if available) to allocate total campus energy consumption to individual buildings. The individual building energy consumption data can then be used to prioritize the team's efforts. A building with higher energy consumption per square foot than the standard range for its specific building type is likely to offer a greater opportunity for improvement and savings.

(4) Establish a target Energy Star rating for the facility.

Like all goals, the target Energy Star rating should be significant, achievable, and measurable. Perhaps most important, all stakeholders (RTL, O&M staff, and C-suite) must accept the target rating. In most cases, the

Area	Average Electricity Consumption (kWh/SF)	
	Minimum	Maximum
Hospital	28	50
Outpatient facility	20	40
Nursing facility	20	40
Administrative and educational areas	15	35
Laboratory and research areas	30	50
Residential facility	15	25

Table 6-2: Typical Health Facility Electricity Consumption

Area	Average Electricity Consumption (kBtu/SF)	
	Minimum	Maximum
Hospital	75	275
Outpatient facility	40	180
Nursing facility	40	150
Administrative and educational areas	25	132
Laboratory and research areas	65	300
Residential facility	25	70

Table 6-3: Typical Health Facility Heating Fuel Consumption

Area	Average Electricity Consumption (gallons/SF)	
	Minimum	Maximum
Hospital	40	100
Outpatient facility	15	60
Nursing facility	50	80
Administrative and educational areas	5	15
Laboratory and research areas	25	35
Residential facility	50	80

Table 6-4: Typical Health Facility Water Consumption

ultimate goal of the retrocommissioning effort should be to earn an Energy Star award. In 2009 only 29 hospitals (out of approximately 6,000 in the United States) earned the Energy Star award, which requires a rating of 75 or higher.

To apply for the Energy Star award, a facility must submit a Statement of Energy Performance (SEP) and a Data Checklist to the EPA. The SEP contains basic building information, site and source energy consumption, and the Energy Star rating. The Data Checklist verifies that the facility's HVAC systems are operating in compliance with applicable codes and that the facility has not reduced energy consumption at the expense of infection control and other environmental requirements. A licensed professional (preferably the RTL) must sign the SEP and the Data Checklist. This individual verifies that the facility has accurately reported all energy use and building characteristics and that facility operation complies with industry standards and applicable regulations. In short, the licensed professional protects the integrity and credibility of the award.

When a health care facility has a baseline Energy Star rating of significantly less than 50, the chance of achieving an Energy Star rating of 75 in the near term is significantly reduced. To keep the team motivated, it is preferable to set an interim goal to strive for rather than a loftier goal that will take much longer to achieve. In the shuffle of day-to-day responsibilities and an overwhelming maintenance workload (many health care facilities have extremely thin O&M staffing levels), it is easy to lose sight of a distant goal and put off the steps needed to achieve it. Thus, a health care facility that likely cannot achieve its primary goal in the near term should begin by pursuing intermediate goals. ASHE established its Energy Efficiency Commitment (E2C) program for this purpose. The E2C program provides awards for improvement in energy efficiency in 5 percent increments, beginning with 10 percent improvement.

Once a health care facility has set its primary and intermediate goals, the RTL and the O&M staff develop a timetable with deadlines. Absent a timetable and a sense of urgency, interest in the retrocommissioning effort will dwindle.

The sample timetable shown in Figure 6-1 indicates a baseline Energy Star rating of 37, a current Energy Star rating of 42, a target Energy Star rating of 75, and intermediate E2C goals of 10 percent, 20 percent, and 30 percent improvement. It also indicates the expected annual energy cost savings associated with each goal—reaching more than $3.5 million per year when the primary goal is achieved.

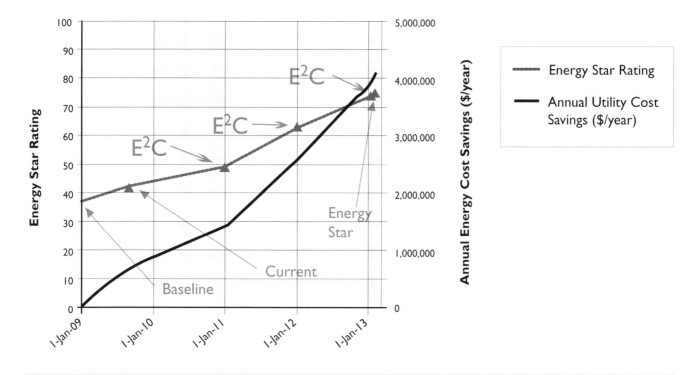

Figure 6-1: Sample Energy Efficiency Goal Timetable

(5) Identify the potential energy cost savings associated with increasing the Energy Star rating from the baseline level to the target level.

Although a successful retrocommissioning effort will yield other benefits as well, achieving energy cost savings is its primary focus. Depending on a facility's baseline Energy Star rating, the energy cost savings resulting from the retrocommissioning effort should range between 5 and 35 percent of baseline energy costs. Savings for facilities with higher baseline Energy Star ratings typically fall at the low end of the range, while savings for facilities with lower baseline ratings typically fall at the high end (since a lower baseline provides a greater opportunity for improvement and savings).

Portfolio Manager will automatically calculate the energy cost savings associated with a target increase in the Energy Star rating (assuming the O&M staff has entered the utility data into the Portfolio Manager account as previously recommended). The savings calculated by Energy Star are based on flat utility unit costs (total consumption divided by total cost). Most utilities, however, use considerably more sophisticated and complex rate structures with customer, demand, and commodity components. Some of these components are fixed, while others vary with consumption.

A comprehensive retrocommissioning effort includes evaluation and implementation of supply-side energy cost reduction measures that affect utility unit costs. A comprehensive retrocommissioning effort may also change a facility's daily and weekly electricity consumption profile. In most applications, retrocommissioning reduces electricity consumption to a greater extent during nights and weekends than during weekdays. This change in the electricity consumption profile reduces the facility's electricity load factor (ratio of average electrical demand to monthly billed demand). Changes in electricity load factor may warrant or possibly even necessitate a change in the facility's electricity rate and rider combination (electric utilities frequently offer standard, time-of-use, and interruptible rate structures). For these reasons, the utility cost savings projected by Portfolio Manager may not be exact. They should be sufficiently accurate, however, for planning purposes. It should also be noted that a more precise estimate is not possible at the onset of the retrocommissioning process because neither the supply-side energy cost reduction measures nor changes in the electricity load profile are known yet.

(6) Obtain and review construction drawings and specifications for the original construction and any renovations to the facility.

The existing conditions at most health care facilities result from a near continuous series of new construction, expansion, and renovation projects. The construction documents for these projects contain information valuable for the retrocommissioning effort. The health care facility should have a current archive of construction documents. Ideally, these documents are organized chronologically by project number in an electronic format (e.g., AutoCAD). If the health care facility does not have a current construction document archive, the retrocommissioning team must develop one. If the health care facility cannot provide construction documents, the RTL should contact the project design team and request copies. If this fails, the RTL should contact the state health department (most state health departments review the documents and may retain copies).

The retrocommissioning team should review each set of construction documents, typically beginning with the oldest project and progressing to the most recent, to discern the design intent of the energy-consuming systems. The review typically focuses on the lighting and HVAC systems with specific attention to equipment schedules and control diagrams. The retrocommissioning team should come away from the construction document review with an understanding of how the original design professionals intended the energy-consuming systems to function. It is important to realize, however, that the energy systems are not likely to be functioning in strict accordance with their design intent.

(7) Obtain and review submittal data and maintenance manuals for the major equipment.

The contractor typically provides submittal data and maintenance manuals to the design team for review at the onset of construction. The submittal data identifies the equipment manufacturer, model number, serial number, performance data, and electrical characteristics of the equipment. The maintenance manuals include detailed instructions for maintaining the equipment, including troubleshooting guides and spare parts lists. The retrocommissioning team needs this information for all major equipment, including water chillers, cooling towers, boilers, pumps, air-handling units, exhaust fans, kitchen hoods, and similar equipment. The retrocommissioning team should also obtain copies of equipment factory test and start-up reports if available.

The health care facility should have a current archive of submittal documents and maintenance manuals, ideally organized chronologically by project number in an electronic format. Some highly progressive health care facilities are now using building information modeling (BIM) as a means to archive documents related to the planning, design, and construction process, including the owner's project requirements (OPR), basis of design (BOD), drawings, submittal documents, shop drawings, installation instructions, maintenance manuals, test results, and so on. If the health care facility cannot provide the submittal documents and maintenance manuals, the RTL should contact the equipment manufacturers, design team, and contractors and request copies. The retrocommissioning team should develop a submittal data and maintenance manual archive if the health care facility does not have a current one.

The retrocommissioning team reviews the submittal data, maintenance manuals, factory test reports, and start-up reports to find the rated capacities and efficiencies of the equipment under the anticipated operating conditions. During the review, equipment nearing the end of its useful life, obsolete equipment, or equipment otherwise in need of replacement is diagnosed. The team also uses the submittal data and start-up reports to identify equipment performance issues. For example, the design flow and water pressure drop for a chilled water coil can be used to determine whether debris is obstructing the coil.

(8) Obtain and review testing, adjusting, and balancing reports for the original construction and renovations.

During project delivery, the TAB contractor documents the results of the TAB process in a written report and submits it to the design team for review. The O&M staff should have an archive of these reports, which the retrocommissioning team obtains and reviews.

The team compares each TAB report to the construction drawings and identifies any significant deviations, which may indicate unresolved installation and performance issues. The team also compares the airflows indicated in the TAB report to the design airflows. If a significant number of discrepancies are found, this indicates the TAB report may not be accurate. A report that has not been properly prepared is sometimes referred to as a "drive-by TAB report."

The TAB reports also contain initial equipment test data that the retrocommissioning team can use as a baseline for comparison to current equipment performance. If the health care facility cannot provide the TAB reports, the RTL should contact the design teams and contractors and request copies. If the health care facility does not have a current TAB report archive, the retrocommissioning team should develop one.

(9) Obtain and review control diagrams for the original construction and any renovations.

(a) The contractor typically provides control diagrams to the design team for review as part of the planning, design, and construction process. The control diagrams generally include schematic equipment and system diagrams, wiring diagrams, sequences of operation, and catalog data sheets for the control equipment and components.

The health care facility should have a current archive of the control diagrams, ideally organized chronologically by project number in an electronic format. If the health care facility cannot provide the control diagrams, the RTL should contact the control system supplier, design team, and contractors and request copies. If the health care facility does not have a current control diagram archive, the retrocommissioning team should develop one.

(b) The retrocommissioning team reviews the control diagrams to determine the intended sequences of operation and setpoints for the equipment and systems as well as to identify potential opportunities for performance optimization. The control diagram review should identify the following aspects of the automatic temperature control system:

(i) **Manufacturer, supplier and installer:** The control diagram review team should identify the manufacturer of the control system equipment and find out which companies served as local supplier and installer.

(ii) **Control system type or types in use:** Common control system types include pneumatic, electric, analog electronic, and direct digital control (DDC), and most health care facilities use a combination of these. DDC control with pneumatic actuation at the air-handling units and either pneumatic or analog electronic controls at the air terminals is a combination often found at health care facilities.

(iii) **Network architecture:** DDC systems utilize hierarchal control networks. Possible networks include enterprise level, building level, floor level, and device level. Many DDC systems use a combination enterprise/building-level network residing on a fiber-optic network and a combination floor/device-level network residing on twisted copper. In facilities that use this type of network architecture, workstations and building level controllers are connected to the building-level network and air terminal controllers and variable frequency drives (VFDs) are connected to floor-level networks.

(iv) **Communication protocol or protocols in use:** DDC systems use either an open or proprietary communication protocol. The most common open communication protocol is BACnet; other types include MODBUS and LON. If the system uses such an open protocol, it may be possible to connect control equipment from different manufacturers to the same system.

(v) **Number and location of operator workstations:** O&M staff use operator workstations to access the control system, monitor equipment performance, change control parameters, and manually control equipment (an act commonly referred to as an "override"). Most health care facilities have operator workstations located in the control shop, maintenance office, facility management office, and central energy plant.

(vi) **Remote access to the control system:** Some DDC systems are accessible from remote locations via the Internet or phone modem, allowing O&M staff to access the system from home and the RTL and other retrocommissioning team members to access it from off-site. This access can significantly expedite the retrocommissioning process. If the system allows remote access, the review team should identify the software and hardware required to use this feature. If the system does not permit remote access, the team should determine the actions required to provide this capability. (In some cases, however, facility IT security protocols may prevent such access.)

(vii) **Intended sequences of operation:** The control diagrams include sequences of operation for equipment and systems. These typically describe in general terms how equipment and systems were intended to be controlled.

(viii) **Design setpoints:** The control diagrams typically indicate design setpoints such as air-handling unit supply air temperature, supply air static pressure, and minimum outside airflow.

(ix) **Data archiving capability:** Nearly all DDC systems have the capability to record data, commonly referred to as "trending." Network speed and system memory often limit trending capability to a select few points for short periods of time. Some DDC systems, however, have the hardware and software required for continuous data archiving of all points, a capability that can greatly benefit the retrocommissioning effort. If the system does not currently allow continuous data archiving, the control system review should identify the actions required to provide this capability.

(x) **Availability of a control system commissioning tool:** A relatively small number of DDC systems have a software commissioning tool that allows users to query the system. For example, the system could be asked for a list of all air terminals with open dampers and little or no airflow. Like continuous data archiving, this type of commissioning tool can greatly benefit the retrocommissioning team. If a commissioning tool is not currently available, the actions required to provide this capability should be determined.

(xi) **Energy conservation opportunities:** The retrocommissioning team should look for obvious energy conservation opportunities such as a supply air temperature setpoint that is too low, a static pressure setpoint that is too high, or overlapping heating and cooling setpoints.

Most health care facilities have some type of energy management system (EMS), also known as a building automation system (BAS). These systems typically include provisions for sophisticated energy conservation and cost reduction strategies such as weekly scheduling of equipment and systems, night setback/setup, demand limiting, automatic setpoint reset, and optimal dispatch of equipment. In many health care facilities, however, O&M staff only use the EMS for monitoring and manual control, and the EMS energy conservation strategies either have been disabled or were never deployed. The frequent underutilization of EMS energy conservation strategies in health care facilities is due to a number of factors, most notably insufficient O&M staff training, both initial and ongoing. In some cases, health care facilities have spent considerable time, effort, and money on EMS training, only to see their newly trained employee leave the health care facility for a more lucrative position in the control system industry.

Tapping the potential of the existing EMS to optimize equipment and system performance and to conserve energy should be a major initiative of the retrocommissioning team. In conjunction with implementing EMS energy conservation strategies, the team should train the O&M staff. Without such training, benefits realized from the retrocommissioning effort will not be sustainable.

(10) Conduct a detailed survey of the facility with a focus on the mechanical rooms, electrical rooms, and energy-consuming equipment and systems (water chillers, boilers, water heaters, air-handling units, exhaust fans, and pumps).

A comprehensive survey of every square foot of floor area in a health care facility would be time-consuming and cost-prohibitive. Since the heating, cooling, and ventilation systems typically account for 60 to 70 percent of a health care facility's annual energy consumption, these systems provide the greatest opportunity for energy conservation. Thus, focusing initial survey efforts on mechanical rooms, electrical rooms, and other energy-consuming equipment (kitchen, laundry, incinerator, etc.) expedites the retrocommissioning process and allows the health care facility to realize energy cost savings at an earlier date. After the initial retrocommissioning work has been completed and the transition to an ongoing retrocommissioning program has begun, the team surveys other areas of the facility (e.g., the building envelope, elevators, food services equipment, and laundry equipment) for further energy conservation opportunities.

(a) To facilitate the initial facility survey, copies of the following documents should be obtained. If the health care facility does not have any of them (e.g., site plan, floor plans, diagrams, etc.), locating these documents should be a goal of the retrocommissioning effort.

(i) **Documentation of previous energy conservation efforts:** Any prior energy audits, master plans, facility condition assessments, studies, and reports will prove useful to the retrocommissioning effort.

(ii) **Equipment inventory:** The facility's equipment inventory should indicate the equipment number, type, manufacturer, model number, serial number, location (building and room number), and year installed for all equipment in the facility. All equipment should bear a nameplate indicating its unique inventory number. Using a computerized maintenance management system (CMMS) that automatically generates preventive maintenance work orders and tracks equipment histories to generate the equipment inventory is a recommended practice. The team then verifies that the equipment information in the CMMS inventory matches the actual equipment nameplate data.

(iii) **Facility site plan:** The current health facility site plan should indicate the location of property lines, roads, drives, parking lots, buildings, major utilities (electricity, natural gas, water, etc.), fuel oil tanks, utility meters, and exterior equipment (bulk oxygen tank, primary transformers, cooling towers, air-cooled condensers, air-cooled chillers, etc.).

(iv) **Building list:** The list of all buildings on the health facility campus should include the name, gross floor area, number of floors, and year constructed for each building.

(v) **Electrical single-line diagrams:** The health care facility's current electrical single-line diagrams should provide a schematic arrangement of electric utility services, utility meters, switchgear, transformers, main panelboards, submeters, branch panelboards, and large motors. Most health care facilities have separate electrical single-line diagrams for their normal power and essential power distribution systems.

(vi) **Floor plans:** A floor plan for each building, indicating room numbers and room names, should be marked to indicate the area served by each air-handling unit.

(vii) **Piping diagrams:** Accurate piping diagrams are needed for the following systems:

1. Chilled water

2. Tower water

3. Heating water

4. Steam and steam return

5. Domestic cold water

6. Domestic hot water

7. Medical gases (oxygen, medical air, medical vacuum, nitrous oxide, nitrogen, etc.)

(viii) **Chemical treatment reports:** The survey team reviews chemical treatment reports for the cooling tower, steam, and closed loop systems (preferably for the most recent 12 consecutive months, if available). Assuming they have been properly completed, these reports provide valuable information such as cycles of concentration, control parameters, make-up rates, blowdown rates, equipment operation, and peak system loads. The survey team notes any discrepancies such as inappropriate chemical treatment processes or control parameters that frequently fall out of acceptable range.

(ix) **Equipment logs:** The survey team reviews recent equipment logs for the cooling and heating equipment (a minimum of 12 consecutive months, if available) to determine maximum loads, minimum loads, average loads, and actual equipment sequencing strategy. The team notes performance improvement opportunities such as low chilled water or heating water temperature difference, inefficient equipment sequencing (e.g., operating more chillers than the load requires), and temperatures or other parameters out of normal range (e.g., chiller condenser entering water temperatures that exceed 85°F).

(x) **Equipment service histories:** The survey team reviews CMMS equipment service histories (work orders, repairs, etc.) to identify chronic maintenance problems such as numerous hot and cold complaints from the same area and frequent equipment failures.

(xi) **Service contracts:** Service contracts for chemical treatment, elevator maintenance, scheduled water chiller maintenance, and other equipment servicing are useful.

(b) During the facility survey, the retrocommissioning survey team notes any discrepancies from the construction documents such as missing equipment, equipment in a different location, different air-handling unit configurations, and equipment that has been replaced. The team takes photographs of major equipment, unsafe conditions, inoperable equipment, damaged insulation, pipe leaks, duct leaks, and other obvious performance improvement opportunities. Also during the survey, the following conditions and information are looked for and recorded:

(i) **Equipment nameplate data:** Each piece of equipment is inspected and the nameplate data recorded, including inventory number, manufacturer, model number, serial number, year manufactured, and electrical characteristics (voltage, full load amps, etc.).

(ii) **Duct leaks:** The exposed ductwork is inspected and any significant leaks (torn flexible duct connections, damaged gaskets at access doors, maintenance openings, ruptured seams, unplugged sensor openings, etc.) are noted.

(iii) **Pipe leaks:** The exposed piping and any leaks noted (e.g., leaks in valves, flanges, pump seals, deaerator overflow, etc.).

(iv) **Damaged insulation:** Exposed piping, ductwork, and equipment is inspected and any torn, damaged, or otherwise missing insulation noted.

(v) **Inoperable equipment:** Any equipment found to be out of service is recorded.

(vi) **Improper equipment operation:** Any equipment that is not operating properly or is otherwise in need of maintenance attention (excessive noise, vibration, loose belts, etc.) is noted.

(vii) **Equipment operating at full capacity:** Equipment operating near its full capacity (indicated by pumps or fans operating at 100 percent speed, water chillers operating at their electrical demand limit, control valves that are 100 percent open, etc.) indicates the possibility of impaired performance, excessive load, unrealistic control setpoint, or control malfunction and should be noted.

(viii) **High-pressure drop or partially closed balancing valves:** Any high-pressure drop balancing valves (globe valves, triple duty valves, etc.) and partially closed valves are noted. Partially closed triple-duty valves (which provide isolation, check, and balancing functions) located at the discharge of pumps controlled by variable frequency drives are common in health care facilities. (A typical arrangement is illustrated in Figure 6-2.)

(ix) **Unnecessary simultaneous heating and cooling:** Obvious simultaneous heating and cooling (e.g., partially open cooling and heating control valves on the same air-handling unit or an air terminal with a 100 percent open damper and a partially open reheat control valve) are noted. Reducing simultaneous heating and cooling is the most significant energy conservation opportunity in many health care facilities.

(x) **Uncomfortable areas:** Occupied areas that are found to be too warm, too cold, too humid, or otherwise uncomfortable are noted.

(xi) **Unsafe conditions:** Unsafe conditions such as missing junction box covers, combustible materials stored in mechanical rooms, missing fan belt covers, exposed electrical conductors, and so on are noted.

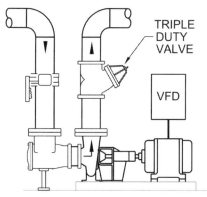

Figure 6-2: Pump with Triple-Duty Valve

(11) Conduct a detailed review of automatic temperature control systems, including those for water chillers, boilers, air terminals, air-handling units, exhaust fans, domestic water heating equipment, and fan coil units. Identify existing sequences of operation and setpoints.

The retrocommissioning team can obtain a significant amount of useful information from a facility's automatic temperature control systems. This is particularly true if the health care facility has a comprehensive EMS with DDC air terminal controls and a workstation with trending or data archiving capabilities. To obtain this information, the RTL and the O&M staff responsible for control system operation and maintenance conduct a detailed review of the entire system. For this review to be effective, the reviewers must be familiar with the system manufacturer and type of system in place. They must be able to log on and off; review graphic displays; review control point details; access and review program language; access and review schedules; access and review setpoints; and access, review, and set up trends.

The control system review should include the following items of work:

(a) **Determine actual sequences of operation:** The team discerns the actual sequences of operation by observing the equipment, establishing and reviewing trends, and accessing and reviewing the actual control programs (in control language). The team cannot discern the actual sequences of operation by simply reading the sequences on the construction documents or the control diagrams. Actual sequences of operation, as programmed by the system installer, can be significantly different from the sequences intended by the system designer. Discrepancies between intended and actual sequences are quite common. These discrepancies are due to a number of factors, including insufficient detail in the construction documents and owner-directed changes as well as a simple language barrier between the designer and the system programmer—the designer understands systems but may not understand control programming; the programmer understands control programming but may not understand systems.

Actual sequences of operation should be determined for the major energy-consuming systems, including the following:

(i) **Single-duct reheat air terminals:** The standard sequence of operation for pressure-independent, single-duct reheat air terminals is to modulate the terminal damper in a pressure-independent manner between a heating airflow setpoint and a cooling airflow setpoint in sequence with the heating water control valve as needed to maintain the space temperature at the thermostat setpoint. The TAB contractor typically obtains the cooling and heating airflow setpoints from the air terminal schedule on the construction documents. In cases where each air terminal is not individually scheduled, the heating airflow setpoint is a default percentage of the cooling airflow setpoint (e.g., 40%). Most air terminal DDC controllers can offer significantly more complex, more energy-efficient sequences. Potential sequence improvements include establishing a deadband (also known as bias) between cooling and heating functions, establishing more airflow setpoints (up to eight), implementing unoccupied and occupied modes of operation, implementing night setback/setup, remotely overriding the thermostat setpoint, and limiting the thermostat setpoint range (e.g., 68° F to 75° F).

(ii) **Dual-duct air terminals:** The standard sequence for dual-duct air terminals is to modulate the hot duct and cold duct airflow settings in sequence as required to maintain the space temperature at the thermostat setpoint. The TAB contractor typically obtains the cooling and heating airflow setpoints from the air terminal schedule on the construction documents. However, most air terminal DDC controllers can support significantly more complex and energy-efficient sequences than are typically programmed. Potential sequence improvements include establishing a deadband between cooling and heating functions, implementing unoccupied and occupied modes of operation, implementing night setback/setup, remotely overriding the thermostat setpoint range, and limiting the setpoint range. Some dual-duct air terminal controllers also offer a "no mixing" sequence for dual-duct air terminals that prevents opening of the hot and cold duct dampers at the same time.

(iii) **Fan coil units:** The standard sequence of operation for fan coil units is to modulate heating and cooling valves in sequence as needed to maintain the space temperature at the thermostat setpoint. The occupant typically controls the fan speed using a manual three-speed selector switch (low, medium, or high). However, most fan coil unit controllers are capable of offering significantly more complex and energy-efficient sequences. Potential sequence improvements include establishing a deadband between cooling and heating functions, implementing unoccupied and occupied modes of operation, implementing night setback/setup, remotely overriding the thermostat setpoint range, and limiting the setpoint range. Some fan coil unit controllers are also able to sequence the fan speed in conjunction with the valves. Operating fan coil units at the lowest possible speed reduces energy consumption and provides superior humidity control.

(iv) **Air-handling units:** Air-handling units can be configured in a nearly infinite number of ways. Standard sequences typically use separate proportional-integral control loops for each heating and cooling component (economizer dampers, preheat control valve, chilled water control valve, etc.). The potential for this arrangement to result in simultaneous heating and cooling due to overlapping setpoints or control loop hunting can be eliminated by instead using a single proportional-integral loop with separate table statements for each controlled device. Other potential sequence improvements include disabling the air-side economizer cycle as the first stage of humidification, automatically resetting the supply air temperature setpoint based on the critical zone (the air terminal requiring the coldest air), automatically resetting the supply air static pressure setpoint based on the critical zone (the air terminal with the most open terminal damper), and automatically resetting the outside airflow setpoint based on the entry-level building pressure. Air-handling units that serve administrative, education, or similar spaces can also be shut down during unoccupied periods. Air-handling units serving large assembly areas (auditoriums, classrooms, etc.) can also be equipped for demand-controlled ventilation (i.e., resetting the outside airflow setpoint based on actual occupancy).

(v) **Exhaust fans:** Exhaust fans in health care facilities typically operate continuously. Many such fans, however, could be shut down during unoccupied periods. Kitchen hood exhaust fans can be equipped for variable volume operation based on actual cooking activity.

(vi) **Chilled water system:** Many types of chilled water systems are available, including constant volume primary, primary/secondary, and variable primary. In many health care facilities, the operator manually sequences the water chillers. Potential sequence improvements include maximum capacity sequencing, chilled water temperature setpoint reset, and chilled water differential pressure setpoint reset. In some applications, conversions to low-flow/high delta T operation or variable primary operation can be cost-effective. Hydronic free cooling systems should be sequenced automatically based on the outdoor air wet bulb temperature (the wet bulb temperature is a relatively accurate predictor of the lowest water temperature a cooling tower can produce). To prevent a disruption of chilled water service during the transitions back and forth between chiller operation and hydronic free cooling, the water chillers should be equipped with refrigerant lift controls that allow the water chillers to operate with very cold entering condenser water temperatures. Thermal storage systems can also be cost-effective in applications with time-of-use electricity rates or high electricity demand rates. Sequencing chilled water pumps using an optimal dispatch approach (the number of pumps in operation is automatically controlled according to the flow requirement, head requirement, number of pumps, and pump performance curves) can significantly reduce direct pump energy consumption (pump motor electricity consumption) as well as indirect pump energy consumption (the refrigeration energy required to transfer the heat produced by the pump from the chilled water to the tower water).

(vii) **Tower water system:** Tower water systems are typically of the constant volume type, in which a specific cooling tower serves a specific water chiller. Some newer facilities have variable volume manifold systems, in which a group of cooling towers (commonly referred to as a tower farm) serves a group of water chillers. Potential sequence improvements for tower water systems include automatically resetting the tower water supply temperature setpoint according to the outdoor air wet bulb temperature and other factors (thus optimizing the balance between cooling tower fan energy consumption and water chiller efficiency), automatically resetting the tower water differential pressure setpoint (in manifold systems only), and implementing refrigerant lift control. Converting constant volume systems to variable volume manifold systems can also be cost-effective in some instances.

(viii) **Heating water system:** Many older heating water systems are constant volume, while newer heating water systems are typically variable volume. Potential sequence improvements for both types of systems include automatically resetting the heating water supply temperature setpoint, automatically resetting the differential pressure setpoint reset, and implementing optimal pump dispatch. Resetting the heating water supply temperature and heating water differential pressure setpoints downward during warmer weather also extends the life of the heating water control valves. Without reset strategies, the heating water control valves operate in nearly closed positions for extended periods. When a valve operates in a nearly closed position at a high water temperature, the water may flash to steam (due to the combination of high velocity, pressure drop, and high temperature) and damage the valve seat (damage commonly referred to as a "wire draw"). Converting constant volume systems to variable volume systems is cost-effective in most applications.

(b) **Check the air terminal calibration:** Pressure-independent air terminals are equipped with airflow-measuring stations. Airflow is typically derived by using this formula:

$$\text{Airflow} = \text{Velocity} \times \text{Area} \times \text{Calibration Constant}$$

Velocity is determined using an average velocity sensor at the inlet of the air terminal. The air terminal controller determines velocity by extracting the square root of the pressure drop across the sensor. The controller automatically calibrates the velocity sensor on a regular basis by closing the damper and resetting the sensor reading to zero. Air terminals serving areas where the airflow cannot be temporarily shut off should be equipped with autozero modules, which allow calibration without shutting off airflow. The testing, adjusting, and balancing contractor typically enters values for the air terminal area (a function of the air terminal size) and calibration constant into the controller during the TAB process. Most air terminal controllers are equipped with a factory default calibration constant, which the TAB contractor adjusts on-site as needed to align the indicated airflow with the actual measured airflow (typically measured using a flow hood).

The retrocommissioning team should review the air terminal programming and ensure the controllers are calibrating the air terminals on a regular basis. The team should also verify that the calibration constants are not set at the factory default values (an indication either that the terminal was not calibrated when installed or that its controller has lost its memory).

(c) **Determine actual setpoints and other settings:** The retrocommissioning team reviews all systems and documents the actual setpoints (which are likely to be different from the setpoints indicated on control diagrams). Related settings for trending and alarms are also identified.

(i) **Actual airflow setpoints:** The retrocommissioning team reviews the air terminal programs and documents the actual airflow setpoints. Most air terminal controllers allow up to eight airflow setpoints (unoccupied and occupied heating and cooling minimums and maximums). Often, however, only two airflow setpoints (cooling maximum and heating maximum) have been entered into the controller because these were the only values indicated on the air terminal schedule in the construction documents. The retrocommissioning team may also discover air terminals with setpoints at the controller default values, another indication that either the terminal was not calibrated when installed or its controller has lost its memory.

(ii) **Overridden control points:** As a general rule, health facility maintenance staff work very hard to resolve and address complaints from patients, staff, and visitors. If the maintenance staff have not received sufficient training or they do not have the time to fully investigate a problem (they receive a complaint at night or on a weekend when staffing levels are limited), their response to a complaint may be to override a control point. Overridden control points, which include damper positions and valve positions, are a frequent cause of simultaneous heating and cooling (reducing simultaneous heating and cooling is nearly always the most significant energy conservation opportunity in a health care facility). The retrocommissioning staff reviews all systems and documents any overridden control points. Many energy management systems can print a standard report that lists the overridden points. The retrocommissioning team discusses each of these with the O&M staff and determines the cause. Where possible, the retrocommissioning team restores automatic operation by releasing the overridden points.

(iii) **Weekly schedules:** Energy management systems are capable of turning equipment on and off based on scheduled occupancy. The retrocommissioning team reviews and documents existing weekly schedules.

(iv) **Deadbands:** A deadband (sometimes referred to as bias) is a temperature range on either side of the setpoint where no heating or cooling takes place. Energy management systems are capable of establishing different deadbands for each space. The retrocommissioning team reviews and documents existing deadbands.

(v) **Minimum and maximum thermostat setpoints:** Energy management systems are capable of establishing minimum and maximum setpoints for each space. Thermostat setpoints outside the range are ignored. The retrocommissioning staff reviews and documents existing minimum and maximum thermostat setpoints.

(vi) **Trend data settings:** Most energy management systems offer two types of data trending. Data can either be recorded at regular time intervals or at each change of valve (COV). The retrocommissioning team reviews and documents existing trends and may also establish trends for additional control points.

(vii) **Alarm settings and alarm messages:** Energy management systems are capable of generating alarms to alert maintenance staff about potential problems. Alarms are typically either change-of-state or analog limit type. The EMS generates change-of-state alarms when equipment or devices that are supposed to be on are off, or vice versa. The EMS generates analog limit alarms when temperatures or pressures (or other analog values) are outside their normal operating range. In many facilities, the EMS generates too many nuisance alarms due to improper setup, and the O&M staff ignore the alarms (much like the shepherds ignored the little boy who "cried wolf"). The retrocommissioning staff sifts through the alarm logs to identify chronic problems that need to be resolved and then modifies alarm setup parameters to reduce nuisance alarms.

(c) Other items of work that are part of the detailed review of automatic temperature control systems include identification of the following:

(i) **Devices not controlling to setpoint:** The retrocommissioning team reviews all systems and documents all devices that are not controlling to setpoint (e.g., supply air setpoint is 55° F and actual supply air temperature is 59° F). The retrocommissioning team also documents all devices with control outputs at 0 percent or 100 percent as these conditions indicate a problem. They could be due to equipment failures, system failures, or unattainable setpoints (e.g., a supply air temperature setpoint of 52° F when the cooling coil was designed for 55° F).

(ii) **Devices not working:** Control devices can fail in a manner that is not readily apparent to the O&M staff. The retrocommissioning team reviews all systems and documents control devices that are not working properly (e.g., chilled water valves that do not fully close, dampers that do not fully open, and inaccurate sensors). Repairing or replacing failed devices can be a significant performance improvement opportunity.

(iii) **Communication errors:** The retrocommissioning team reviews the entire system and documents energy management system network communication errors and failed control points (points that are not reporting properly to the automatic temperature control system).

(iv) **Software revision:** The retrocommissioning identifies the current software revision in place and the most current version available from the manufacturer. Upgrading the software to the most recent version may need to be part of the retrocommissioning effort.

(v) **Hardware limitations:** The retrocommissioning team documents hardware limitations caused by the use of older or obsolete automatic temperature control panels and energy management system workstations. Upgrading such hardware may need to be included in the retrocommissioning effort.

(vi) **Network speed:** The retrocommissioning team assesses the network speed (how long it takes before commands take effect and sensors update). In many cases, network speed can be improved by modifying the control programming (e.g., relocating programming to the controller serving the equipment).

(vii) **Password access:** The retrocommissioning team identifies the individuals authorized to use the control system and their access level. Each user should have a unique password. The permitted actions for each user should be tailored to their level of training. Individuals with limited knowledge or training should have read-only capability. Individuals with moderate training should be allowed to change setpoints. Only individuals with extensive training should be allowed to override setpoints or change programming.

(viii) **Obvious energy conservation opportunities:** The retrocommissioning team documents obvious energy conservation opportunities discovered during review of the control systems.

(12) Obtain and evaluate utility rate structures for natural gas, electricity, and water. Identify and evaluate potential supply-side measures to reduce energy costs.

Supply-side energy cost reduction measures reduce the unit cost of energy, or the "energy rate." Possible supply-side energy cost reduction measures for health care facilities include, but are not limited to, those discussed in this section.

(a) **Electricity master metering:** Many health care facilities have multiple electricity meters. When each meter is separately metered and billed, the total billed demand is the sum of the individual meter peak demands. The installation of a single master meter to serve an entire campus will reduce billed demand as a result of meter diversity. Meter diversity is equal to 1 minus the ratio of the sum of the individual meter peak demands to the peak coincident sum of the meter demands (the peak coincident sum is always less than the sum of the individual peaks because each meter does not experience its peak demand at the same time). The reduction in billed electricity demand costs is equal to the meter diversity multiplied by the current demand costs. Meter diversity typically varies from 8 to 25 percent, with facilities having only two meters at the low end of the range and facilities having five or more meters at the high end of the range. Master metering can also achieve savings by eliminating meter charges (also known as customer charges) and by qualifying the meter for a more cost-effective rate schedule (eligibility requirements for lower unit cost rate schedules frequently include minimum demands or consumption).

(b) **Electricity combined billing:** Electricity combined billing (sometimes referred to as electronic master metering) is the electronic combination of consumption data from multiple meter points prior to the application of rates. Electricity combined billing is restricted in some areas due to concerns about "cost-shifting," which occurs when changes in rate schedules, rate design, or customer metering arrangements shift costs from one customer or group of customers to another. Electricity combined billing yields the same savings as electricity master metering. The cost of implementing combined billing is generally lower than the cost of implementing master metering because the customer does not have to purchase building transformers or install a campus-wide electrical distribution system. Combined billing also preserves a record of individual building consumption, which allows effective management of energy consumption and cost.

(c) **Electricity rate analysis:** Electric utilities typically offer many types of rates, including small general service, large general service, time-of-use (TOU), interruptible, and real-time pricing. Each available rate offers different customer charges, energy charges, and demand charges. Electricity rate analysis is the process of evaluating the rates offered by a utility company according to actual or expected energy consumption and billed demands and then identifying the most cost-effective rate for each meter. For a specific meter, which rate is most cost-effective typically depends on the meter load factor (ratio of average demand to average monthly billed demand). Since load factors for health care facilities are typically in the range of 70 to 80 percent, the most cost-effective rates are typically those with the lowest energy charges and the highest demand charges (i.e., time-of-use rates). The graph shown in Figure 6-3 illustrates a comparison of the available electricity rates for a health care facility.

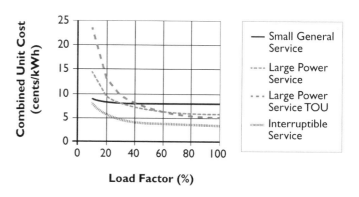

Figure 6-3: Sample Electricity Rate Analysis

(d) **Primary electricity metering:** Electric utilities generally offer a lower rate or a demand credit to facilities with meters located on the primary side (higher voltage side) of the building transformers. Typically, the utility offers a reduction in metered consumption and demands to account for the transformation losses. Actual transformation losses are typically in the range of 0.8 to 1.2 percent of the transformer load. If the credit offered by the utility exceeds the losses, the primary metering will reduce energy costs. If the credit offered by the utility is less than the actual losses, primary metering will increase energy costs.

(e) **Electricity delivery voltage:** Electric utilities generally offer a lower rate to facilities that accept service at a higher distribution level or transmission level voltage. Accepting service at a higher voltage requires the facility to own and maintain building transformers. If the rate reduction is sufficient to offset the cost of owning, operating, and maintaining the building transformers, accepting a higher delivery voltage is cost-effective. If the rate reduction is not sufficient to offset these costs, accepting a higher delivery voltage is not cost-effective.

(f) **Interruptible electricity rates and distributed generation:** Many electric utilities offer reduced rates for customers that agree to reduce their electrical demand during peak demand periods. These rates are commonly known as interruptible or curtailable rates. Interruptible rates generally involve two demand rates, on-peak and off-peak. The on-peak demand rate is applied to the highest demand that occurs during a period of peak utility demand. The off-peak demand is applied to the highest demand that occurs at any time during the billing month. Interruptible rates are typically in the range of 25 to 35 percent lower than standard rates (see Figure 6-3). For a health care facility to be eligible for an interruptible rate, it must have the capacity to generate all or a major portion of its electricity requirements on-site. The use of on-site generators is commonly referred to as

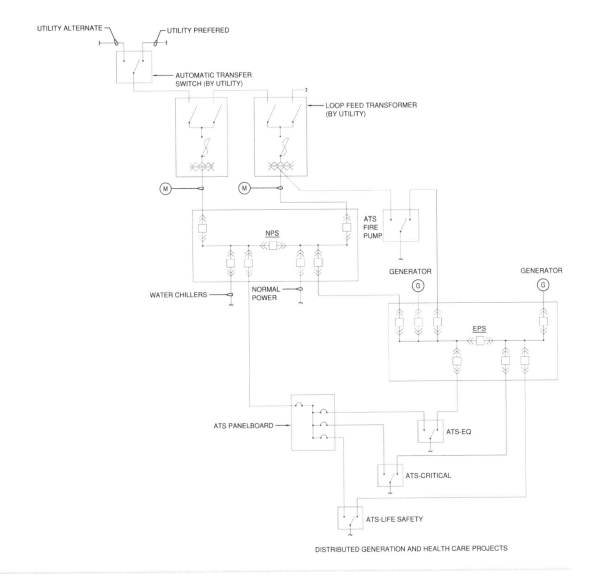

Figure 6-4: Distributed Generation

distributed generation. In recent years, many health care facilities have installed distributed generation equipment in order to quality for interruptible rates. Distributed generation also yields other benefits, including an increase in overall power system reliability and the ability to operate air-conditioning equipment during a utility outage. However, current health care codes and regulations do not require any portion of the air-conditioning system to be connected to the essential/standby power system, and most health care facilities do not have sufficient generator capacity to operate their air-conditioning equipment. A schematic diagram illustrating a distributed generation system in a health care facility is provided in Figure 6-4.

(g) **Power factor correction:** Facilities consume both real power (kW) and reactive power (kVAr). The real and reactive power components combine to form apparent power (kVA). Power factor is the ratio of real power to apparent power. (These relationships are illustrated in Figure 6-5.) If the power factor is unity (100 percent), the real power is equal to the apparent power. If the power factor is less than unity, the real power is less than the apparent power. In other words, it takes more apparent power to transmit the same amount of real power when the power factor is less than unity. The power factor for a purely resistive load, such as electric resistance heat, is unity (100 percent). Due to the presence of large induction motors, the uncorrected power factor for most health care facilities is 82 to 85 percent.

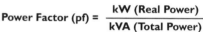

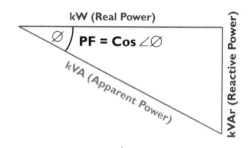

Figure 6-5: Power Factor

Power factor can also be described in terms of the relationship between voltage and current waveforms. When the power factor is unity, the voltage and current waveforms are perfectly aligned. When the power factor is less than unity, the current waveform "lags" the voltage waveform. The lag amount is expressed in degrees. Power factor is equal to the cosine of the lag angle. Power factor is also equal to the ratio of kW (real power) to kVA (apparent power). The typical relationship between the current and voltage waveforms is illustrated in Figure 6-6.

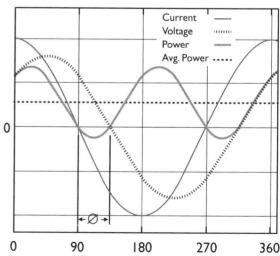

Figure 6-6: Current and Voltage Waveforms

Utility distribution losses are dependent on apparent power or current. The energy losses in watts in an electrical distribution system are proportional to the square of the current in amps. To reduce these losses, utilities typically offer their customers incentives to reduce apparent power by increasing power factor. These incentives can be in the form of a penalty for low power factor or use of apparent power as the basis for determining billed demand (commonly referred to as a kVA meter). Power factor is increased by installing capacitor banks, which provide a local source of reactive power, reducing the reactive power required from the electric utility. The capacitor banks are typically installed at large induction motors and/or at the electrical service entrance.

However, capacitor banks also reduce the natural frequency of the circuit. If the natural frequency is reduced to the same level as a harmonic current found within the electrical circuit, resonance will occur, which can cause damage to electrical distribution system components. In health facility electrical systems, harmonic frequencies with sufficient amplitude to be of concern typically are fifth order (five times the base frequency) and seventh order (seven times the base frequency). In most cases, the source of these harmonics is variable frequency drives. Resonance can be avoided by installing a harmonic filter tuned to the specific frequency of the harmonic current at the capacitor. (The harmonic currents in a typical electrical distribution system are illustrated in Figure 6-7.) Installation of a capacitor bank that

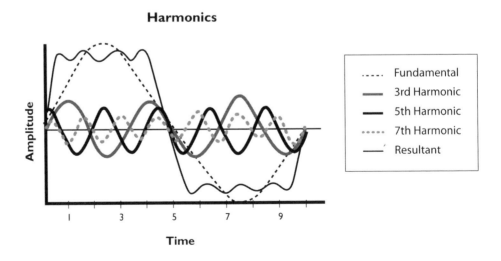

Figure 6-7: Typical Electrical Distribution System Harmonic Currents

generates too much reactive power can also cause problems in the form of a "leading" power factor (the current wave leads the voltage wave). Leading power factors are prevented by installing a switching capacitor bank that varies the amount of capacitance in use as required to maintain the power factor at unity.

(h) **Negotiated electricity rate:** Electric utilities frequently offer special rates to large customers to defer the installation of combined heating and power systems. These rates are frequently referred to as "cogeneration deferral" rates. In most areas, the Public Service Commission must approve cogeneration deferral rates. To assure the deferral rates do not adversely affect other ratepayers, the rates must be high enough to cover the utility's variable costs and contribute to fixed costs. To secure these rates, a facility must develop a credible analysis of cogeneration viability demonstrating the facility has sufficient incentive to implement the cogeneration system at the standard electricity rates.

(i) **Natural gas master metering:** Many health care facilities have multiple natural gas meters. When each meter is separately metered and billed, the total billed contract demand is the sum of the individual meter maximum daily quantities. The installation of a single master meter to serve an entire campus will reduce the contract demand due to meter diversity. The typical meter diversity for a health care facility with numerous meters can vary from 3 percent up to 10 percent. Master metering can also achieve savings by eliminating customer charges and by qualifying the facility for more cost-effective rate schedules.

(j) **Natural gas combined billing:** Natural gas combined billing (sometimes referred to as electronic master metering) is the electronic combination of consumption data from multiple meter points prior to the application of rates. Natural gas combined billing yields the same savings as natural gas master metering. The implementation cost for combined billing is typically lower than the implementation cost for master metering because combined billing does not require installation of a natural gas distribution system.

(k) **Natural gas transportation rates:** Natural gas utilities typically offer both bundled sales rates and unbundled transportation rates. If the customer elects the bundled sales rate option, the local distribution company (LDC) provides all services required to supply the customer with natural gas, including purchasing the gas at the wellhead; gathering and transporting the natural gas through an interstate natural gas pipeline to the LDC; and distributing the gas to the customer's meter. If the customer elects the unbundled transportation option, the customer is responsible for purchasing the natural gas and transporting it from the wellhead through an interstate pipeline to the city gate—the point at which custody is transferred from the pipeline to the LDC. The LDC retains responsibility for distributing the gas from the city gate to the customer's meter. In most cases, unbundled rates are considerably lower than bundled rates. The savings are due to a reduced natural gas commodity unit cost, reduced pipeline transportation rates, and lower municipal franchise taxes (with the unbundled transportation rate, only the LDC portion of the cost is subject to municipal franchise taxes). In some areas, transportation rates are available to large customers only. To achieve the savings, a health care facility must elect unbundled transportation service, purchase the natural gas, and make arrangements with a pipeline to transport the natural gas to the city gate. If a health care facility does not have the expertise to provide these services, the RTL or other outside consultant can provide them.

(l) **Natural gas purchasing group:** Natural gas commodity costs are typically dependent on the NYMEX index, basis differential, and supplier margin. The NYMEX index represents the spot and contract prices at the Henry Hub in Louisiana. The basis differential is the difference between the NYMEX index and the actual cost of natural gas at the delivery point. The basis differential for Centerpoint Energy Gas Transmission (CEGT) East, for example, typically varies from a few cents per MMBtu negative to more than $3 per MMBtu negative. Natural gas pipeline rates are affected by contract demand and volumetric consumption. Health care facilities that elect unbundled natural gas transportation rates can elect to participate in a natural gas purchasing group. Typically, these groups include other large natural gas consumers such as universities, other health care facilities, and industrial plants. The purchasing groups use the leverage associated with larger volumes to negotiate reductions in supplier margins and pipeline transportation rates.

(m) **Hedging natural gas costs:** Natural gas commodity costs are quite volatile, as illustrated in Figure 6-8. Facilities that purchase their own natural gas can typically use the spot and futures markets to hedge their natural gas costs for up to 18 months in

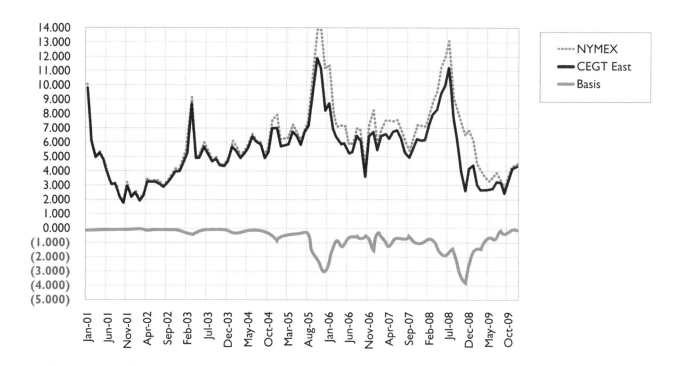

Figure 6-8: Natural Gas Cost Volatility

advance. Hedging can take many forms, including establishing a fixed price, an index not to exceed a cap, or a variable rate that floats between a cap and floor (commonly referred to as a "collar"). Both the index and the basis differential components of the price can be hedged. It should be noted that the purpose of hedging is to manage risk; hedging activities over a long period does not reduce costs. Hedging natural gas costs involves pooling, nominations, balancing, and cash-in/cash-out activities and requires significant knowledge and expertise. Improper nominations and balancing can yield significant penalties. Many health care facilities do not have the in-house expertise to hedge natural gas costs. Under these circumstances, the facility can outsource hedging activities to the RTL or other consultant.

(n) **Interruptible natural gas rates:** Natural gas pipeline charges typically depend on contract demand. Facilities that have dual fuel boilers can elect contract demand levels that are lower than the amount of natural gas the facility needs under worst case cold weather conditions (frequently referred to as the maximum daily quantity or MDQ). If they do so, a portion of their gas is then "interruptible." During extremely cold weather, when natural gas consumption is high, the utility can issue an operational flow order (OFO) that instructs their customers to reduce natural gas consumption below their contract demand. Facilities with contract demands lower than their MDQ react to the OFO and reduce natural gas consumption by switching their boilers to the alternate fuel. The monthly energy cost savings achieved by electing a lower contract demand are equal to the reduction in contract demand multiplied by the pipeline demand rate. Facilities that do not have dual fuel capability can take advantage of this option by installing synthetic natural gas (SNG) storage facilities on-site (mixing LPG with air creates a natural gas substitute).

(o) **Pipeline bypass:** Large health care facilities can eliminate local distribution charges by installing a direct connection to the pipeline. The installation of an LDC bypass requires Federal Energy Regulatory Commission approval and a large capital investment.

(p) **Sanitary sewer diversion credits:** Many wastewater utilities offer a sanitary sewer diversion credit mechanism. Under these arrangements, the customer installs diversion meters on the boiler makeup water and cooling tower makeup water supplies (these water uses are typically diverted from the sanitary sewer). The diversion meters are then read monthly by the O&M staff or the water utility. The water utility generates the monthly water bills in the standard manner using the total water consumption recorded by the water meter. The wastewater utility, however, generates the monthly sewer bills on the total water consumption minus the diversion meter consumption. The savings are equal to the diversion meter consumption multiplied by the sewer charge. Sewer charges typically account for a majority of the total water cost.

(13) Identify and evaluate demand-side energy cost reduction opportunities. Develop estimates of implementation cost, annual savings, and simple payback for each demand-side energy cost reduction opportunity.

Demand-side energy cost reduction measures are typically grouped into these categories: lighting, steam, chilled water, heating water, air distribution, plumbing, automatic temperature controls, electrical, and building envelope.

(a) **Lighting.** In a health care facility, lighting accounts for 12 to 20 percent of total energy costs. Possible demand-side energy cost reduction measures for lighting in health care facilities are discussed below:

(i) **Replace T-12 lamps with T-8 lamps.** Many different types of high-efficacy fluorescent lamps are available on the market (lighting efficacy is typically expressed as lumens per watt). Although T-5 lamps are currently available, the general consensus is that the "super T-8" lamps are more cost-effective (T-5 lamps are 5/8" diameter and T-8 lamps are 1" diameter). Replacement of existing T-12 lamps with T-8 lamps can reduce lighting energy consumption by up to 40 percent.

(ii) **Replace magnetic ballasts with electronic ballasts.** Electronic ballasts are more efficient and quieter than magnetic ballasts. The replacement of magnetic ballasts can reduce lighting energy consumption by up to 20 percent.

(iii) **Replace older interior light fixtures with high-efficiency interior fixtures.** Older light fixtures tend to be less efficient than new fixtures. The new fixtures produce a higher illumination level at the work space using fewer lamp lumens and power input because they are more efficiently constructed, have better lenses, and have cleaner, more reflective surfaces. Replacement of existing fixtures with new fixtures can reduce lighting energy consumption by up to 10 percent. When the new fixtures are equipped with T-8 lamps and electronic ballasts, replacement of existing fixtures can reduce lighting energy consumption by up to 50 percent.

(iv) **Install reflectors in existing fixtures.** The installation of specular reflectors in existing fixtures can increase light fixture efficiency, permitting a reduction in the number of fixtures and lamps. Specular reflectors, however, may change fixture spacing requirements and necessitate relocating the fixtures.

(v) **Conduct a delamping audit.** Many areas of a health care facility typically have excessive illumination levels. The retrocommissioning team should perform a comprehensive lighting audit in which the illumination level at the work surface in each space within the facility is measured and recorded in footcandles. The team then compares current illumination levels to Illumination Engineering Society (IES) recommendations and recommends removal of lamps (commonly referred to as delamping) in areas where existing illumination levels significantly exceed IES recommendations.

Refer to Appendix 6-1 for a sample lighting audit spreadsheet.

(vi) **Regularly relamp and clean fixtures.** Lighting designers determine the number of light fixtures required for certain areas of a health care facility based on the desired illumination level, fixture efficacy, lamp lumen output, number of lamps per fixture, lamp lumen depreciation factor, and lamp dirt depreciation factor. The age of the lamp and the cleanliness of the fixture affect the lamp lumen depreciation factor and the lamp dirt depreciation factor. Recommended illumination levels can be maintained using fewer fixtures if relamping and cleaning of fixtures are conducted regularly. Some facilities use a computerized maintenance management system (CMMS) to automatically generate work orders to relamp and clean fixtures in groups (commonly referred to as "group relamping").

(vii) **Employ daylighting.** Daylighting is the automatic adjustment of light fixture output (artificial light) in response to variations in natural light as required to maintain the recommended illumination level. In addition to energy savings, maximizing the use of natural light improves the healing environment.

(viii) **Employ occupancy sensors.** Occupancy sensors are available in infrared, ultrasonic, and dual technology types. The infrared type detects occupancy by measuring subtle increases in temperature. The ultrasonic type detects occupancy through motion. The dual technology type uses both infrared and ultrasonic detection methods. The installation of occupancy sensors in areas of intermittent occupancy such as conference rooms, toilet rooms, and offices can significantly reduce lighting energy consumption in these areas.

(ix) **Replace incandescent lamps with compact fluorescent lamps.** Incandescent lamps provide relatively low efficacy and have short life compared to fluorescent lamps (the average life of an incandescent lamp is approximately 2,000 hours compared to 20,000 hours for a compact fluorescent lamp). The replacement of incandescent lamps with compact fluorescent lamps can significantly reduce lighting energy consumption. (In 2007 the U.S. Congress passed the Energy Independence and Security Act, which provides for the phaseout of most incandescent lightbulbs beginning with the 100-watt lamp in 2012 and ending with the 40-watt lamp in 2020.)

(x) **Replace older exit lights with LED exit fixtures.** Older exit lights are typically equipped with incandescent lamps. Replacing these with new LED fixtures will reduce lighting power consumption from approximately 40 watts per fixture to approximately 9 watts per fixture. The LED lamps also offer a considerably longer lamp life.

(xi) **Employ photocells to control exterior lights.** Using photocells to control lighting for surface parking lots and parking decks will significantly reduce the number of hours of light fixture operation. Photocells turn off exterior lights when a sufficient level of natural light is available. Time clocks and energy management systems are not as effective for this purpose due to the number of factors they do not consider, such as daylight savings time, cloud cover, time of year, etc.

(xii) **Use high-efficiency exterior light fixtures:** Metal halide, LED, high-pressure sodium, and low-pressure sodium exterior fixtures are considerably more efficient than other types of fixtures, including quartz halogen and incandescent.

(xiii) **Reduce exterior light levels:** Many parking lots and other exterior spaces are over-illuminated. A reduction in illumination to accepted levels will reduce lighting energy costs.

(xiv) **Consider using solar exterior light fixtures:** Several lighting manufacturers have developed solar-powered exterior light fixtures, which require no external power connection.

(b) **Steam.** In a typical health care facility, steam generation and distribution accounts for 15 to 30 percent of total energy costs. Possible demand-side energy cost reduction measures for health facility steam systems include, but are not limited to, the following:

(i) **Reduce steam pressure.** Autoclaves and other sterilizing equipment typically require 50 to 60 psig steam pressure, while many health facility steam systems operate at pressures of 100 psig or higher. Reducing the steam pressure to the minimum level required will reduce operating temperatures, heat loss, and steam loss. The steam pressure at the boilers must exceed the sterilizer steam pressure requirement by 5 to 10 psig because sterilizers require high-quality (little or no liquid) steam and pressure must be reduced at the sterilizer to create sufficient steam superheat to evaporate all liquid.

(ii) **Install high-turndown burners.** Standard burners have a turndown capability of 3 to 1. If the steam requirement is less than the minimum burner capacity, the burners will cycle on and off as required to maintain the steam pressure at setpoint. Before the boiler cycles back on, however, it and its associated stack are purged to remove all combustibles. The repeated cooling and heating of the boiler and stack significantly decreases boiler efficiency. Replacing standard 3-to-1 turndown burners with high-turndown burners (typically with a capability of 10 to 1) can eliminate burner cycling and substantially increase average fuel-to-steam efficiency.

(iii) **Consider disconnecting standby boilers.** Standby boilers that remain connected to the main steam header continue to radiate and convect heat to the mechanical room space when not in use. Heat losses from this activity are typically in the range of 2 percent of the design heat input to the boiler. Disconnecting standby boilers from the main steam header can create savings but will increase the amount of time required to place a standby boiler in operation in the event of a primary boiler failure.

(iv) **Repair and replace steam traps.** A typical health facility steam system has steam trap losses of approximately 8 to 10 percent of total steam flow. These losses increase boiler makeup, blowdown, and chemical treatment requirements. The losses can be reduced to 2 to 3 percent of total steam flow if steam traps are regularly tested and repaired. Absent proactive testing and repair, steam traps generally fail in 1 to 5 years (more frequently for high-pressure traps than low-pressure traps). Traps can fail either open or closed. When they fail open, the devices they serve continue to function, which means the failure can go undetected by O&M staff.

(v) **Employ a steam trap monitoring system.** Several steam trap manufacturers have developed monitoring systems that automatically detect steam trap failures. The installation of a steam trap monitoring system will ensure that steam trap failures are immediately detected and repaired.

(vi) **Employ a boiler stack heat recovery system.** A standard steam boiler has a fuel-to-steam efficiency of 82 percent. The losses comprise 10 percent latent combustion efficiency losses (heat required to change water from liquid to vapor), 6 percent sensible combustion efficiency losses (heat associated with the difference in temperature between the boiler stack and the combustion air), and 2 percent boiler radiation and convection losses (heat transferred through the boiler surfaces to the boiler room). Boiler stack heat recovery systems can either be condensing or non-condensing. A non-condensing heat recovery system transfers sensible heat only from the boiler stack to either the combustion air or the boiler feedwater (in the latter case, it is commonly referred to as a "feedwater economizer"). Non-condensing heat recovery systems can increase boiler fuel-to-steam efficiency by 4 to 5 percent. A condensing heat recovery system transfers both sensible and latent heat from the boiler stack to a lower temperature water system such as boiler makeup water or domestic hot water (the water temperature must be less than the stack dewpoint). Condensing heat recovery systems can increase boiler fuel-to-steam efficiency by 8 to 12 percent. Due to the presence of CO_2 and SO_2 in the boiler stack, condensing heat recovery equipment must be resistant to acid corrosion, making condensing heat recovery systems more expensive than non-condensing systems. A non-condensing feedwater economizer is shown in Figure 6-9.

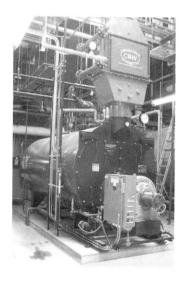

Figure 6-9: Feedwater Economizer

(vii) **Use oxygen trim controls to regulate boiler combustion air levels.** Boiler combustion air levels are typically adjusted at equipment start-up to the minimum amount needed to assure complete combustion based on stack oxygen content. However, combustion air requirements at part load conditions can vary significantly from combustion air requirements at full load conditions. As a result, combustion air levels that have been set manually may be excessive at part load conditions. An oxygen trim system automatically regulates combustion air levels according to the amount of excess oxygen in the boiler stack. Reducing combustion air levels while still maintaining complete combustion reduces stack losses and increases boiler efficiency.

(viii) **Employ automatic blowdown controls.** Boiler blowdown typically removes dissolved solids from the mud drum (commonly referred to as bottom blowdown) and from the boiler water surface (commonly referred to as surface blowdown). The mud drum blowdown is manual. The surface blowdown can be controlled either manually using a needle valve or automatically using a modulating valve with an electronic or pneumatic actuator. The amount of blowdown required for a facility depends on the desired number of cycles of concentration and the total steam system loss. The cycles of concentration (sometimes called the concentration ratio) is the ratio of the concentration of chemicals in the water in the boiler to the concentration of chemicals in the makeup water. The number of cycles required to keep the level of dissolved solids low enough to avoid damaging the boiler can vary from three to 20 depending primarily on the makeup water chemistry. Boiler blowdown is equal to the cycles of concentration multiplied by the quantity of total boiler makeup water (equal to system losses plus blowdown). The desired number of cycles depends on the chemistry of the makeup water and the maximum permissible limit on dissolved solids for the boiler. Standard limits for fire tube boilers are 300 ppm total hardness ($CaCO_3$), 180 ppm silica (SiO_2), 900 ppm total alkalinity ($CaCO_3$), and 3,500 mmhos/cm conductivity. Standard limits for water tube boilers are the same except the total hardness limit is 500 ppm. With an automatic blowdown system, the surface blowdown rate is varied as required to maintain the correct steam conductivity. An automatic blowdown system can reduce blowdown levels and increase overall steam efficiency.

(ix) **Use a variable frequency drive to control the boiler draft fan.** Combustion air levels are typically modulated using fan inlet vanes. The use of a variable frequency drive (VFD) to control fan speed is more efficient than using inlet vanes.

(x) **Use variable speed boiler feedwater pumps.** Boiler feedwater pumps are typically constant speed pumps, and fixed opening orifices are typically used to provide a minimum feedwater flow. Use of a VFD to control pump speed as required to maintain boiler feedwater pressure is more efficient than using constant speed pumps.

(xi) **Use a deaerator with a condensing vent.** Steam systems typically use deaerators to process the boiler feedwater. The function of a deaerator is to remove oxygen by a combination of mechanical, chemical, and thermal means. The feedwater is processed by heating to a near saturation temperature, vigorous mechanical scrubbing, and chemical treatment with an oxygen scavenger such as sodium sulfite. Deaerators can be either pressurized or atmospheric. They have a vent for the removal of oxygen, which allows a certain level of steam to escape. Newer deaerators are equipped with condensing vents located close to the makeup water and condensate return inlet, and the makeup water and condensate return spray into the deaerator. This spray condenses the water vapor in the vent, minimizing water loss from the system.

(xii) **Include a condensate surge tank in the steam system.** Steam flow rates in health care facilities can vary substantially due to volatile steam requirements associated with laundry equipment, food service equipment, sterilizers, and humidifiers. Large fluctuations in steam flow requirements can cause the deaerator to overflow. Installation of a condensate surge tank can capture any overflow, eliminating this source of water loss.

(xiii) **Reduce humidification setpoints and eliminate unnecessary humidification.** The 2005 edition of NFPA 99: *Health Care Facilities* establishes a minimum relative humidity level of 35 percent for anesthetizing locations. By addendum, ANSI/ASHRAE/ASHE Standard 170-2008: *Ventilation of Health Care Facilities* establishes a minimum relative humidity level of 20 percent for anesthetizing locations. These documents also establish minimum relative humidity levels for emergency department, surgery, and recovery areas. Humidifiers are required to maintain these humidity levels. Reducing humidification setpoints and eliminating humidification in administrative areas can achieve significant cost savings.

(xiv) **Modify flash tank vents to recover flash steam.** High-pressure steam condensate is typically returned to the condensate return unit through a flash tank. The purpose of the flash tank is to cool the condensate enough to keep it from flashing to steam as it enters the return unit. Flash tanks have a vent to remove any flash steam. This vent can be modified so the flash steam is recovered to a low-pressure steam main. Flash steam recovery reduces boiler steam flow, boiler makeup, and chemical treatment requirements. A flash steam recovery system is illustrated in Figure 6-10.

(xv) **Keep piping insulation repaired.** Over time, construction and maintenance activities damage insulation covering steam, steam return, and condensate return piping. Repairing any damaged insulation will reduce heat loss from steam piping.

(xvi) **Use high-efficiency fan and pump motors.** High-efficiency motors can reduce motor power requirements. In constant

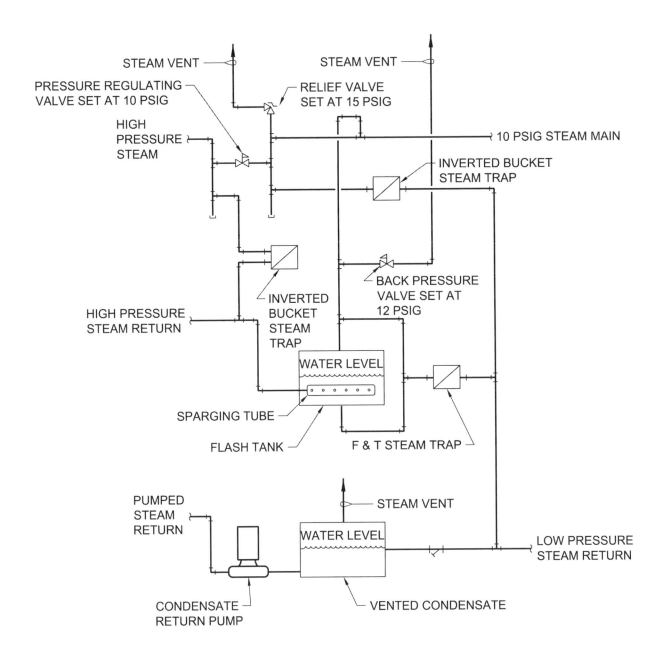

Figure 6-10: Flash Steam Recovery System

speed applications, however, replacing standard efficiency motors with high-efficiency motors can actually increase electrical power requirements due to an unintended increase in motor speed. The difference between the motor synchronous speed and the actual speed is commonly referred to as motor slip. The amount of slip is a function of the motor characteristics and the amount of torque required by the motor. In general, high-efficiency motors have less slip than standard efficiency motors. A comparison of the efficiency of standard and high-efficiency motors is illustrated in Figure 6-11.

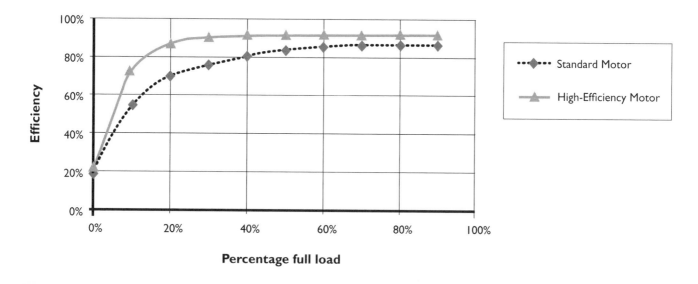

Figure 6-11: Comparison of Standard and High-Efficiency Motors

(xvii) **Institute remote boiler monitoring.** Most states require high continuous attendance by a licensed operator for high-pressure steam boilers. It may be possible, however, to secure approval for remote boiler monitoring by installing controls to remotely monitor steam pressure; boiler status; and high-water, low water, and boiler alarms. Remote boiler monitoring can significantly reduce maintenance staffing requirements.

(c) **Chilled water.** In a typical health care facility, chilled water generation and distribution accounts for 20 to 30 percent of total energy costs. Possible demand-side energy cost reduction measures for health facility chilled water systems include, but are not limited to, the following:

(i) **Replace older water chillers with newer models.** Newer water chillers are typically more efficient than older chillers due to advances in technology. Selection of a replacement chiller should be based on consideration of many factors, including capacity, design efficiency, part load efficiency, minimum load, and space requirements. The most common refrigerant choices for new water chillers are HFC-134a and HCFC-123. Refrigerants containing chlorine (e.g., HCFC-123 and HCFC-22) are being phased out due to concerns regarding ozone depletion in the upper atmosphere. The current phaseout schedule for HCFC-123 is indicated in Figure 6-12.

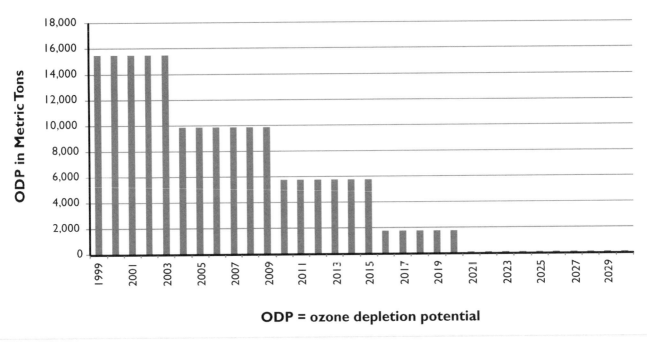

ODP = ozone depletion potential

Figure 6-12: HCFC-123 Refrigerant Phaseout Schedule

(ii) **Switch from air-side economizer cycles to hydronic free cooling.** Air-side economizer cycles typically yield mixed results in health care facilities. The energy cost savings associated with reduced water chiller operation (when outside air is cool enough to provide free cooling) are partially offset by higher humidification costs (during cold weather, the specific humidity or water content of the outside air is significantly less than the specific humidity of the return air). Therefore, hydronic free cooling systems, which use a plate-and-frame heat exchanger to transfer heat directly from the chilled water system to the tower water system, are typically recommended for health care facilities. Hydronic free cooling systems can produce chilled water approximately 1,800 to 3,000 hours per year depending on the facility location (more hours of hydronic free cooling are available in northern climates). A graph comparing the potential energy cost savings for air-side economizer cycles and hydronic economizer cycles as a function of indoor relative humidity for a health care facility is shown in Figure 6-13.

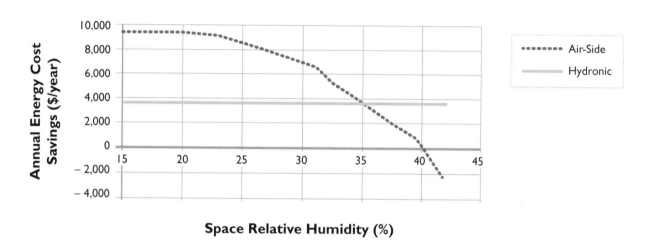

Figure 6-13: Comparison of Air-Side and Hydronic Free Cooling Savings

(iii) **Replace air-cooled chillers with water-cooled water chillers.** Water-cooled chillers are considerably more efficient than air-cooled chillers due to a lower refrigerant lift. Refrigerant lift is the difference between the condenser and evaporator refrigerant pressures. Water chiller power requirements are dependent on refrigerant lift, theoretical refrigerant cycle efficiency, compressor efficiency, and drive efficiency. Replacing air-cooled chillers with high-efficiency water-cooled chillers can reduce water chiller electrical demand and energy consumption by up to 40 percent.

(iv) **Install a heat pump chiller/heater.** A heat pump chiller/heater produces chilled water and heating water simultaneously. Health care facilities are ideal applications for this technology due to their continuous need for heating and cooling. Depending on natural gas and electricity rates, a heat pump water chiller can produce heating water for as little as 20 to 30 percent of the cost associated with high-efficiency natural gas-fired boilers. The annual energy cost savings achieved by a recent heat pump chiller/heater application are illustrated in Table 6-5.

Item	Units	Value
Chiller capacity	tons	350
Average load	%	60
Leaving chilled water temperature	°F	44
Leaving heating water temperature	°F	140
Standard chiller efficacy	kW/ton	0.65
Average electricity unit cost	cents/kWh	3.40
Average natural gas cost	$/MMBtu	12
Boiler combustion efficiency	$/MMBtu	82
Net annual savings	$/year	398,807

Table 6-5: Heat Pump Chiller/Heater Annual Energy Cost Savings

A heat pump chiller/heater can also be operated as a standard water chiller. This requires installation of a heat exchanger to transfer heat to the cooling towers. The same heat exchanger can also be used for hydronic free cooling. When equipped in this manner, a heat pump chiller/heater can also function as a standby water chiller. A typical heat pump chiller/heater piping diagram is illustrated in Figure 6-14.

(v) **Perform a life cycle cost analysis to determine whether a variable speed or constant speed water chiller is preferable.** Variable speed water chillers are more efficient than constant speed water chillers at reduced loads and reduced refrigerant lift. Constant speed water chillers, however, are more efficient at design conditions than variable speed water chillers. A

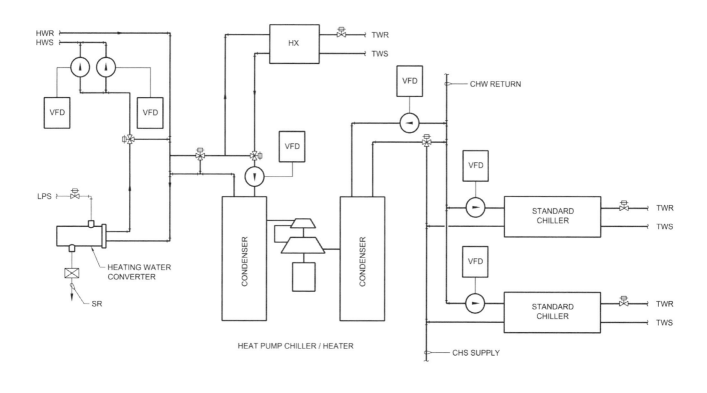

Figure 6-14: Heat Pump Chiller/Heater Piping Diagram

comparison of variable speed and constant speed water chiller alternatives for a new chiller plant is illustrated in Figure 6-15.

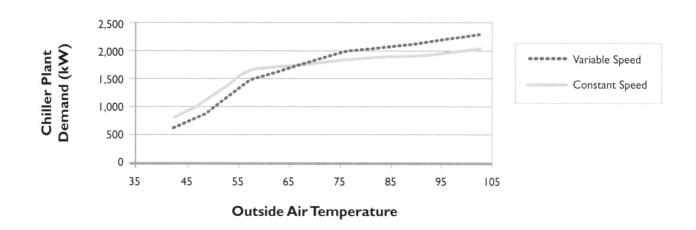

Figure 6-15: Comparison of Constant Speed and Variable Speed Chillers

As indicated in Figure 6-15, the variable speed chillers are more efficient and use less electricity at lower loads and lower condenser water temperatures than constant speed chillers. At higher loads and higher condenser water temperatures, however, constant speed chillers are more efficient and use less electricity. Health care facilities should select water chillers based on a life cycle cost analysis that considers water chiller efficiencies at anticipated loads and entering condenser water temperatures. The analysis should consider constant speed and variable speed chillers of comparable cost. The analysis should not compare a constant speed chiller to the same chiller equipped with a VFD. Variable speed chillers are generally more efficient than constant speed chillers at part loads and are generally less efficient than constant speed chillers at full load (due to the inefficiency of the VFD). When the demand component of the electricity rate is relatively low compared to the energy component, variable speed water chillers are more cost-effective than constant speed water chillers. When the demand component of the rate is relatively high compared to the energy component, constant speed water chillers are more cost-effective than variable speed water chillers.

(vi) **Use a variable volume chilled water system.** Water chillers and cooling towers remove all of the heat generated by the chilled water pump from the chilled water system; this is commonly referred to as the refrigeration effect. Variable volume chilled water systems use less pumping energy than constant volume systems, and thus reduce pumping, water chiller, and cooling tower energy requirements.

(vii) **Convert a constant speed chilled water system to a variable primary operation.** Variable primary chilled water systems are now feasible due to advances in water chiller technology that permit chillers to operate reliably with a wide range of rapidly changing evaporator flow rates. A trend line indicating the reaction of a modern water chiller to a sudden reduction in evaporator flow is provided in Figure 6-16.

Variable primary chilled water systems are more energy efficient than primary/secondary systems because they eliminate constant speed primary chilled water pumps and excess water flow through the decoupler. A typical variable primary chilled water system is illustrated in Figure 6-17.

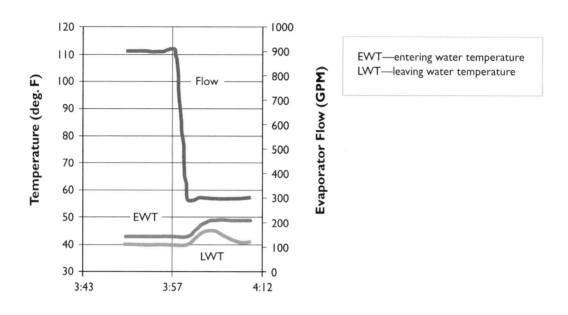

Figure 6-16: Water Chiller Reaction to Sudden Change in Evaporator Flow

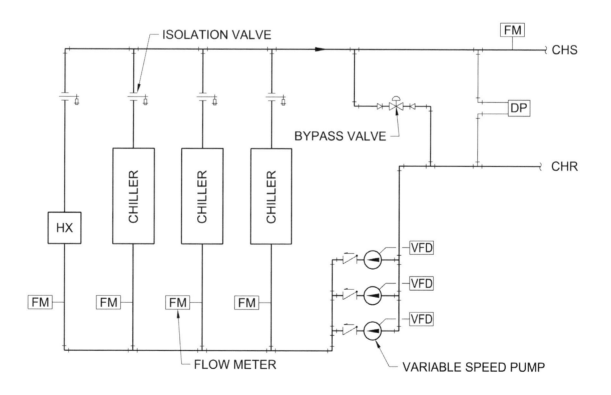

Figure 6-17: Variable Primary Chilled Water System

(viii) **Convert the chilled water system to high delta T/low-flow operation.** Most health facility chilled water systems operate with a 42 to 45° F chilled water supply temperature, typically with a 10° F temperature difference (or delta T) between the chilled water return and the chilled water supply. If the control valves are working properly, reducing the chilled water supply temperature to 38° F will increase the chilled water temperature difference to approximately 16° F. The relationship between entering water temperature and temperature difference for a chilled water coil originally selected for a 10° F delta T with 45° F entering chilled water temperature is illustrated in Figure 6-18.

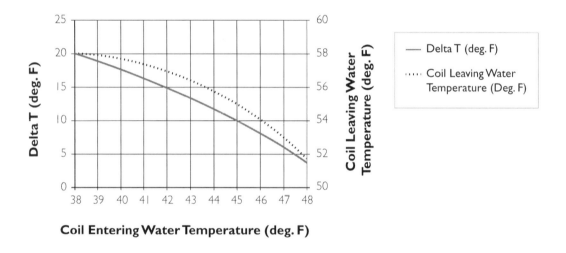

Figure 6-18: Typical Cooling Coil Delta T

As indicated in Figure 6-18, reducing the coil entering water temperature (chilled water supply temperature) from 45° F to 38° F doubles the coil delta T from 10° F to 20° F. Doubling the coil delta T cuts the chilled water flow requirement by 50 percent. A 50 percent reduction in flow will yield an 87.5 percent reduction in theoretical pump energy (in theory, pump energy is directly proportional to the cube of the flow). Due to changes in pump, motor, and VFD efficiencies, the actual reduction in pumping energy will be somewhat less than the theoretical reduction. The actual reduction in chilled water pump power requirements, however, more than offsets the associated increase in water chiller power requirements caused by the higher chiller refrigerant lift (reducing the chiller leaving water temperature reduces the evaporator refrigerant pressure and increases the difference between the compressor suction and discharge pressures). Conversions to high delta T/low-flow operation also increase the capacity of the existing chilled water distribution system. The relationship between chilled water distribution capacity, pipe size, and delta T is illustrated in Figure 6-19.

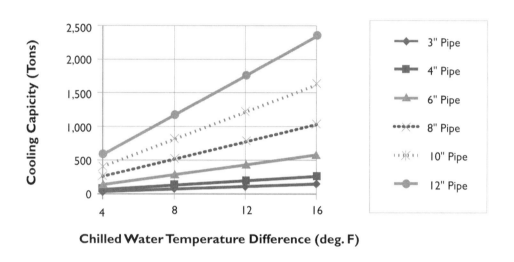

Figure 6-19: Relationship between Delta T and Pipe Capacity

(ix) **Convert a constant speed tower water system to variable volume operation.** Most tower water systems consist of dedicated systems for each water chiller. Each system includes a constant speed tower water pump and a cooling tower. The use of variable speed systems with manifold pumps and manifold towers offers greater reliability, lower capital costs, and lower energy costs. With a variable volume tower water system, a tower water control valve at each water chiller is modulated to maintain the condenser water flow rate at setpoint. The flow setpoint is automatically adjusted as required to prevent the refrigerant lift from decreasing below a minimum setpoint. Maintaining a minimum refrigerant lift allows the water chillers to operate at colder tower water supply temperatures. The tower water pumps and cooling towers are sequenced according to the tower water flow rate.

A schematic diagram for a typical variable volume water system is shown in Figure 6-20.

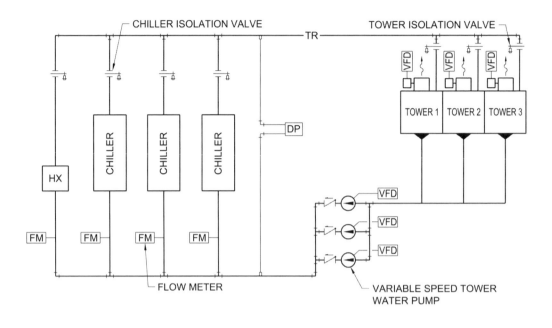

Figure 6-20: Variable Volume Tower Water System

(x) **Use variable speed cooling tower fans.** Using variable speed drives to modulate the capacity of cooling tower fans is considerably more efficient than using blending valves.

(xi) **Install a booster water chiller for operating room HVAC systems.** Most health care chilled water systems are operated and sequenced according to the requirements of the air-handling units that serve the operating rooms. Most surgeons prefer operating room conditions in the range of 60 to 62° F and 50 percent relative humidity. Achieving these conditions requires the air leaving the cooling coil to have a dewpoint in the range of 41 to 43° F. The relationship between temperature, relative humidity, and required cooling coil dewpoint is illustrated in Figure 6-21.

Installing a booster water chiller to produce the colder water required by operating room air-handling units makes it possible to increase the central plant water chiller leaving water temperature setpoints, thus requiring less power. The booster water chiller can also be connected to the essential power system so that operating room cooling can

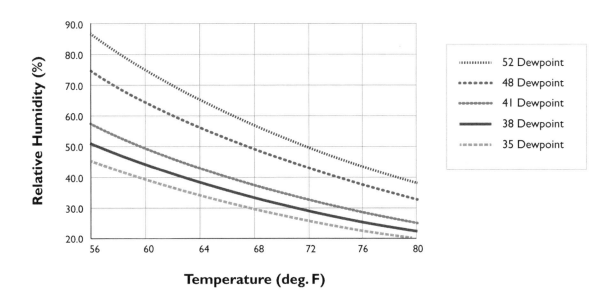

Figure 6-21: Operating Room Dewpoints

be maintained in the event of a long-term power outage. A typical booster water chiller application is illustrated in Figure 6-22.

(xii) **Implement an automatic reset program for the tower water supply temperature setpoint.** Water chillers operate more efficiently at lower tower water supply temperatures. Each one-degree (F) reduction in entering tower water temperature reduces the chiller power requirement by

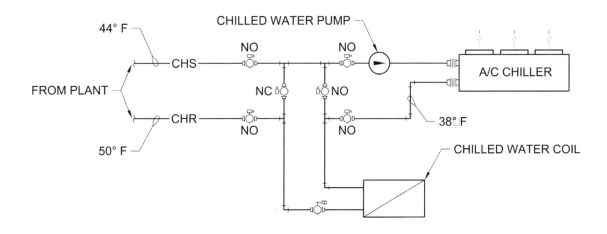

Figure 6-22: Booster Water Chiller

approximately 0.5 to 1.5 percent according to the type of water chiller. Reducing the tower water supply temperature setpoint to a level that cannot be attained by the cooling tower, however, wastes tower fan energy. Water chillers have minimum entering tower water temperatures and refrigerant lifts to assure proper oil circulation and motor cooling (in refrigerant-cooled hermetic motors). Water chillers also have maximum entering tower water supply temperatures and refrigerant lifts to prevent compressor surge (alternating refrigerant flow reversals in the chiller compressor), which may damage the compressor. The typical refrigerant compressor map in Figure 6-23 indicates the design refrigerant volume and head selection, surge line, and unloading at various entering condenser water temperatures.

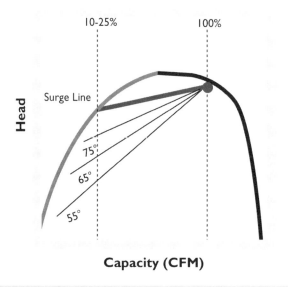

Figure 6-23: Water Chiller Compressor Map

Minimum entering water temperatures are typically in the range of 55 to 70° F and maximum entering water temperatures are typically in the range of 80 to 85° F, depending on specific chiller characteristics. A tower water reset strategy automatically adjusts the tower water supply temperature setpoint between minimum and maximum setpoints according to the water chiller load and the outside air dry bulb and wet bulb conditions. An optimized reset strategy automatically adjusts the tower water supply temperature setpoint as required to minimize the total water chiller and cooling tower fan energy required. Using a variable volume tower water system that controls the tower water flow to each water chiller at setpoint with a minimum refrigerant lift override, combined with an optimized tower water supply temperature setpoint reset strategy is good practice.

(xiii) **Consider resetting the chilled water supply temperature setpoint.** Water chiller power requirements can be reduced by increasing the chilled water supply temperature setpoint. A chilled water reset strategy automatically adjusts the chilled water supply temperature setpoint according to the outside air conditions and the load. Chilled water reset strategies must be examined closely, however, as an increase in chilled water supply temperature can cause elevated relative humidity in the space being cooled and increase chilled water pumping energy requirements.

(xiv) **Install a maximum capacity chiller sequencing program.** Water chillers are typically most efficient when operated at 60 to 80 percent of their capacity. Overall system efficiency, however, typically peaks when water chillers are operating at full load due to their auxiliary power requirements (i.e., tower water pump, chilled water pump, and cooling tower fan). A maximum capacity chiller sequencing program starts the water chillers in a specific user-selected order when the chilled water supply temperature increases above setpoint. The program stops the water chillers when the load decreases below the capacity of the water chillers that will remain in operation.

(xv) **Install a cooling tower fan optimal dispatch sequencing program.** If a variable volume tower water system is used, the control system should sequence the cooling towers in an optimal dispatch manner based on the total tower water flow requirement or load. The sequencing program should consider specific cooling tower minimum and maximum flow requirements. If the flow through a cooling tower is too low, dry areas in the fill may result, significantly reducing overall tower efficiency.

(xvi) **Install a chilled water pump and tower water pump optimal dispatch sequencing program.** The control system should sequence the chilled water pumps and tower water pumps in an optimal dispatch manner based on total flow and head requirements. The sequencing program should maximize pumping efficiency (commonly referred to as wire-to-water efficiency). Ideally, all of the pumps in a manifold pumping system should be identical. Sequencing dissimilar pumps is difficult because different pumps, even when operated at the same speed and head, will have different flows. In some cases, one of the pumps may have little or no flow (a condition commonly referred to as deadheading), which will damage the pump. The sequencing program should consider each pump's performance curve, which is a graphic illustration of the relationship between flow and head. A performance curve for two identical pumps connected in parallel is illustrated in Figure 6-24.

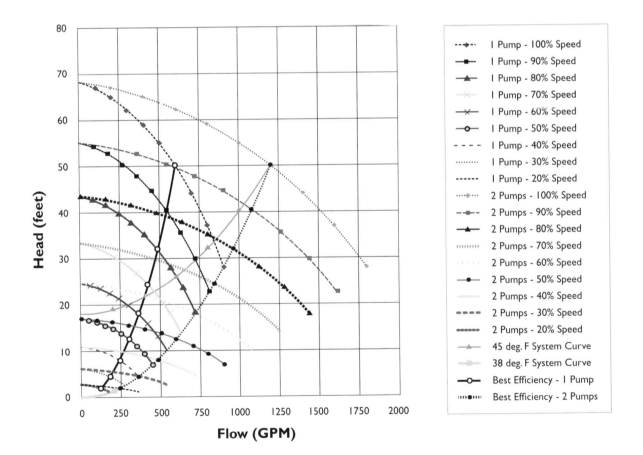

Figure 6-24: Duplex Pumping System Performance Curves

(xvii) **Control tower water valves to maintain minimum refrigerant lift.** If a variable volume tower water system is used, control of the tower water control valves should be overridden as required to maintain sufficient refrigerant lift for normal water chiller operation. Control in this manner will allow the water chiller to operate at cold condenser water temperatures and greatly simplify the transition from water chiller operation to hydronic free cooling operation. Without refrigerant lift controls, the water chiller must be shut down for approximately 20 minutes at the onset of hydronic free cooling (when the tower water is being cooled) and for approximately 20 minutes at the end of hydronic free cooling (when the tower water is being warmed). This disruption in chilled water service frequently yields patient and staff discomfort, which makes the O&M staff reluctant to use the hydronic free cooling system.

(xviii) **Regularly clean condenser and evaporator tube bundles.** Fouling in the tube bundles adversely impacts water chiller efficacy. As a result, regular cleaning of the tube bundles can reduce water chiller power consumption.

(xix) **Institute automatic chiller monitoring.** A remote chiller monitoring system monitors approach temperature differences, refrigerant pressures, power requirements, overall system efficacy, and other factors. When a problem occurs, the monitoring system alerts the operator and suggests a resolution. Maintaining the equipment and system in peak operating condition improves overall system efficacy and reduces annual energy consumption and costs. For example, automatic chiller monitoring can detect the presence of non-condensables (typically air) in the chiller condenser (typically caused by a faulty purge unit). The presence of non-condensables causes an increase in the condenser refrigerant and compressor discharge pressures. Repairing the chiller purge equipment and removing the non-condensables reduces the compressor discharge pressure and power requirements.

(xx) **Implement an automatic reset program for the chilled water differential pressure setpoint.** The automatic temperature control system modulates the chilled water pump speed to maintain the remote differential pressure at setpoint (this is typically the differential pressure at a location two-thirds the distance to the most hydraulically remote circuit). The actual differential pressure required to provide adequate flow, however, varies based on a number of factors, including the current flow requirement. Automatically adjusting the differential pressure setpoint as required to maintain the critical chilled water control valve at 95 percent open ensures the differential pressure setpoint is at near optimum level. The control system selects the critical valve from a defined list of valves selected for consideration as part of the reset strategy. In smaller systems with 10 or fewer valves, the critical valve can be the most open valve. In larger systems, the critical valve should be the 10th percentile valve (e.g., in a system with 50 valves, the critical valve is the 5th most open; in a system with 200 valves, the critical valve is the 20th most open).

(xxi) **Regularly repair chilled water system piping.** Construction and maintenance activities damage insulation covering chilled water supply and return piping over time. Repair of damaged insulation will reduce chilled water piping heat losses.

(xxii) **Employ high-efficiency pump, fan, and chiller motors.** High-efficiency motors can reduce motor power requirements.

(xxiii) **Verify that cooling towers have adequate capacity.** Cooling towers should be capable of providing the design leaving water temperature at the highest reasonably anticipated outside air wet bulb temperature (typically, the ASHRAE 0.4 percent wet bulb temperature for health facility location) and load. The tower leaving water temperature should be consistent with the maximum entering condenser water temperature for the chillers it serves. Higher condenser entering water temperatures caused by inadequate cooling tower capacity reduce water chiller efficiency and increase water chiller power requirements.

(xxiv) **Use high-performance cooling towers.** Cooling towers equipped with variable speed fans, velocity reduction cylinders, efficient PVC fill, and automatic cleaning systems are more energy-efficient than standard cooling towers. A high-performance cooling tower is illustrated in Figure 6-25.

(xxv) **Replace air-cooled DX cooling equipment with water-cooled equipment.** Air-cooled direct expansion (DX) cooling equipment is less efficient than water-cooled equipment.

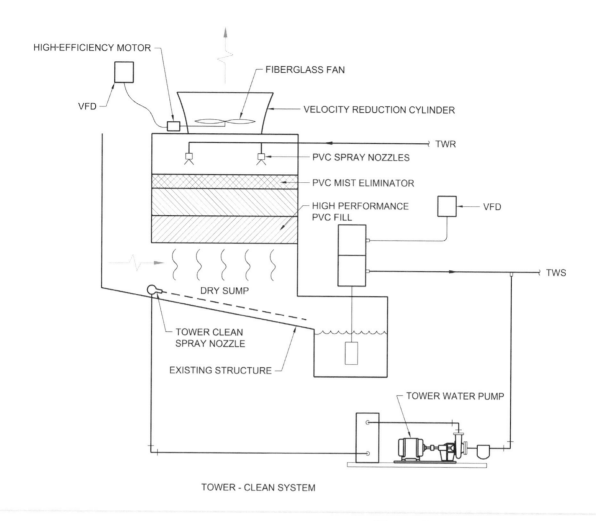

Figure 6-25: High-Performance Cooling Tower

Replacing DX systems with chilled water equipment can reduce electricity consumption and demand.

(xxvi) **Employ a thermal storage system.** When electricity demand charges are high or time-of-use electricity rates are in effect, using thermal storage systems can yield significant savings. The water chillers produce excess cooling during non-peak hours and store it in the thermal storage facility. During on-peak hours, cooling in the thermal storage facility cools the facility. Common thermal storage systems are ice banks and open chilled water storage tanks. A typical chilled water storage tank is illustrated in Figure 6-26.

(xxvii) **Install profile pumps in chilled water systems serving multiple buildings.** In large chilled water systems serving

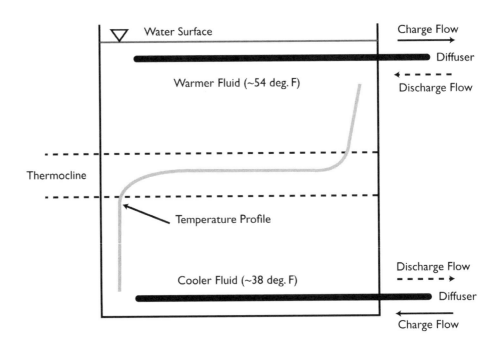

Figure 6-26: Vertical Stratified Chilled Water Storage Tank

multiple buildings, the main chilled water pumps should not be selected to meet the pressure requirements of the most hydraulically remote circuit. When the most remote circuit has sufficient differential pressure, the buildings and valves that are hydraulically closer to the main pumps have too much pressure. In response to the higher differential pressure, the closer coil control valves modulate closed, which wastes energy. In some cases, the excess differential pressure may actually force the valves open (if the pressure exceeds the valve close-off rating), which wastes even more energy due to excess flow, reduced delta T, increased pumping energy, increased cooling, and increased heating (in a variable volume reheat system a colder air-handling unit supply temperature increases reheat). A better alternative is to select the main pumps for the hydraulically closer buildings and coils and to install profile pumps in each building. The automatic temperature control system automatically sequences each building's profile pump to maintain the building differential pressure at setpoint. A typical profile pumping installation is illustrated in Figure 6-27.

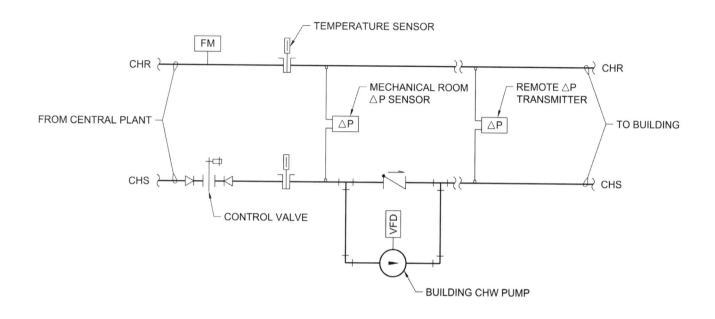

Figure 6-27: Profile Pumping

(d) **Heating water.** In a typical health care facility, heating water distribution accounts for 2 to 3 percent of total energy consumption (excluding the cost of steam, natural gas, and other heating fuels). Possible demand-side energy cost reduction measures for health facility heating water systems include, but are not limited to, the following:

(i) **Use a heat pump water chiller/heater to produce heating water.** A heat pump water chiller/heater, which is equipped with two compressors in series, produces both chilled water and heating water. Depending on natural gas and electricity rates, heat pump water chillers can produce heating water for as little as 20 to 30 percent of the cost associated with high-efficiency natural gas-fired boilers.

(ii) **Use a combination of condensing and dual fuel boilers to save energy.** Condensing boilers can provide fuel-to-heat efficiencies as high as 96 percent (the efficiency is significantly affected by the boiler entering water temperature) as compared to standard boiler efficiencies in the range of 82 percent. Condensing boilers, however, are not readily available in dual-fuel arrangements, and dual-fuel capability with fuel oil storage on-site is required for health care facilities in many areas. These requirements can be met by using either a synthetic natural gas system, a parallel steam-fired heating water converter served by dual-fuel steam boilers, or a combination of condensing and non-condensing dual-fuel boilers. An example of the latter is illustrated in Figure 6-28.

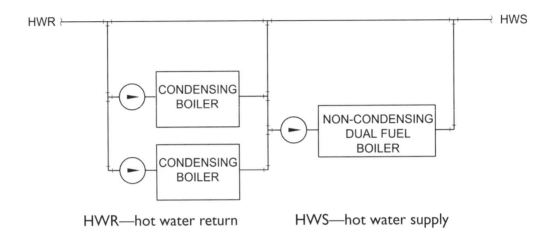

Figure 6-28: Combination of Condensing and Non-Condensing Boilers

(iii) **Use a hybrid boiler plant to gain fuel choice flexibility.** Depending on natural gas and electricity rate structures and boiler efficiencies, electric boilers can be more cost-effective than natural gas boilers. A progressively designed boiler plant includes both electric and natural gas boilers to provide fuel choice flexibility. If interruptible rates are in effect, the electric boilers are used during off-peak periods and the natural gas-fired boilers are used during on-peak periods. The use of both types of boilers also satisfies health facility regulations requiring dual-fuel capability. A hybrid boiler plant is particularly cost-effective when a heat pump chiller/heater is used. The graph in Figure 6-29 indicates the most cost-effective heating equipment for a hybrid boiler plant with a heat pump chiller/heater (HPCH) as a function of natural gas and electricity rates.

(iv) **Consider converting heating water systems to variable volume operation.** Variable volume heating water systems are typically more cost-effective than constant speed heating water systems because variable volume systems require less pumping energy. However, variable volume heating water

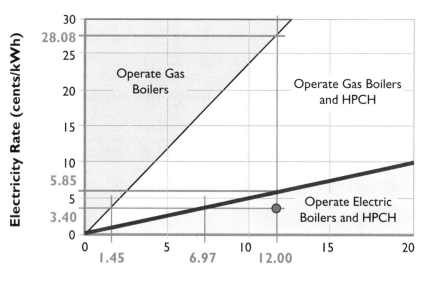

Figure 6-29: Hybrid Plant Heating Equipment Operation

systems are typically not as cost-effective as variable volume chilled water systems because excess heating water pumping energy actually reduces the heating fuel requirement. When electricity rates are extremely low relative to the cost of heating fuel, constant speed heating water systems can actually be more cost-effective than variable volume systems. Variable volume heating water systems also require provisions for minimum flow to prevent pump and control valve damage. Provisions may include a small number of three-way valves or a bypass control valve. Use of a bypass control valve is more efficient, as it can be closed when system flow exceeds the minimum flow requirement.

(v) **Implement an automatic reset program for the heating water differential pressure setpoint.** The automatic temperature control system modulates the heating water pump speed to maintain the remote differential pressure at setpoint (this is typically the differential pressure at a location two-thirds the distance to the most hydraulically remote circuit). The actual differential pressure required to provide adequate flow, however, varies according to a number of factors, including the current flow requirement. Automatically adjusting the differential pressure setpoint as required to maintain the critical heating water control valve at 95 percent open ensures the differential pressure setpoint is at near optimum level. The control system selects the critical valve from a defined list of valves selected for consideration in the reset strategy. In smaller systems with 10 or fewer valves, the critical valve can be the most open valve. In larger systems, the critical valve should be the 10th percentile valve (e.g., in a system with 50 valves, the critical valve is the 5th most open; in a system with 200 valves, the critical valve is the 20th most open).

(vi) **Implement an automatic reset program for the heating water supply temperature setpoint.** Automatically adjusting heating water supply temperatures downward during warmer weather reduces heat loss from system piping. Heating water supply temperature reset strategies also increase valve controllability, increase valve seat life, and reduce the potential for wire draw valve damage. Wire draw is damage to the seat of a control valve caused when water flashes into steam due to the reduction in pressure. Wire draw typically occurs when a valve is modulated at nearly closed positions. The acceleration of the water through the small opening reduces the residual pressure below the saturation pressure at the water temperature. Wire draw can be prevented by reducing the differential pressure or reducing the supply water temperature. A typical heating water supply temperature setpoint reset strategy is illustrated in Figure 6-30.

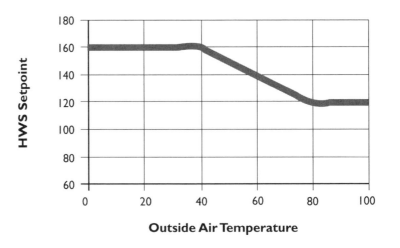

Figure 6-30: Heating Water Reset Strategy

(vii) **Regularly repair heating system piping insulation.** Heating water supply and return piping insulation is typically damaged over time due to maintenance and repair activities. Repairing damaged insulation will reduce heating water piping heat losses.

(viii) **Use high-efficiency pump motors.** Use of high-efficiency motors can reduce motor power requirements.

(ix) **Use distributed pumping in heating water systems serving multiple buildings.** Distributed pumping saves energy in large district heating water systems that serve multiple buildings by locating the system pumps at the buildings as well as in the central energy plant. Each building pump or set of building pumps is selected for head and flow requirements that match the needs of the buildings it serves. Distributed pumping can also reduce capital costs in new installations as it eliminates the need for two sets of pumps (one at the plant and one in each building). A typical heating water distributed pumping arrangement with constant speed boiler pumps at the central energy plant and variable speed profile pumps at the buildings is illustrated in Figure 6-31.

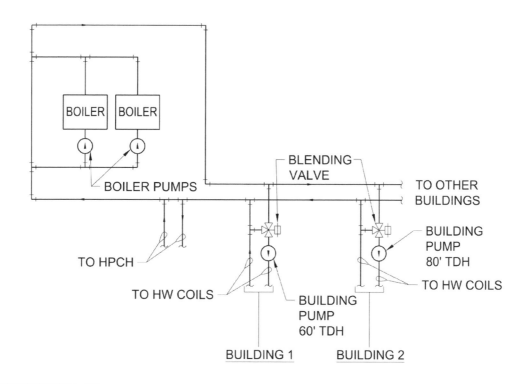

Figure 6-31: Distributed Heating Water Pumps

(e) **Air distribution.** In a typical health care facility, air distribution accounts for 12 to 20 percent of total energy costs. Possible demand-side energy cost reduction measures for health facility air distribution systems include, but are not limited to, the following:

(i) **Use VAV systems in areas where the cooling airflow requirement exceeds minimum ACH:** Variable air volume (VAV) systems should be used for all areas where the cooling airflow requirement exceeds the minimum air change rate (measured in air changes per hour, or ACH). These areas include operating rooms, offices, treatment rooms, patient rooms, etc. Variable volume systems reduce fan energy requirements, fan heat gain, and simultaneous heating and cooling. Typically, heating water reheat coils are used to maintain the space temperature at setpoint. These systems require simultaneous heating (reheat coil) and cooling (chilled water coil) to function properly. Although some amount of simultaneous heating and cooling is necessary for dehumidification, it should be minimized.

(ii) **Use occupancy sensors and weekly scheduling to control air distribution systems during unoccupied periods.** Occupancy sensors and weekly schedules can be used to reduce minimum airflow requirements and modify the heating and cooling space temperature setpoints during unoccupied periods.

(iii) **Increase deadband between cooling and heating setpoints.** A deadband is the difference between the space temperature heating and cooling setpoints. Increasing the deadband will reduce heating and cooling energy consumption. Increasing the deadband during unoccupied periods is commonly referred to as a night setback/setup arrangement.

(iv) **Automatically reset supply air temperature setpoints.** Simultaneous heating and cooling in variable volume reheat, double-duct, and multi-zone air-handling systems can be significantly reduced by implementing a supply air temperature reset strategy in which the supply air temperature setpoints are automatically reset as required by space temperatures. Cooling setpoints are reset as required to maintain the warmest space temperature at a maximum level. To ensure proper dehumidification, the supply air temperature is overridden as required to maintain return air relative humidity at a maximum level.

(v) **Automatically reset supply air static pressure setpoints.**
Supply fan speeds are typically modulated as required to
maintain the supply air duct pressure at setpoint. The actual
static pressure required to provide adequate flow, however,
varies according to a number of factors, including the current
airflow requirement. Automatically adjusting the static
pressure setpoint as required to keep the most open terminal
damper nearly completely open (typically 95 percent) ensures
the static pressure setpoint remains at the optimum level.

(vi) **Reduce air change rates during unoccupied periods.**
The minimum air change rates established by health
care regulations typically apply to occupied periods only.
Reducing the air change rate during unoccupied periods can
significantly reduce fan energy requirements, fan heat gain,
and simultaneous heating and cooling. Occupancy is typically
detected by occupancy sensors. Unoccupied/occupied air
change switching is particularly cost-effective for operating
rooms, LDRP rooms, cath labs, airborne infection isolation
(AII) rooms, and other areas with high minimum occupied
air change rates. Health care regulations require air change
switching arrangements to include provisions for maintaining
the proper pressure relationship during unoccupied periods.
An unoccupied/occupied air change rate system for an
operating room with a modulating return air damper for
pressure control is illustrated in Figure 6-32.

An ASHE monograph discussing
operating room HVAC setback
strategies can be found on the
ASHE website at www.ashe.org/
management_monographs.

(vii) **Reduce AII room airflow setpoints when rooms are not
occupied by potentially airborne infectious patients.**
Airborne infection isolation rooms must be fully exhausted
with a negative pressure relationship to adjacent spaces. AII
rooms also require 12 air changes per hour as compared to
only six air changes per hour for a standard patient room.
(In some jurisdictions, AII rooms must be equipped with an
anteroom.) Because AII rooms are rarely used for airborne
infection isolation patients in most health care facilities,
equipping these rooms with controls to reduce the minimum
airflow setpoint to six air changes per hour when the room
is not occupied by an airborne infectious patient can achieve
significant energy cost savings. When the room is being used
in isolation mode, the exhaust fan speed is modulated to
maintain 12 air changes per hour and the supply air terminal
is modulated to maintain the supply airflow at setpoint. The

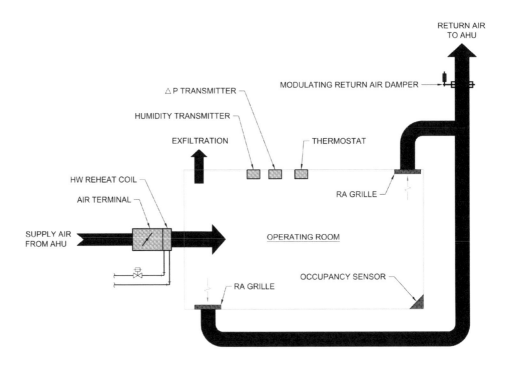

Figure 6-32: Operating Room Unoccupied/Occupied Air Change Rates

supply airflow setpoint is equal to the exhaust airflow minus the airflow offset (the difference between the exhaust and supply flow rates). The airflow offset provides a negative pressure relationship between the AII room and the corridor. (The airflow offset required to provide the correct pressure relationship is dependent on the effective leakage area of the AII room.) When the room is being used in normal mode, the exhaust fan speed is modulated to maintain a minimum of six air changes per hour and the supply terminal functions in the same manner as described for the isolation mode (i.e., the negative pressure relationship is maintained during normal mode). A typical AII isolation/normal system is illustrated in Figure 6-33.

(viii) **Use demand-controlled ventilation control where appropriate.** Ventilation rates depend on a number of factors, including whether a space is occupied, floor area, contaminant generation rates, and acceptable contaminant concentration rates. In many areas in a health care facility (e.g., offices, conference rooms, classrooms, and auditoriums), the most significant of these factors is occupancy. Demand-

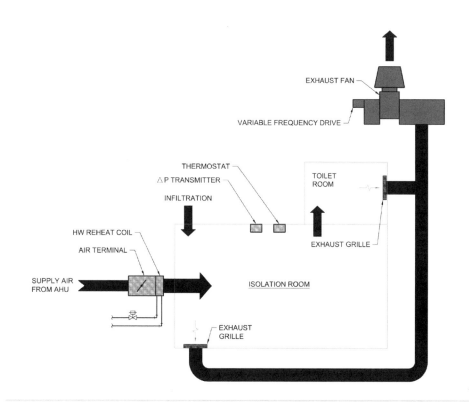

Figure 6-33: All Isolation/Normal System

controlled ventilation arrangements vary the ventilation airflow according to actual room occupancy, which is typically determined using space and outdoor CO_2 sensors (the space CO_2 concentration is maintained at 700 ppm higher than the outdoor CO_2 concentration). Reducing the ventilation rates reduces cooling and heating energy requirements.

(ix) **Make sure existing and new ductwork is well-sealed.** Current SMACNA standards establish default duct leakage and sealing classifications for ductwork based on the operating pressure requirement. If the drawings and specifications for a project do not stipulate the desired classification, the default levels are presumed to apply. Consequently, it is imperative that project specifications clearly establish the duct leakage and sealing classifications for all ductwork. Existing ductwork is also prone to leakage, and leakage rates in the range of 8 to 20 percent are not uncommon. For this reason, sealing existing ductwork can significantly reduce fan energy requirements and fan heat gain.

(x) **Use filters with a low air pressure drop.** Air-handling units serving inpatient care and treatment areas must be equipped with both pre-filters and final filters. The total air pressure drop of these filters is a function of the filter size, face velocity, type, and allowance for filter loading. Installing large filters with low initial pressure drops (either a larger face area or a different type of filter) and replacing them at regular intervals can significantly reduce fan energy requirements and fan heat gain.

(xi) **Monitor filter air pressure drop to detect dirty filters.** The air pressure drop across filters should be continuously monitored (typically accomplished by the energy management system) so that dirty filters are promptly detected and replaced.

(xii) **Select heating and cooling coils with low air pressure drops.** The air pressure drop that occurs across heating and cooling coils is a function of several factors, including coil area, face velocity, number of rows, and fin spacing. Selecting coils with larger areas, lower face velocities, fewer rows, and fewer fins can achieve lower air pressure drops and significantly reduce fan energy requirements and fan heat gain.

(xiii) **Install exhaust air energy recovery equipment.** Average ventilation rates in health care facilities are typically in the range of 20 to 40 percent of the total airflow requirement. Recovering energy using exhaust air energy recovery equipment can significantly reduce peak heating and cooling requirements. Enthalpy wheels can recover up to 80 percent of the sensible and latent heat in the exhaust air. The operation of an enthalpy wheel is illustrated in Figure 6-34.

A schematic diagram of an energy recovery air-handling unit with an enthalpy wheel for exhaust air energy recovery is shown in Figure 6-35.

The performance of various types of exhaust air energy recovery equipment is compared in Table 6-6.

The impact of using an enthalpy wheel with recirculation on the annual operating costs and life cycle cost of a typical health facility HVAC system is illustrated in Table 6-7.

(xiv) **Modulate ventilation rates to control building pressure.** Due to high exhaust requirements, the building pressures in health care facilities are typically negative to the outside at the entry level. A negative building pressure at the entry level

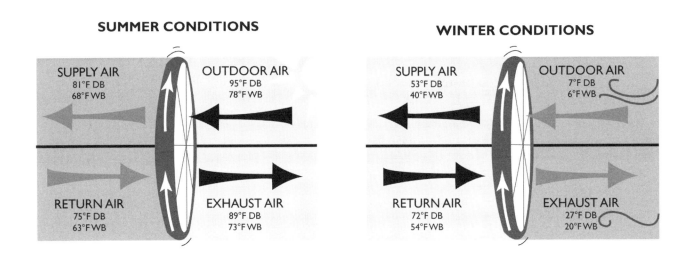

SUMMER CONDITIONS

SUPPLY AIR
81°F DB
68°F WB

OUTDOOR AIR
95°F DB
78°F WB

RETURN AIR
75°F DB
63°F WB

EXHAUST AIR
89°F DB
73°F WB

WINTER CONDITIONS

SUPPLY AIR
53°F DB
40°F WB

OUTDOOR AIR
7°F DB
6°F WB

RETURN AIR
72°F DB
54°F WB

EXHAUST AIR
27°F DB
20°F WB

Figure 6-34: Exhaust Air Energy Recovery Using an Enthalpy Wheel

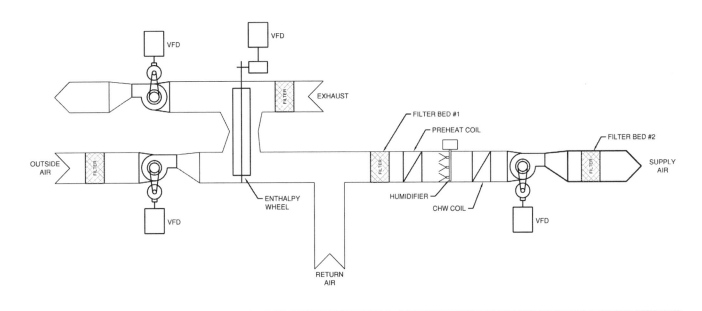

Figure 6-35: Energy Recovery Air-Handling Unit with an Enthalpy Wheel

can cause excessive amounts of infiltration, exfiltration, low relative humidity, high relative humidity, and other problems. Due to the stack effect, which is created by the buoyancy of warm air, these problems are particularly pronounced in taller buildings. In the winter, the building temperature is warmer than outside. The warm air rises to the top of the building, creating a negative pressure at the bottom of the building

Type	Sensible Effectiveness (%)	Latent Effectiveness (%)
Air-to-air heat exchanger	60	0
Refrigerant migration coils	60	0
Glycol runaround system	60	0
Enthalpy wheel	75	75

Table 6-6: Exhaust Air Energy Recovery Equipment Performance

Item	Recirculation without exhaust air energy recovery	100% outside air with enthalpy wheel	20% outside air with enthalpy wheel
Cooling load (tons)	346	352	295
Heating and humidification load (HP)	63	42	38
Capital cost ($)	1,957,642	2,223,398	1,937,975
Annual electricity cost ($/year)	113,919	118,781	113,231
Annual natural gas cost ($/year)	91,752	85,743	82,604
Annual maintenance cost ($/year)	200,000	205,000	208,000
Life cycle cost ($)	8,458,760	8,779,623	8,390,629

Table 6-7: Exhaust Air Energy Recovery Cost Comparisons

(below the neutral plane) and positive pressure at the top of the building (above the neutral plane). In the summer, when the building temperature is colder than outside, the cold air drops to the bottom of the building, creating negative pressure at the top of the building and positive pressure at the bottom. A building pressure control system that modulates ventilation airflows to maintain the building pressure at a neutral relationship to the outside at the entry level can minimize these problems. Due to the stack effect, all buildings have areas of positive pressure and negative pressure relative to the outside. The goal is to minimize these pressure differences. A diagram of a tall building illustrating its pressure relationship relative to the outside on a cold day is provided in Figure 6-36.

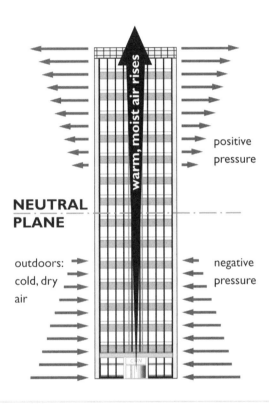

Figure 6-36: Building Pressure Relationships on a Cold Winter Day

(xv) **Replace traditional single-fan double-duct units with separate heating and cooling units.** Double-duct and multi-zone air-handling systems generally require significant amounts of simultaneous heating and cooling. Traditional double-duct and multi-zone air-handling units use a single supply air fan to blow air through a heating coil into a hot duct and separately through a cooling coil into a cold duct. Double-duct air terminals or zone dampers are modulated to mix the hot air and the cold air together as required to maintain space temperatures at setpoint. The use of an air-side economizer with this type of unit reduces cooling requirements while simultaneously increasing heating requirements. Replacing traditional single-fan double-duct and multi-zone units with separate draw-through heating and cooling units, however, will reduce both heating and cooling requirements. The ventilation air is introduced into the cooling unit only. Both the heating and cooling units are typically of the variable volume type, so the zone dampers (for a multi-zone system) and double-duct terminals (for a double-duct system) are typically replaced with new variable volume arrangements. The hot and cold terminal dampers are modulated in sequence to maintain the space temperature at the respective heating and cooling setpoints (the hot damper is fully closed before the cold damper begins to open). Consequently, simultaneous heating and cooling is significantly reduced (due to minimum ACH and dehumidification requirements, a certain amount of simultaneous heating and cooling cannot be avoided).

(xvi) **Use two-fan double-duct air-handling units with neutral deck for ORs.** The 2010 edition of the FGI *Guidelines for Design and Construction of Health Care Facilities*, which incorporates ASHRAE 170-2008 and its addenda, recommends a minimum of 20 to 25 air changes per hour for operating rooms. These minimums are based on the results of a detailed investigation of the relationship between air changes and the likelihood of a surgical site infection (see references provided in the sidebar). For a number of reasons, including thermal comfort for operating room (OR) staff, most operating rooms are designed for space temperatures in the range of 58 to 62° F, with a maximum relative humidity of 55 percent. (In Table 2.1-2, footnote 14 in the 2006 edition of the FGI *Guidelines*, HVAC system designers are required to consult with the OR staff when establishing the design conditions for operating rooms.) Achieving these conditions requires the use of low temperature supply air (42–44° F) or a desiccant. With conventional variable air volume (VAV) reheat systems, the combination of a high minimum air change requirement and low temperature supply air is extremely inefficient as it causes extraordinarily high levels of simultaneous heating and cooling. The use of a two-fan double-duct system with a cold deck and a "neutral deck" in these applications can yield significant savings. Some have estimated annual savings of as much as $15,000 to $20,000 per operating room when compared to the use of a constant volume reheat system. Schematic diagrams of the air-handling equipment and air terminals used with a two-fan double-duct system with neutral deck are provided in Figures 6-37 and 6-38.

Research into the Relationship Between Air Changes and Surgical Site Infections

Memarzadeh F and Manning A. 2002. Comparison of operating room ventilation systems in the protection of the surgical site. ASHRAE *Transactions* 108, Pt. 2.

Memarzadeh F and Jiang Z. 2004. Effects of operating room geometry and ventilation system parameter variations on the protection of the surgical site, in IAQ 2004: Critical Operations: Supporting the Healing Environment through IAQ Performance Standards.

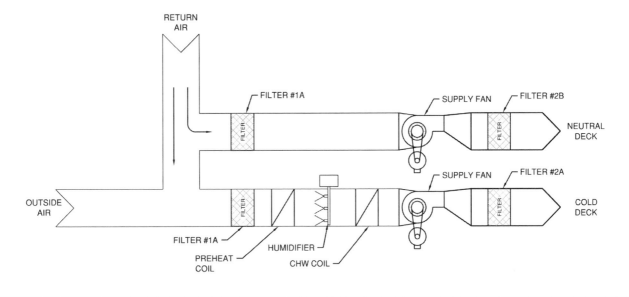

Figure 6-37: Two-Fan Double-Duct AHU with "Neutral Deck"

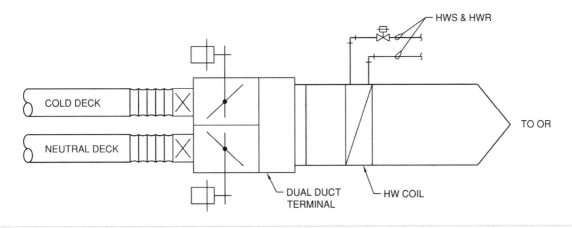

Figure 6-38: Dual-Duct Terminal with Reheat Coil

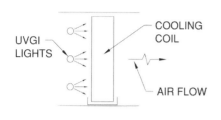

Figure 6-39: UVGI Lighting at Cooling Coil

(xvii) **Use high-efficiency fan motors in variable volume air distribution systems.** High-efficiency motors can reduce fan motor power requirements in variable volume systems.

(xviii) **Install UVGI lights at cooling coils.** In recent years, several manufacturers have introduced UVGI (ultraviolet germicidal irradiation) lights intended for installation in air-handling units. The primary purpose of these lights is to prevent mold and mildew growth on the cooling coil, which reduces the coil air pressure drop, fan energy requirements, and fan heat gain. Proper installation of UVGI lights at a cooling coil is illustrated in Figure 6-39.

(xix) **Use air-side economizer cycles in air-handling systems that do not serve areas requiring humidification.** In facilities that are not humidified, air-side economizer cycles can significantly reduce cooling energy requirements. During colder weather, an air-side economizer cycle uses outside air for cooling rather than mechanical refrigeration. Air-side economizer cycles should not be used in air systems serving areas requiring humidification because the additional humidification costs (required because the outside air specific humidity is lower than the return air specific humidity) more than offset the cooling savings. A typical air-side economizer cycle is illustrated in Figure 6-40.

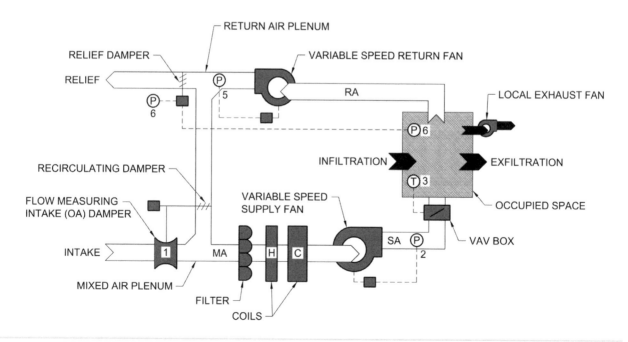

Figure 6-40: Air-Side Economizer Cycle

(xx) **Use variable speed drives to balance exhaust fan airflows.** Variable speed exhaust fans permit a reduction in exhaust flow requirements based on actual occupancy or use. Variable speed exhaust fans also simplify balancing requirements. Since variable frequency drives are not significantly more expensive than constant speed motor starters, the use of variable speed exhaust fans does not significantly affect project costs.

(xxi) **Regularly repair air distribution system duct insulation.** Over time, maintenance and repair activities typically damage duct insulation. Repairing damaged insulation will reduce air distribution system heat gains and losses.

(xxii) **Install master/slave programming for rooms served by multiple heating and cooling equipment units to prevent simultaneous heating and cooling.** When multiple heating and cooling units (fan coil units, air terminals, unit heaters, etc.) serve a single room, the equipment is commonly regulated using multiple independent thermostats, which can lead to simultaneous heating and cooling. Depending on the thermostat setpoints, one air terminal may be in cooling mode and one in heating mode at the same time. To prevent this, a master/slave arrangement (one of the thermostats is the "master" and all other thermostats are "slaves") should be used to control all heating and cooling units serving a single room. Most energy management systems can be easily programmed for master-slave control of multiple air terminals serving a single room.

(xxiii) **Use variable volume kitchen hood exhaust systems.** Many kitchen hoods are of the constant volume type, which operates the hood exhaust fan and makeup air unit continuously at constant speed. New sensing technology now makes it possible to automatically vary exhaust airflow in response to the amount of cooking activity under the hood. Variable volume kitchen hood exhaust systems reduce fan, cooling, and heating energy consumption. A typical variable volume kitchen hood exhaust system is illustrated in Figure 6-41.

(xxiv) **Pressure test rooms that require a positive or negative pressure differential.** Airflow offsets (differences between supply and return/exhaust airflows) are used to create desired pressure differences in patient care areas in order to promote infection control. Operating rooms and similar areas are

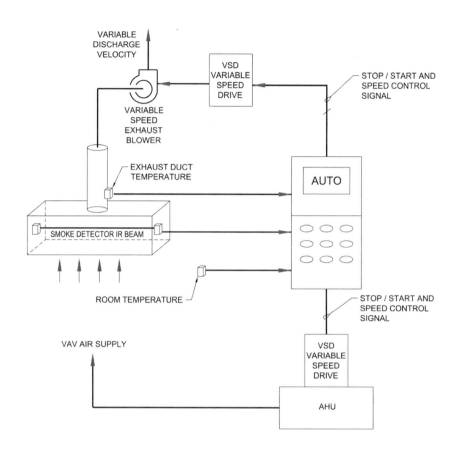

VARIABLE
DISCHARGE
VELOCITY

VSD
VARIABLE
SPEED
DRIVE

STOP / START AND
SPEED CONTROL
SIGNAL

VARIABLE
SPEED
EXHAUST
BLOWER

EXHAUST DUCT
TEMPERATURE

AUTO

SMOKE DETECTOR IR BEAM

ROOM TEMPERATURE

STOP / START AND
SPEED CONTROL
SIGNAL

VAV AIR SUPPLY

VSD
VARIABLE
SPEED
DRIVE

AHU

Figure 6-41: Variable Volume Kitchen Hood

maintained with a positive pressure relationship to adjacent spaces. AII rooms and other similar spaces are maintained at a negative pressure relationship to adjacent spaces. The amount of airflow offset required to create a pressure difference is a function of the effective leakage area of the space. Minimizing the airflow offset by minimizing the effective leakage area reduces fan energy requirements. To ensure optimum equipment performance, all areas requiring a positive or negative pressure relationship should be pressure tested.

(xxv) **Balance the exhaust system so it provides the correct total amount of exhaust air.** Health facility exhaust fan airflows are often significantly higher than the sum of the design exhaust air requirements for the individual air devices (grilles and registers). Excess exhaust is typically caused by a combination of exhaust duct leakage and improper exhaust system balancing. Excess exhaust increases the amount of outside air required to maintain building pressure. This situation can be remedied by installing variable frequency drives at the exhaust fans (or replacing their fan sheaves) and reducing the fan speeds to obtain the correct total exhaust airflow. The exhaust system is then rebalanced to ensure that each air device has the proper flow. In some cases, sections of the exhaust ducts may have to be sealed to reduce leakage.

(f) **Plumbing.** In a typical health care facility, water and sewer consumption accounts for 2 to 5 percent of total energy costs. Possible demand-side energy cost reduction measures for health facility plumbing systems include, but are not limited to, the following:

   (i) **Use variable volume domestic hot water recirculation systems.** Most domestic hot water recirculation systems are constant volume. Variable volume systems use variable speed return pumps and automatic control valves to regulate domestic hot water return flows. Each control valve is modulated to maintain the associated domestic hot water return temperature at setpoint. Variable volume systems also greatly expedite identification and resolution of domestic hot water return problems, which are common in health care facilities due to the complexity and size of their hot water systems. Domestic hot water return problems often frustrate O&M staff as they are difficult to resolve.

   (ii) **Reduce medical vacuum pump cutout settings.** The airflow capacity of a medical vacuum pump varies with the vacuum level. At higher vacuum levels, the pump capacity is greatly diminished. Higher vacuum levels also increase system leaks. Consequently, a reduction in medical vacuum pump cutout settings reduces pump run times and associated electrical consumption.

   (iii) **Reduce medical air compressor cutout settings.** The airflow capacity of a medical air compressor varies with the pressure level. At higher pressures, the compressor capacity is greatly diminished. Higher pressures also increase system leaks. Consequently, a reduction in compressor cutout settings reduces compressor run times and associated electrical consumption.

   (iv) **Use condensing water heaters rather than standard ones.** Condensing water heaters are more efficient than standard water heaters.

(v) **Consider use of solar water heaters.** Solar water heaters can reduce purchased energy requirements.

(vi) **Use low-flow plumbing fixtures.** Low-flow faucets, shower heads, water closets, and urinals reduce water consumption.

(vii) **Use electronic flush valves and faucets.** Electronic flush valves and faucets reduce water consumption.

(g) **Automatic temperature controls.** The design, installation, maintenance, and operation of an automatic temperature control system can significantly affect the energy costs of a health care facility. It should also be noted that a well-designed, installed, and maintained automatic temperature control system can accomplish many of the potential energy cost reduction measures described above, including supply air temperature reset, chilled water temperature reset, tower water supply temperature reset, optimal dispatch of equipment, differential pressure reset, static pressure reset, night setback/setup, unoccupied/occupied air change rates, and so on. Possible demand-side energy cost reduction measures for health facility automatic temperature control systems include, but are not limited to, the following:

(i) **Tune control loops.** Control valves, dampers, pump speeds, and fan speeds are typically controlled by automatic temperature control systems using proportional-integral (PI) control loops. In theory, a PI control loop provides stable control with no offset from setpoint. The PI control loop output has both a proportional component based on deviation from setpoint and an integral component based on the period in which the deviation occurred. Under steady-state conditions (i.e., stable loads and setpoints), the integral component eliminates any deviation from setpoint. Proper setup of a PI control loop, however, requires adjustment of the proportional and integral gains, which should initially be "tuned" by the control system installer.

Tuning typically requires review of a close interval trend showing the output, setpoint, and controlled variable (supply air temperature, supply air static pressure, chilled water differential pressure, etc.) followed by an adjustment of the proportional and integral gains. The proportional gain is the ratio of the change in control loop output to the difference between the controlled variable and the setpoint (commonly referred to as the "error term"). Increasing the proportional gain will increase the control system's initial response to a deviation from setpoint. The integral gain is the ratio of the change in control loop output to the cumulative (integral) error term over time. Increasing the integral gain will increase the speed of the control system's response to a sustained deviation from setpoint.

In most cases, the tuning process must be repeated several times to obtain stable control. In the real world, though, proportional and integral values are rarely tuned. The result is that many valve, damper, fan speed, and pump speed control systems are either "hunting" (continuously undershooting and overshooting the setpoint on a cyclical basis) or not controlling precisely to the setpoint, commonly referred to as "offset." From a distance, these systems seem to be working because they often do not trigger occupant complaints. On closer inspection, however, they are wasting energy and reducing the life of control components. Several control system manufacturers have developed self-tuning software programs that automatically adjust the proportional and integral gain setpoints for a specific application. These programs are relatively new, however, and their functionality has not been sufficiently tested.

The stability gained by tuning a control loop is illustrated in Figure 6-42.

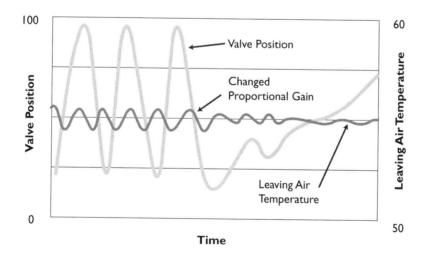

Figure 6-42: Control Loop Tuning

(ii) **Use weekly scheduling to shut off equipment and systems serving unoccupied spaces.** Automatic temperature control systems connected to a central energy management system with an operator workstation typically include a function referred to as "weekly scheduling." The weekly schedules automatically shut off equipment such as air-handling units and air terminals during unoccupied periods. Weekly schedules are most commonly used for equipment and systems serving administrative areas with no regular night or weekend occupancy. Weekly schedules can also be used to change setpoints and other control parameters during unoccupied periods (e.g., night setback/setup of space temperature setpoints).

(iii) **Institute automated metering and cost allocation.** Many larger health care facilities have recently implemented automated metering and cost allocation (AMCA) systems. These systems allocate the cost of owning, operating, and maintaining district energy systems to the various buildings and departments using cost-of-service-based rates with customer charge, demand, and commodity components in a manner similar to that of a regulated utility. In some cases, the district energy systems serve commercial, retail, and residential customers not associated with the health care facility. The AMCA system can reduce the costs of the health care organization by allocating the fixed costs associated with the district energy system (e.g., the cost of capital, depreciation, maintenance, and insurance) over a larger rate base. An AMCA system combined with a decentralized utility budget (allocating utility costs to each department, building, or area) also provides significant incentive for energy savings by placing financial responsibility for the energy costs directly in the hands of the energy user. A schematic diagram of a typical AMCA system is provided in Figure 6-43.

(iv) **Properly sequence air terminal damper and reheat control valves.** With variable volume hydronic reheat systems, the heating water control valve should be modulated open before the airflow is increased from the minimum heating setpoint to the maximum heating setpoint. This procedure minimizes airflow, fan energy, and reheat (simultaneous heating and cooling).

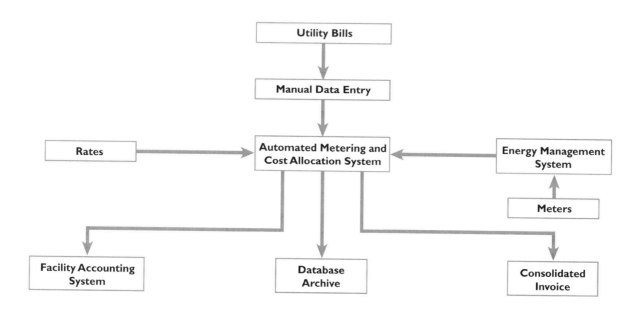

Figure 6-43: Automated Metering and Cost Allocation System

(v) **Use a single loop to control AHU supply air temperature.**
To the extent possible, air-handling unit supply air
temperatures should be controlled by a single PI loop with
table statements for each controlled device. The single-loop
method of control eliminates the possibility of an inadvertent
overlap of heating and cooling. The single-loop control
method for supply air temperature control is illustrated in
Figure 6-44.

(vi) **Set fan coil unit controls to the lowest possible fan speed.**
Most fan coils have multiple fan speed capability. However,
fan coils with multiple speeds should be operated at the
lowest possible fan speed to minimize fan energy and provide
better humidity control. The recommended sequence of
operation for fan coil units is illustrated in Figure 6-45.

(vii) **Employ a demand limiting program to shut down non-
essential electrical loads during peak hours.** When the
cost of electrical demand represents a significant portion of
the overall electricity rate, a demand limiting program can
achieve significant cost savings. A demand limiting program
shuts down non-essential loads during periods of peak use as

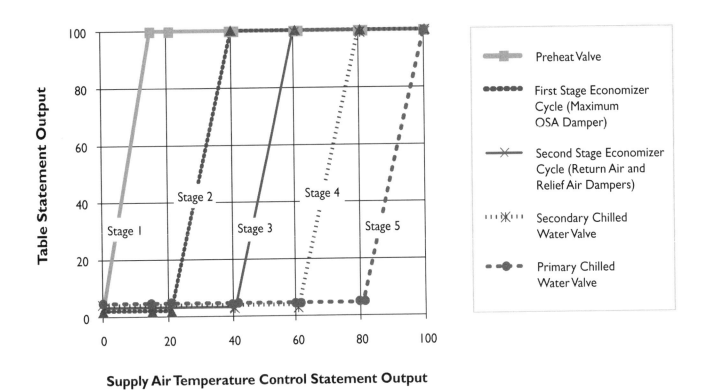

Figure 6-44: Single-Loop AHU Temperature Control

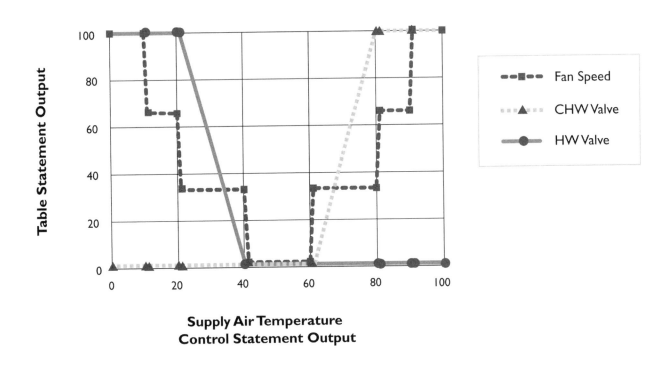

Figure 6-45: Fan Coil Unit Sequence of Operation

required to prevent the electrical demand from exceeding a threshold value.

(viii) **Reduce airflow settings:** Perhaps the most significant energy cost reduction measure for many health care facilities is to assure that HVAC system airflow settings are correct. The minimum settings should be as low as possible to minimize simultaneous cooling and heating. Eight airflow settings should be verified:

1. Occupied—minimum cooling

2. Occupied—maximum cooling

3. Occupied—minimum heating

4. Occupied—maximum heating

5. Unoccupied—minimum cooling

6. Unoccupied—maximum cooling

7. Unoccupied—minimum heating

8. Unoccupied—maximum heating

A diagram indicating the proper airflow settings for an occupied patient care HVAC zone appears in Figure 6-46.

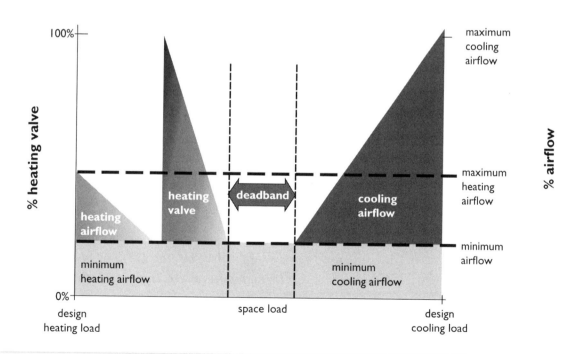

Figure 6-46: Energy-Efficient Air Terminal Operation

(h) **Electrical.** In a typical health care facility, electrical distribution losses account for less than 1.5 percent of total energy costs. Possible demand-side energy cost reduction measures for health facility electrical systems include, but are not limited to, the following:

   (i) **Specify and install low-impedance transformers.** Specifying and installing lower impedance transformers (those with less than a 5 percent voltage drop when supplying at full current of an electrical load) will reduce transformation losses and electricity consumption.

   (ii) **Specify and install 277-volt lighting.** Specifying and installing 277-volt lighting instead of 120-volt lighting reduces both transformation and distribution electrical losses.

   (iii) **Use a PV grid to generate electricity on-site.** A photovoltaic (PV) grid is a system of solar panels and transmission equipment that uses sunlight to generate electricity. Major advances in PV technology have made it possible to use PV grids to provide a significant portion of the electricity a health care facility consumes.

   (iv) **Consider using a combined heating and power (CHP) system.** Depending on natural gas and electricity rates, combined heating and power systems (also known as cogeneration) that generate both power and thermal energy from a single fuel can yield significant energy cost savings. The relative difference between the cost of electricity and the cost of natural gas (commonly referred to as the "spark spread"), and the stability of the difference over time, is the single most important factor in determining the economic viability of a combined heating and power system.

(i) **Building envelope.** In a typical health care facility, approximately 40 percent of the total cooling load and 50 percent of the total heating load are due to heat gain and heat loss through the building envelope. The other portion of the cooling load is due to ventilation, fan heat gain, duct heat gain, piping heat gain, and internal loads (from lights, people, equipment, etc.). The other portion of the heating load is due to ventilation, steam losses, steam piping heat losses, boiler radiation and convection losses, and boiler combustion losses. Sources of envelope heat gain include infiltration, water vapor transfer, solar heat gain through windows, and heat transfer by conduction through the walls, windows, and roof. Sources of envelope heat loss include infiltration, water vapor transfer, and heat transfer by conduction through walls, windows, and roof. Possible demand-side energy cost reduction measures for the health facility building envelope include, but are not limited to, the following:

(i) **High-efficiency glazing:** The windows in many health care facilities have a single pane. The replacement of older windows with new insulated windows equipped with shading features can dramatically reduce heating and cooling loads. Better windows also improve patient and staff comfort. A comparison of the performance of various window types is provided in Table 6-8.

Type	U-Value	Solar Heat Gain Coefficient
Single-pane—Clear	1.02	0.80
Single-pane—Tinted	1.02	0.62
Double-pane—Clear	0.48	0.70
Double-pane—Low E	0.48	0.36
Triple-pane—Clear	0.30	0.60
Triple-pane—Low E	0.30	0.31

Table 6-8: Comparison of Window Performance

The heat transfer characteristics of a high-performance window are illustrated in Figure 6-47. U-value is a measure of heat transmission (SHGC) through a building part. The solar heat gain coefficient is the fraction of heat from the sun that enters through a window. Visible transmittance (VT) is the percentage of visible light transmitted.

(ii) **Increase wall insulation.** Adding additional insulation to walls can reduce heating and cooling loads.

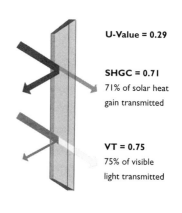

U-Value = 0.29

SHGC = 0.71
71% of solar heat gain transmitted

VT = 0.75
75% of visible light transmitted

Figure 6-47: High-Performance Window

(iii) **Increase roof insulation.** Adding additional insulation to roofs can reduce heating and cooling loads.

(iv) **Assess the need for vapor barriers and the quality and location of existing vapor barriers.** Properly located vapor barriers are needed to prevent condensation within the exterior building envelope. In hot and humid climates, the vapor barrier is typically located on the exterior side of the insulation. In cold climates where the building is humidified, the vapor barrier is typically located on the interior side of the insulation. A less than adequate vapor barrier or an improperly located vapor barrier can allow condensation to form within the wall, and the resulting mold and mildew can cause catastrophic damage. A vapor barrier analysis plots temperature and dewpoint throughout the wall from the interior surface (point 0) to the exterior surface. If the temperature decreases below the dewpoint at any point in the wall (indicating the potential for condensation), the vapor barrier is either inadequate or improperly located. Figure 6-48 shows a vapor barrier analysis for a 12-inch thick wall

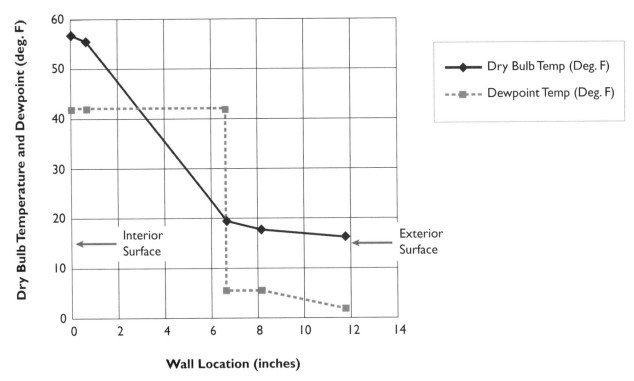

Figure 6-48: Vapor Barrier Analysis

in a cold climate under winter conditions that indicates an improper vapor barrier location.

(14) Discuss supply-side and demand-side energy cost reduction opportunities with the facility manager. Develop a long-range plan to implement changes proposed to reduce energy expenditures and costs.

(a) The RTL should meet with the health facility O&M staff. The meeting agenda should cover the following topics:

  (i) **Baseline Energy Star rating:** The RTL discusses the baseline rating for the health care facility and its underlying assumptions (floor area, type of facility, number of beds, etc.).

  (ii) **Primary and intermediate goals:** The RTL discusses the primary goal (target Energy Star rating) and the intermediate goals (e.g., E2C awards). The primary and intermediate goals must be significant, attainable, positively stated, timely (to inspire a sense of urgency), measurable, and most importantly, accepted by all parties.

  (iii) **Construction drawings and specifications review:** The RTL discusses the conclusions from the review of construction documents and specifications, including performance improvement opportunities.

  (iv) **Submittal document and maintenance manual review:** The RTL discusses the conclusions from the review of submittal documents and maintenance manuals, including performance improvement opportunities.

  (v) **TAB report review:** The RTL discusses the conclusions from the review of TAB reports, including performance improvement opportunities.

  (vi) **Control diagram review:** The RTL discusses the conclusions from the review of control diagrams, including performance improvement opportunities.

  (vii) **Facility survey:** The RTL discusses the conclusions from the facility survey, including performance improvement opportunities.

  (viii) **Control system review:** The RTL discusses the conclusions from the review of the automatic temperature control system, including performance improvement opportunities.

  (ix) **Supply-side energy cost reduction opportunities:** The RTL provides a list of potential supply-side energy cost reduction measures. The list indicates the estimated cost, projected savings, and simple payback for each measure. The RTL and the O&M staff review the list and identify the most cost-effective measures.

(x) **Demand-side energy cost reduction opportunities:** The RTL provides a list of potential demand-side energy cost reduction measures. The list indicates the estimated cost, projected savings, and simple payback for each measure. The RTL and the O&M staff review the list and identify the most cost-effective measures.

(xi) **Available labor:** The RTL and the O&M staff discuss and determine the O&M staff labor that can be used to implement selected performance improvement measures. The discussion addresses the current skills and knowledge level of these individuals and the amount of additional training that may be required.

(xii) **Sources of capital:** The RTL and the O&M staff discuss potential sources of capital for implementing the energy cost reduction measures, including external funding and future utility and deferred maintenance budgets. In many health care facilities, external funding must be obtained through a specific capital budget process (in other words, discretionary capital is not available). In these facilities, funding for energy conservation and related infrastructure projects must compete for funding with medical equipment upgrades, physician recruitment, and expansion projects that are directly aligned with the health care facility's core mission. When external capital is not available, the RTL should investigate and evaluate other potential funding sources, including utility energy efficiency programs, performance contracts, and shared savings contracts.

(b) After the meeting, the RTL and the O&M staff collaboratively develop a long-range plan (typically five to 10 years) for implementing the selected supply-side and demand-side energy cost reduction measures. The plan is structured to meet the primary and intermediate goals and must be achievable within the limitations of available labor and capital. For the reasons previously cited, the O&M staff should implement the bulk of the work. To the extent possible, the plan should be "self-funded" from future annual utility and deferred maintenance budgets. Improvements with the shortest payback measures should be implemented first. The accumulated savings from these measures can then be reinvested in projects with longer payback periods. Self-funded plans typically require external funding (funding in excess of the annual deferred maintenance and utility budgets) during the first few years only; this funding is commonly referred to as "seed capital." An example of a self-funded plan is illustrated in Figure 6-49 and Figure 6-50.

Work Category	Project	Cost ($)	Savings ($/year)	Duration (days)	Start Date	Stop Date
	Program Grand Total	10,842,000	1,936,500	2404	1-Jul-10	29-Jan-17
Retrocommissioning	Ward Tower	182,000	53,000	274	1-Jul-10	1-Apr-11
	ACRC	176,000	46,000	274	2-Apr-11	1-Jan-12
	Biomedical Research Center 1	183,000	110,000	274	2-Jan-12	3-Oct-12
	Biomedical Research Center 2	169,000	108,000	274	4-Oct-12	5-Jul-13
	JTSNSI	181,000	51,000	274	6-Jul-13	7-Apr-14
	IOA	88,000	27,500	157	8-Apr-14	11-Sep-14
	OPC/OPDC	72,000	24,500	157	12-Sep-14	16-Feb-15
	Barton	80,000	38,500	157	17-Feb-15	24-Jul-15
	JEI	70,000	24,500	157	25-Jul-15	29-Dec-15
DDC Retrofit and Network Upgrade	Main Plant, JTSNSI Plant, and IOA Plants	194,000	108,000	798	1-Jul-10	6-Sep-12
	Shorey	495,000	82,500	729	1-Jul-10	29-Jun-12
	Physical Plant	310,000	82,500	477	30-Jun-12	20-Oct-13
	Central Building	760,000	82,500	813	21-Oct-13	13-Jan-16
	Upgrade Networks and Workstations	995,000	0	381	14-Jan-16	29-Jan-17
Lighting Retrofit	Campus Lighting Audit	100,000	0	120	1-Jul-10	16-Dec-10
	IOA	20,000	5,000	40	16-Dec-10	10-Feb-11
	JTSNSI	20,000	5,000	40	10-Feb-11	7-Apr-11
	BRC I	205,000	60,000	180	7-Apr-11	15-Dec-11
	BRC II	20,000	5,000	40	15-Dec-11	9-Feb-12
	Barton	100,000	31,000	90	9-Feb-12	14-Jun-12
	Main Plant	20,000	4,000	40	14-Jun-12	9-Aug-12
	Physical Plant	120,000	34,000	40	9-Aug-12	4-Oct-12
	Central Building	450,00	125,000	180	4-Oct-12	13-Jun-13
	ACRC	250,000	68,000	150	13-Jun-13	9-Jan-14
	OPC/OPDC	100,000	26,000	40	9-Jan-14	6-Mar-14
	JEI	100,000	26,000	40	6-Mar-14	1-May-14
	COPH	25,000	7,000	40	1-May-14	26-Jun-14
	ED II	350,000	88,000	120	26-Jun-14	11-Dec-14
	Shorey	200,000	54,000	120	11-Dec-14	28-May-15
	Ward	50,000	13,000	40	28-May-15	23-Jul-15
	CHRP	50,000	13,000	40	23-Jul-15	17-Sep-15
District Energy and HVAC Retrofits	PXH at WCEP	413,000	59,000	210	1-Jul-11	20-Apr-12
	Connect Distribution to WCEP	285,000	35,000	210	20-Apr-12	8-Feb-13
	ACRC, JTSNSI, Family Medical, and IOA	1,109,000	155,000	400	8-Feb-13	22-Aug-14
	ED II HVAC Retrofit	2,900,000	285,000	400	22-Aug-14	4-Mar-16

Figure 6-49: Sample Self-Funded Long-Range Plan

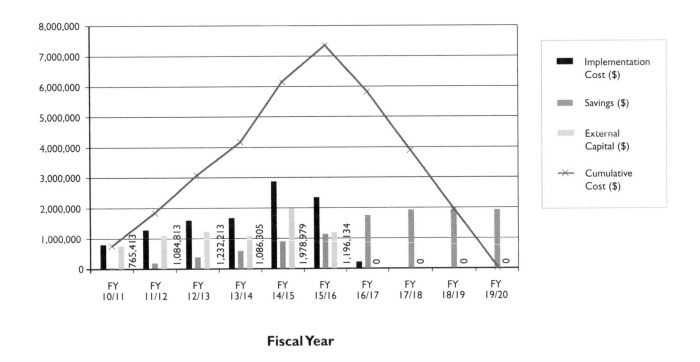

Figure 6-50: External Funding Requirements for Sample Long-Range Plan

As indicated in Figure 6-49, the sample self-funded plan requires seed capital only for six years. After 10 years, when all projects have been implemented, all of the seed capital has been returned and the health care facility is saving nearly $2 million per year in annual utility costs. The results are sustainable because O&M staff have been trained in proper operation as a result of their involvement in project implementation.

For a self-funded plan to be viable, health care facilities must set future utility budgets according to current energy use intensity and future utility rates. When utility costs go down because of declining energy use intensity, annual utility budgets must remain at current levels (adjusted only for utility rate escalation and new construction) to provide the funding needed to implement additional energy cost reduction measures. The RTL must be certain the health facility C-suite understand this concept and have accepted it.

(15) Develop a scorecard to track and record actual energy cost savings (i.e., progress toward reaching the energy cost reduction target).

Progress toward intermediate and primary energy cost reduction goals should be tracked monthly. An Energy Star scorecard is

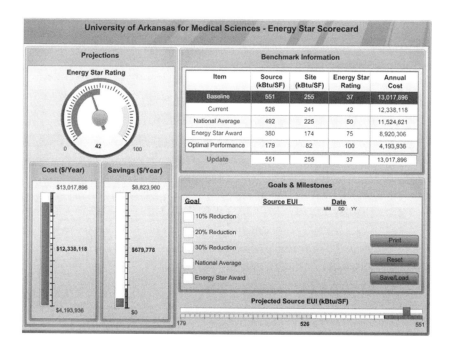

Figure 6-51: Sample Energy Star Scorecard

particularly useful for this purpose. The sample Energy Star scorecard shown in Figure 6-51 indicates the baseline rating, current rating, current energy cost savings, target energy cost savings, and progress toward the facility's intermediate and primary goals. The current energy cost savings should be the actual energy cost savings resulting from the facility's energy conservation program. The actual savings are the sum of the supply-side and demand-side cost savings. The supply-side savings are equal to the savings realized by changes in utility rates or procurement. The demand-side savings are calculated by multiplying any reductions in billing determinants (customer charges, demand, consumption, etc.) by the current rate. Calculating the savings in this manner ensures the reported savings are accurate and credible. The O&M staff should update the Energy Star scorecard each month and display it in a prominent location. Using LCD flat screens connected to the facility energy management system to display the most current version of the Energy Star scorecard is a recommended practice. The screens should be installed in prominent locations such as the main facility lobby and the O&M shop.

The retrocommissioning team should use the scorecard to publicize the retrocommissioning program and maintain facility awareness, focus, and vigilance. The O&M staff should use the scorecard to forecast energy consumption and costs in future years (utility budgeting) and predict monthly natural gas consumption for hedging purposes (nominations and balancing).

(16) Conduct detailed testing of water chillers, cooling towers, chilled water pumps, and tower water pumps. Measure and record pressures, temperatures, flows, and power consumption.

(a) The recommended test procedures for an air-cooled water chiller are listed below:

(i) Measure and record the chilled water pump strainer water pressure drop. If the pressure drop is more than expected (e.g., 3 psig), remove and clean the strainer. Measure and record the water pressure drop after the strainer has been cleaned.

(ii) Verify that the chilled water pump is operating at 100 percent speed (if controlled by a variable frequency drive).

(iii) Measure and record the condenser ambient temperature.

(iv) Measure and record the water chiller discharge, condensing, evaporator, and suction refrigerant temperatures and pressures.

(v) Measure and record the volts, amps, kVA, and kW for each compressor motor. Compare the results to nameplate data.

(vi) Measure and record the volts, amps, kVA, and kW for each condenser fan motor. Compare the results to nameplate data.

(vii) Measure and record the evaporator water pressure drop. Compare the results to the manufacturer's design pressure drop.

(viii) Calculate the apparent evaporator flow rate in GPM using the formula below:

$$CEF = DEF \times (MEWPD/DEWPD)^{1/2}$$

where:

CEF = Calculated evaporator flow rate

DEF = Design evaporator flow rate

MEWPD = Measured evaporator water pressure drop in feet w.g.

DEWPD = Design evaporator water pressure drop in feet w.g.

(ix) Turn off the water chiller, and then close a valve at the discharge of the chilled water pump. Measure and record pump suction and discharge pressures.

(x) Calculate the pump shutoff head using the formula below. The pump shutoff head is the maximum head generated by a centrifugal pump.

CSH = (MSDP – MSSP) x 2.31

where:

CSH = Calculated shutoff head in feet w.g.

MSDP = Measured shutoff discharge pressure in psig

MSSP = Measured shutoff suction pressure in psig

(xi) Compare the calculated pump shutoff head to the design pump shutoff head as indicated on the pump performance curve supplied by the manufacturer. Verify that the pump impeller is the correct size and is working properly. A typical pump performance curve indicating the shutoff head is illustrated in Figure 6-52. The figure shows the pump shutoff head for an 8-in. diameter impeller is 250 feet w.g.

(xii) Open the valve and the discharge of the chilled water pump, and measure and record the pump suction and discharge water pressures.

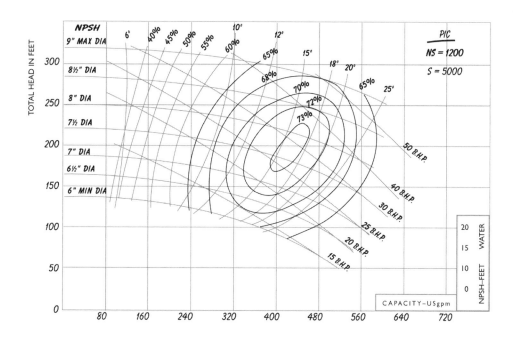

Figure 6-52: Typical Pump Performance Curve

(xiii) Measure and record the chilled water pump balancing valve water pressure drop.

(xiv) Measure and record the pump motor volts, amps, kW, and kVA. Compare results to nameplate data.

(xv) Calculate the pump total dynamic head using the formula below. The pump total dynamic head is the total pressure drop through the piping system expressed in feet of water.

CTDH = (MODP – MOSP) x 2.31

where:

CTDH = Calculated total dynamic head in feet w.g.

MODP = Measured operating discharge pressure in psig

MOSP = Measured operating suction pressure in psig

(xvi) Determine the apparent chilled water flow rate using the pump performance curve. Use of the performance curve to determine the flow rate is illustrated in Figure 6-53. As

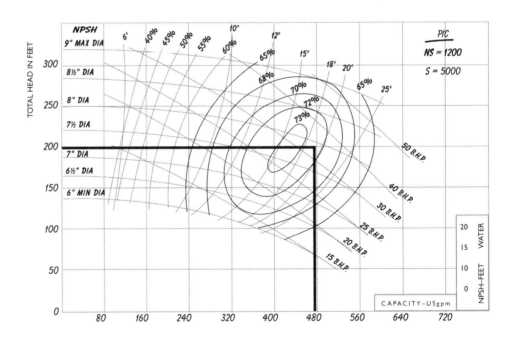

Figure 6-53: Using a Performance Curve to Determine Flow Rate

indicated in the figure, the flow rate corresponding to a CTDH of 200 feet w.g. with an 8-in. impeller is 460 GPM.

(xvii) Compare the measured evaporator flow rate calculated using the evaporator water pressure drop to the evaporator flow rate determined using the pump performance curve. The measured flows should be approximately equal (within 5 percent). If the flows are not approximately equal, the evaporator may be obstructed or the pump may not be functioning properly.

(xviii) Measure and record the evaporator entering and leaving water temperatures.

(xix) Calculate the water chiller cooling production using the formula below:

$$CCP = (EEWT - ELWT) \times CEF / 24$$

where:

CCP = Calculated chiller production in tons

EEWT = Evaporator entering water temperature in °F

ELWT = Evaporator leaving water temperature in °F

CEF = Calculated evaporator flow rate in GPM

(xx) Calculate the water chiller efficacy using the formula below:

$$CCE = Power/CCP$$

where:

CCE = Calculated chiller efficacy in kW/ton

Power = Chiller electrical power consumption in kW

CCP = Calculated chiller production in tons

(xxi) Compare the calculated chiller efficacy to the design efficacy. The calculated efficacy should be approximately the same as the design efficacy (or lower if the ambient temperature at the time of the testing is significantly lower than the design ambient temperature).

(xxii) Calculate the evaporator approach temperature difference using the formula listed below:

$$CEATD = ELWT - ERT$$

where:

CEATD = Calculated evaporator approach temperature difference in °F

ELWT = Evaporator leaving water temperature in °F

ERT = Evaporator refrigerant temperature in °F

(xxiii) Design evaporator approach temperatures are typically in the range of 1 to 3° F, with newer chillers typically at the lower end of the range and older chillers typically at the higher end of the range. Approach temperature differences are theoretically proportional to load. Compare the design evaporator approach temperature difference—adjusted according to the measured chiller production—to the measured evaporator approach temperature difference. If the measured approach temperature difference is significantly greater than the adjusted design approach temperature difference, the evaporator heat transfer surfaces may be fouled, the expansion device may not be working properly, or the refrigerant charge may be incorrect.

(b) The recommended test procedures for a water-cooled water chiller are listed below:

   (i) Measure and record the chilled and tower water pump strainer water pressure drops. If a pressure drop is more than expected, remove and clean the strainer. Measure and record the water pressure drop after the clean strainer is in place.

   (ii) Verify that the chilled water pump and tower water pump are operating at 100 percent speed (if a pump is controlled by a variable frequency drive).

   (iii) Measure and record the water chiller discharge, condensing, evaporator, and suction refrigerant temperatures and pressures.

   (iv) Measure and record the volts, amps, kVA, and kW for each compressor motor. Compare the results to nameplate data.

   (v) Measure and record the evaporator and condenser water pressure drops. Compare measured evaporator and condenser water pressure drops to the manufacturer's design pressure drops.

(vi) Calculate the apparent evaporator and condenser flow rates using the formula provided below:

$$CEF = DEF \times (MEWPD/DEWPD)^{1/2}$$

where:

CEF = Calculated evaporator flow rate

DEF = Design evaporator flow rate

MEWPD = Measured evaporator water pressure drop in feet w.g.

DEWPD = Design evaporator water pressure drop in feet w.g.

$$CCF = DCF \times (MCWPD/DCWPD)^{1/2}$$

where:

CEF = Calculated condenser flow rate

DEF = Design condenser flow rate

MEWPD = Measured condenser water pressure drop in feet w.g.

DEWPD = Design condenser water pressure drop in feet w.g.

(vii) Turn off the water chiller. Close a valve at the discharge of the chilled water and tower water pumps. Measure and record pump suction and discharge pressures.

(viii) Calculate the pump shutoff heads using the following formula:

$$CSH = (MSDP - MSSP) \times 2.31$$

where:

CSH = Calculated shutoff head in feet w.g.

MSDP = Measured shutoff discharge pressure in psig

MSSP = Measured shutoff suction pressure in psig

(ix) Compare the measured pump shutoff heads to the design pump shutoff heads indicated on the pump performance curve supplied by the manufacturer. Verify that the pump impellers are the correct size and are working properly.

(x) Open the valve and the discharge of the chilled water pump and tower water pump and measure and record the pump suction and discharge water pressures.

(xi) Measure and record the chilled water pump and tower water pump balancing valve water pressure drops.

(xii) Measure and record the chilled water pump and tower water pump motor volts, amps, kW, and kVA. Compare the results to nameplate data.

(xiii) Calculate the chilled water pump and tower water pump total dynamic heads using the following formula:

CTDH = (MODP – MOSP) x 2.31

where:

CTDH = Calculated total dynamic head in feet w.g.

MODP = Measured operating discharge pressure in psig

MOSP = Measured operating suction pressure in psig

(xiv) Determine the apparent chilled water and tower water flow rates using the pump performance curves.

(xv) Compare the measured evaporator and condenser flow rates calculated using the water pressure drop to the flow rates determined using the pump performance curves. The measured flows should be approximately equal (within 5 percent). If they are not, the heat transfer surface may be obstructed or the pump may not be functioning properly.

(xvi) Measure and record the evaporator and condenser entering and leaving water temperatures.

(xvii) Calculate the water chiller cooling production using the following formula:

CCP = (EEWT – ELWT) x CEF /24

where:

CCP = Calculated chiller production in tons

EEWT = Evaporator entering water temperature in °F

ELWT = Evaporator leaving water temperature in °F

CEF = Calculated evaporator flow rate in GPM

(xviii) Calculate the condenser heat transfer using the formula below:

CHT = CCF x (CLWT − CEWT) x 500

where:

CHT = Condenser heat transfer in BTUH

CCF = Calculated condenser flow rate in GPM

CLWT = Condenser leaving water temperature in deg. F

CEWT = Condenser entering water temperature in deg. F

(xix) Calculate the heat balance using the formula below. The heat balance should be in the range of 0.9 to 1.1. If the heat balance is not within this range, one or more of the measurements is incorrect.

$$HB = \frac{(CCP \times 12{,}000) + (Power \times 3413)}{(CHT/100)}$$

where:

HB = Heat balance in percent

CCP = Calculated chiller production in tons

Power = Chiller electrical power consumption in kW

CHT = Condenser heat transfer in BTUH

(xx) Calculate the water chiller efficacy using the following formula:

CCE = Power/CCP

where:

CCE = Calculated chiller efficacy in kW/ton

Power = Chiller electrical power consumption in kW

CCP = Calculated chiller production in tons

(xxi) Compare the calculated chiller efficacy to the design efficacy. The calculated efficacy should be approximately the same as the design chiller efficacy (or lower if the condenser leaving water temperature at the time of the testing is significantly lower than the design condenser leaving water temperature).

(xxii) Calculate the evaporator approach temperature difference using the following formula:

$$CEATD = ELWT - ERT$$

where:

CEATD = Calculated evaporator approach temperature difference in °F

ELWT = Evaporator leaving water temperature in °F

ERT = Evaporator refrigerant temperature in °F

(xxiii) Calculate the condenser approach temperature difference using the formula below:

$$CCATD = CLWT - CRT$$

where:

CCATD = Calculated condenser approach temperature difference in °F

CLWT = Condenser leaving water temperature in °F

CRT = Condenser refrigerant temperature in °F

(xxiv) Design evaporator and condenser approach temperatures are typically in the range of 1 to 3 °F, but newer chillers are typically at the lower end of the range and older chillers are typically at the higher end. Approach temperature differences are theoretically proportional to load. Compare the design evaporator and condenser approach temperature differences—adjusted according to the measured chiller production—to the measured evaporator and condenser approach temperature differences. If a measured approach temperature difference is significantly greater than the adjusted design approach temperature difference, the heat transfer surfaces may be fouled or the refrigerant charge may be incorrect. A high evaporator approach temperature difference could also be caused by a malfunctioning thermal expansion device. If the water chiller uses a negative pressure refrigerant (CFC-11 or HCFC-123), a high condenser approach temperature could also be caused by the presence of non-condensibles in the condenser (i.e., the purge equipment is malfunctioning).

(c) The recommended test procedures for a cooling tower are listed below:

(i) Verify that the cooling tower bypass valve (if present) is fully closed (so that all water flows over the cooling tower).

(ii) Observe and document the position of the cooling tower flow balancing valves.

(iii) Observe and record the cooling tower water level.

(iv) Measure and record the ambient wet bulb temperature.

(v) Measure and record the cooling tower entering and leaving water temperatures.

(vi) Measure and record the volts, amps, kVA, and kW for each tower fan motor, and compare the results to nameplate data.

Sample water chiller, cooling tower, and pump test forms are included in Appendix 6-2.

(17) Conduct detailed testing of boilers and heating water pumps. Measure and record pressures, temperatures, flows, and power consumption.

(a) The recommended test procedures for a heating water boiler are listed below:

(i) Measure and record the heating water pump strainer water pressure drop. If the pressure drop is more than expected (e.g., 3 psig), remove and clean the strainer. Measure and record water pressure drop again once the clean strainer is in place.

(ii) Verify that the heating water pump is operating at 100 percent speed (if controlled by a variable frequency drive).

(iii) Measure and record the outside air temperature.

(iv) Measure and record the boiler fuel consumption (e.g., consumption of electricity, natural gas, propane, fuel oil).

(v) Measure and record the boiler combustion efficiency. Boiler combustion efficiency is the calculated efficiency of the combustion process at steady-state conditions. It is stated as the ratio of the actual amount of usable heat gained by the combustion process to the theoretical fuel heating value under ideal conditions (when the exact amount of combustion air required to completely react with the fuel—commonly referred to as stoichiometric combustion air—is present and the stack temperature is no warmer than the incoming combustion air). The theoretical fuel heating value used in the calculation is the "high heating value," which assumes the water vapor in the stack is in the liquid state. In practice, combustion conditions are never ideal, and additional or "excess" air is needed to assure complete combustion. Boiler combustion efficiency is directly affected by the amount of excess combustion air being used and the boiler stack temperature. It should be noted that boiler combustion efficiency does not demonstrate the fuel-to-usable heat efficiency of the system as it does not consider other losses, such as blowdown losses and radiation/convection heat losses from exterior boiler surfaces and piping. Boiler combustion efficiency is typically determined using a boiler combustion efficiency analyzer that measures the stack oxygen content (used to determine the amount of excess air) and the stack temperature.

(vi) Measure and record the boiler water pressure drop.

(vii) Compare the measured boiler water pressure drop to manufacturer's design pressure drop. Calculate the apparent boiler flow rate in GPM using the formula below:

$$MBF = DBF \times (MBWPD/DBWPD)^{1/2}$$

where:

MBF = Measured boiler flow rate

DBF = Design boiler flow rate

MBWPD = Measured boiler water pressure drop in feet w.g.

DBWPD = Design boiler water pressure drop in feet w.g.

(viii) Turn off the boiler. Close a valve at the discharge of the heating water pump. Measure and record pump suction and discharge pressures.

(ix) Calculate the pump shutoff head using the formula below:

$$MSH = (MSDP - MSSP) \times 2.31$$

where:

MSH = Measured shutoff head in feet w.g.

MSDP = Measured shutoff discharge pressure in psig

MSSP = Measured shutoff suction pressure in psig

(x) Compare the measured pump shutoff head to the design pump shutoff head indicated on the pump performance curve supplied by the manufacturer. Verify that the pump impeller is the correct size and working properly.

(xi) Open the valve and the discharge of the heating water pump and measure and record the pump suction and discharge water pressures.

(xii) Measure and record the heating water pump balancing valve water pressure drop.

(xiii) Measure and record the pump motor volts, amps, kW, and kVA, and compare the results to nameplate data.

(xiv) Calculate the pump total dynamic head using the formula below:

> CTDH = (MODP – MOSP) x 2.31
>
> where:
>
> CTDH = Calculated total dynamic head in feet w.g.
>
> MODP = Measured operating discharge pressure in psig
>
> MOSP = Measured operating suction pressure in psig

(xv) Determine the apparent boiler flow rate using the pump performance curve.

(xvi) Compare the measured boiler flow rate calculated using the boiler water pressure drop to the boiler flow rate determined using the pump performance curve. Both flows should be approximately equal (within 5 percent). If the flows are not approximately equal, the boiler may be obstructed or the pump may not be functioning properly.

(xvii) Measure and record the boiler entering and leaving water temperatures.

(xviii) Calculate the boiler heating production using the formula below:

> CBP = (BEWT – BLWT) x MBF x 0.5
>
> where:
>
> CBP = Calculated boiler production in MBH (1,000 Btu/hour)
>
> BEWT = Boiler entering water temperature in °F
>
> BLWT = Boiler leaving water temperature in °F
>
> MBF = Measured boiler flow rate in GPM

(xix) Calculate the boiler efficiency using the formula below:

> CBE = CBP/Fuel
>
> where:
>
> CBE = Calculated boiler efficiency (%)

CBP = Calculated boiler production in MBH

Fuel = Boiler fuel consumption in MBH

(xx) Compare the measured boiler efficiency to the design efficiency. The measured efficiency should be approximately the same as the design efficiency.

(b) The recommended test procedures for a steam boiler are listed below:

(i) Measure and record the outside air temperature.

(ii) Measure and record the boiler feedwater temperature.

(iii) Measure and record the boiler makeup water temperature.

(iv) Determine the boiler makeup water and blowdown flow rates using the chemical treatment reports.

(v) Measure and record the boiler steam pressure.

(vi) Measure and record the boiler stack temperature.

(vii) Measure and record the boiler fuel consumption (consumption of electricity, natural gas, propane, fuel oil).

(viii) Calculate the boiler efficiency using the formula below:

$$CBE = \frac{[SF \times (SF - FWE)]/1000}{Fuel}$$

where:

CBE = Calculated boiler efficiency (%)

SF = Steam flow in lbs./hour

SE = Steam enthalpy in Btu/lb.

FWE = Feedwater enthalpy in Btu/lb.

Fuel = Fuel input in Btu/hour

Sample heating water boiler and steam boiler test forms are included in Appendix 6-3.

(ix) Compare the measured boiler efficiency to the design efficiency. The measured efficiency should be approximately the same as the design efficiency.

(18) Conduct detailed testing of each large air-handling unit. Measure and record outside airflow, return airflow, and supply airflow. Measure and record static pressure drops in each section. Measure and record dry bulb and wet bulb temperatures in each section. Measure and record fan speeds, fan motor currents, and fan motor electrical demand.

The recommended test procedures for a large air-handling unit are listed below:

(a) Observe and record all control damper positions.

(b) Observe and record all control valve positions.

(c) Measure and record the static pressure in the main supply and return air ducts on each floor.

(d) Observe and record supply and return (if applicable) fan speeds.

(e) Measure and record the water pressure drop through heating water and chilled water coils in the air-handling unit. Determine the apparent flow rate using the design flow and design water pressure drop using the following formula:

$$MF = DF \times (MWPD/DWPD)^{1/2}$$

where:

MF = Measured flow rate

DF = Design flow rate

MWPD = Measured water pressure drop in feet w.g.

DWPD = Design water pressure drop in feet w.g.

(f) Measure and record the air pressure drop across filters, dampers, and coils.

(g) Measure and record outside air, return air, mixed air, preheat, cooling coil, and supply air dry bulb temperature and relative humidity.

(h) Measure and record the supply fan suction and discharge pressures.

(i) Measure and record the supply fan RPM.

(j) Measure and record the supply fan motor, volts, amps, kW, and kVA.

(k) Measure and record the return fan suction and discharge pressures.

(l) Measure and record the return fan RPM.

(m) Measure and record the return fan motor, volts, amps, kW, and kVA.

(n) Determine the apparent supply fan and return fan airflow rates using fan performance curves supplied by the AHU manufacturer.

(o) Compare measured values to submittal data, and identify discrepancies.

(19) Conduct detailed testing of each large exhaust fan. Measure and record airflow, fan static pressure, fan speed, fan motor current, and fan motor electrical demand.

The recommended test procedures for an exhaust fan are listed below:

(a) Measure exhaust airflow rates at each exhaust air inlet. Compare measured flow to the design flow.

(b) Measure and record exhaust duct static pressures in main exhaust ducts on each floor served by the exhaust fan, creating a static pressure profile for each exhaust system.

(c) Measure and record exhaust fan motor volts, amps, kW, and kVA.

(d) Measure and record the fan RPM.

(e) Measure and record fan suction and discharge pressures.

(f) Measure and record the exhaust airflow using a duct traverse.

(g) Determine the apparent exhaust airflow rate using the exhaust fan performance curve supplied by the manufacturer.

A sample exhaust fan test form is included in Appendix 6-4.

(h) Compare the measured exhaust fan airflow rate, sum of exhaust grille flow rates, and the exhaust airflow rate indicated by the fan performance curve to the design exhaust flow rate.

(20) Compare actual equipment performance to the manufacturers' rated performance data. Identify and document discrepancies.

After completing the equipment testing, the retrocommissioning team compares all the test results to the design conditions indicated on the submittal documents. The team identifies and documents discrepancies (e.g., diminished capacity or lower efficiency) and discusses them with the O&M staff. The team and the O&M staff plan and implement corrective actions.

(21) Establish and review trends for key equipment operating parameters.

Trends are either the change of value (COV) or the timed interval type. COV trends record data each time the measured value changes more than a designated amount or the control point status changes (e.g., from on to off). Timed interval trends record data at pre-established intervals (e.g., 1 minute, 15 minutes, etc.). The number of trends in use at the same time depends on the data storage capacity of the energy management system. COV trends generally require less data storage than timed interval trends. In some cases, the retrocommissioning team may need to upgrade the EMS or install a BACnet commissioning tool to increase trend capability and capacity. The team uses trend data to analyze the system sequence of operations, identify energy savings opportunities, troubleshoot the system, and assess system or building energy performance.

(a) The retrocommissioning team establishes and reviews trends for the following equipment and systems:

  (i) **Water chillers.** Recommended trends include entering and leaving evaporator and condenser water temperatures, evaporator flow or water pressure drop, condenser flow or water pressure drop, electrical power, evaporator refrigerant pressure, and condenser refrigerant pressure.

  (ii) **Cooling towers.** Recommended trends include entering water temperature, leaving water temperature, outside air temperature, outside air relative humidity, tower bypass valve position, tower fan status, and tower fan speed.

  (iii) **Steam boilers.** Recommended trends include feedwater temperature, feedwater flow rate, makeup water temperature, makeup water flow rate, steam pressure, steam flow rate, fuel consumption, and stack temperature.

  (iv) **Heating water boilers.** Recommended trends include entering and leaving water temperature, stack temperature, boiler heating water flow rate, and fuel consumption.

  (v) **Pumps.** Recommended trends include flow rate, suction pressure, discharge pressure, pump status, pump speed, differential pressure, and differential pressure setpoint.

  (vi) **Air-handling units.** Recommended trends include return fan speed, return fan status, supply fan speed, supply fan status, damper positions, valve positions, outside airflow rate, filter pressure drop, return air temperature, mixed air temperature, preheat temperature, cooling coil discharge temperature, supply air temperature, and supply air static pressure.

  (vii) **Air terminals.** Recommended trends include space temperature, thermostat setpoint, space temperature setpoint, terminal damper position, heating valve position, airflow rate, airflow setpoint, discharge air temperature, mode of operation (occupied or unoccupied), and discharge air temperature.

(b) The team uses these trends for troubleshooting, tuning control loops (this requires a timed interval trend with an interval of 15 to 30 seconds), and measuring and verifying results. Trends can also be used for energy submetering. Instantaneous chilled water, heating water, steam, domestic water, and electrical demands for each building are stored at 15- to 30-minute intervals in a spreadsheet and then totaled to determine consumption.

Sample trends for a double-duct air-handling unit (Figure 6-54), a chilled water pump (Figure 6-55), boiler steam

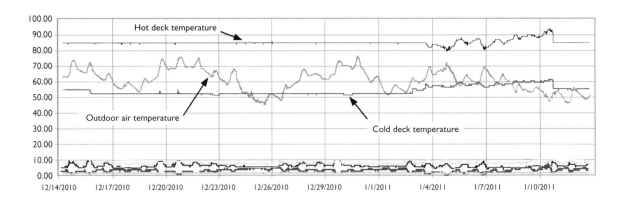

Figure 6-54: Sample Double-Duct Air-Handling Unit Trend

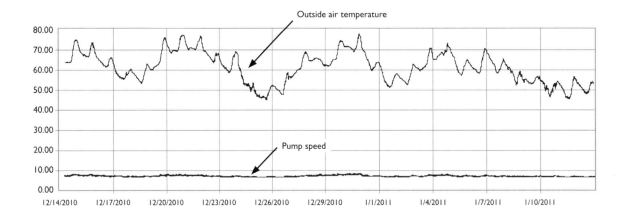

Figure 6-55: Sample Chilled Water Pump Trend

consumption and steam pressure (Figure 6-56), and boiler efficiency and steam pressure (Figure 6-57) are illustrated.

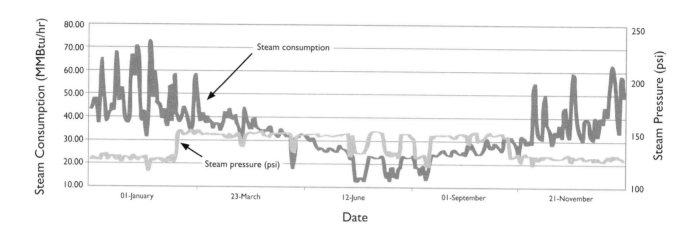

Figure 6-56: Sample Boiler Steam Consumption and Steam Pressure Trend

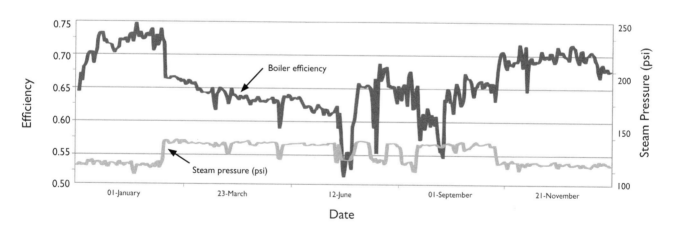

The chart indicates that boiler efficiency declines as steam pressure increases. Consequently, an effective retrocommissioning strategy would be to reduce steam pressure to the extent possible.

Figure 6-57: Sample Boiler Steam Pressure and Efficiency Trend

(22) Develop a detailed room ventilation schedule for the facility. The schedule should identify floor area, ceiling height, room volume, outdoor air change requirement, total air change requirement, pressure relationships, existing airflow setpoints, and proposed airflow setpoints.

The retrocommissioning team uses a spreadsheet to prepare the room ventilation schedule (RVS), including data for all rooms in the facility. The RVS calculates airflow requirements based on room function, occupancy, floor area, ceiling height, room volume, outdoor air change requirement, total air change requirement, pressure relationship, exhaust air requirement, space sensible cooling load, space heating load, and other factors in accordance with applicable regulations.

The team obtains the room names and floor areas from the most recent and accurate floor plans. If the plans are available in electronic drawing format, the floor areas can be calculated using the program's area command. In some cases, the room names on the plans may not match one of the space types listed in the applicable regulations. Room names also may be inconsistent with how rooms are currently being used. The retrocommissioning team reviews these discrepancies with the O&M staff and verifies that the space type indicated for each room in the RVS is an accurate indication of its current function.

The team obtains the room outdoor air change, total air change, and pressure relationship requirements from applicable state and local codes. In most cases, the applicable code is either the FGI *Guidelines for Design and Construction of Health Care Facilities* or ASHRAE Standard 170 (incorporated into the 2010 edition of the *Guidelines*). The desired pressure relationships are created by airflow offsets (differences between the amount of air supplied to the room and the amount of air exhausted or returned from the room). The offset required to create the desired pressure relationship is dependent on the room effective leakage area. In rooms with positive or undefined pressure relationships, the total air change requirement governs the supply airflow requirement. In rooms with negative pressure relationships, the total air change requirement governs the exhaust airflow requirements.

The completed RVS identifies the supply, return, and exhaust airflow requirements for each room under each of the following conditions:

1. Occupied—minimum cooling
2. Occupied—maximum cooling
3. Occupied—minimum heating

4. Occupied—maximum heating

5. Unoccupied—minimum cooling

6. Unoccupied—maximum cooling

7. Unoccupied—minimum heating

8. Unoccupied—maximum heating

The RVS also identifies the air-handling unit and exhaust fan (if applicable) serving each space. The RVS should include a summary page that identifies the supply, return, and minimum outside air (ventilation) airflow requirements for each air-handling unit as well as the exhaust airflow requirement for each exhaust fan. The summary page should also indicate the total facility supply, return, and exhaust airflow requirements.

A sample room ventilation schedule is included in Appendix 6-5.

(23) Develop weekly occupied/unoccupied or on/off schedules for air-handling units and other equipment.

It is a common misconception that all health facility equipment and systems must operate continuously. In reality, a significant amount of equipment can be turned off during unoccupied periods. The only air-handling units that can never be turned off are those serving areas that are continuously occupied or have mandatory pressure relationships. Lighting systems serving intermittently occupied areas can also be turned off during unoccupied periods. The retrocommissioning team develops and implements weekly schedules based on the expected occupancy start and stop times.

(24) Develop revised air-handling unit sequences of operation and setpoints for optimum energy efficiency (supply air temperature control, humidity control, economizer cycles, damper sequencing, supply air temperature setpoint reset, and supply air static pressure setpoint reset).

Many different types of air-handling unit systems are used in health care facilities, including double-duct variable air volume (DDVAV), single-duct variable air volume (SDVAV), multi-zone (MZ), and single zone (SZ) systems. The optimum sequence of operation for a specific air-handling unit depends on the type of unit and its specific configuration. The retrocommissioning team develops and implements energy-efficient strategies for each air-handling unit. Commonly used strategies are described in this section.

(a) **Air-side economizer cycle.** Air-side economizer cycles are designed to eliminate mechanical cooling during cold weather. A typical air-side economizer cycle is illustrated in Figure 6-58.

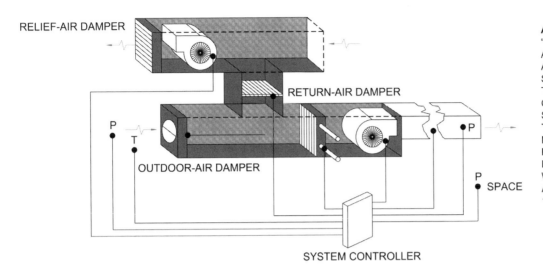

RELIEF-AIR DAMPER

RETURN-AIR DAMPER

P

T

OUTDOOR-AIR DAMPER

P

P SPACE

SYSTEM CONTROLLER

AIRSIDE ECONOMIZER: "A DUCT AND DAMPER ARRANGEMENT AND AUTOMATIC CONTROL SYSTEM THAT, TOGETHER, ALLOW A COOLING SYSTEM TO SUPPLY OUTDOOR AIR TO REDUCE OR ELIMINATE THE NEED FOR MECHANICAL COOLING DIURING MILD OR COLD WEATHER." (FROM ASHRAE STANDARD 90. 1-2004, SECTION 3)

Figure 6-58: Typical Air-Side Economizer Cycle

Economizer cycles are typically enabled and disabled based on dry bulb temperature or enthalpy (total heat content of moist air). Dry bulb economizers are activated when the outdoor air dry bulb temperature is less than the return air dry bulb temperature (for the standard dry bulb type) or when the outdoor air temperature is less than a fixed setpoint (for the differential dry bulb type). Enthalpy economizers are activated when the outdoor air enthalpy is less than the return air enthalpy (for the standard enthalpy type) or when the outdoor air enthalpy is less than a fixed setpoint (for the differential enthalpy type). Economizer cycle controls are termed "integrated" if economizer cycle operation and mechanical cooling can occur simultaneously. If mechanical cooling is locked out when the economizer cycle is enabled, the controls are termed "non-integrated." Enthalpy economizers theoretically yield more energy savings than other economizer types, but they are generally less reliable due to complexity and humidity sensor issues.

Several methods of improving economizer cycle operation are listed here:

+ If a dry-bulb economizer cycle is used, tailor the outdoor air dry bulb temperature enable-and-disable setpoints to the climate. In dry climates, these setpoints should be 60 and 65°F, respectively. In more humid climates, they should be 55 and 60°F, respectively.

• Disable economizer cycles in hot and humid climates (e.g., Miami, Houston, etc.).

• Disable economizer cycles in single-fan double-duct systems (because the heating energy penalty offsets the cooling savings).

• Install accurate and reliable temperature and humidity sensors (enthalpy economizers only).

(b) **Double-duct variable air volume systems.** DDVAV systems, which simultaneously deliver both heated and cooled air to the air terminals, are commonly used in health care facilities. Their advantages include exceptional thermal comfort and reduced risk of a water leak above clinical areas. Their disadvantages include limited dehumidification capability (the hot deck airflow is not dehumidified), reduced benefit from an air-side economizer cycle (cold deck cooling savings are offset by increased hot deck heating requirements), increased potential for wet final filters (either from cooling coil water carryover or condensation), and the need for two sets of final filters. The air-side economizer cycle and dehumidification disadvantages can be avoided by using a two-fan DDVAV system, in which separate supply fans are used for the hot and cold decks. The duct configuration in this type of system prevents outside air from entering the hot deck. DDVAV systems are also generally less efficient than other systems due to an increased potential for simultaneous heating and cooling (mixing of heated and cooled air). A schematic diagram for a typical DDVAV system appears in Figure 6-59.

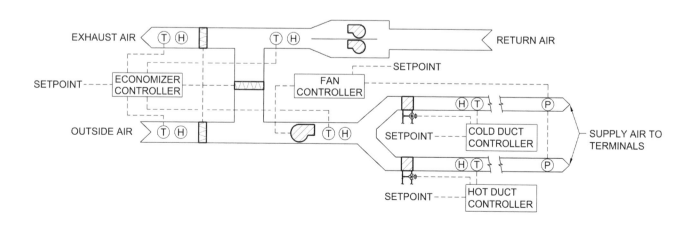

Figure 6-59: Typical DDVAV System

Potential energy-conserving sequence modifications can be applied to DDVAV systems. These include separate hot deck and cold deck static pressure control loops and setpoints, static pressure setpoint reset, hot deck temperature setpoint reset, and cold deck temperature setpoint reset.

Supply air static pressure should be controlled using separate proportional-integral control loops and setpoints for the hot and cold decks. The EMS control output to the variable frequency drive should be equal to the higher of the hot and cold deck control loops. The hot and cold deck static pressure setpoints should be automatically reset according to terminal damper position, outdoor air temperature, and/or occupancy schedule. The most efficient reset method is based on terminal damper position. A proportional-integral control loop resets the hot deck static pressure setpoint between reasonable limits that are based on the most open hot deck terminal damper position and a target maximum hot deck terminal damper position setpoint (e.g., 95 percent). A separate proportional-integral control loop resets the cold deck static pressure setpoint between reasonable limits that are based on the most open cold deck damper position and a target maximum cold deck damper position setpoint (e.g., 95 percent). The upper and lower limits are established during the TAB process (e.g., 0.5 to 1.5 inches w.g.).

The hot deck and cold deck temperature setpoints should be automatically reset according to terminal heating and cooling requirements, outdoor air temperature, and/or occupancy schedule. The most efficient setpoint reset method is based on terminal heating and cooling requirements. A proportional-integral control loop resets the hot deck temperature setpoint between reasonable limits that are based on the highest terminal heating requirement (heating loopout) and a target maximum terminal heating requirement (e.g., 95 percent). A separate proportional-integral control loop resets the cold deck temperature setpoint between reasonable limits that are based on the highest terminal cooling requirement (cooling loopout) and a target maximum terminal cooling requirement (e.g., 95 percent). The upper and lower limits for each loop are based on the design heating and cooling conditions.

Resetting the hot and cold deck temperature setpoints according to the outdoor air temperature is less complex and easier for O&M staff to understand. As a result, it may provide more sustainable results. A sample hot deck and cold deck temperature setpoint reset schedule based on outdoor air temperature (OAT) is illustrated below:

Cold deck setpoint: 6° F if OAT <= 50° F, 55° F if OAT >= 90° F and reset between 61° F and 55° F if OAT is between 50° F and 90° F

Hot deck setpoint: 90° F if OAT <= 50° F, 75° F if OAT >= 78°F, and reset between 90° F and 75° F if OAT is between 50° F and 90° F

The cold deck supply air temperature setpoint reset strategy should include a maximum return air (or space) humidity limit override. A reverse-acting proportional-integral control loop (a loop in which output decreases when input increases) generates an output between the upper and lower cold deck temperature setpoint limits based on the return air humidity level and a maximum return air humidity setpoint (e.g., 60% RH). The cold deck temperature setpoint is equal to the lower of the setpoint reset and humidity override control loop outputs.

(c) **Single-duct variable air volume systems.** SDVAV systems, which deliver only cooled air to the air terminals for reheating by terminal heating water coils, are also commonly used in health care facilities. The advantages of these systems include exceptional thermal comfort and less ductwork. Their major disadvantage is increased risk of a water leak above clinical areas. A schematic diagram for a typical SDVAV system appears in Figure 6-60.

Potential energy-conserving sequence modifications for SDVAV systems include supply air static pressure setpoint reset, humidifier economizer cycle override, optimum outside air and return air damper sequencing, single control loop for supply air temperature control, and supply air temperature setpoint reset.

When an air-side economizer cycle is used in a system that requires humidification, the first stage of humidification should be to automatically disable the economizer cycle (otherwise the cooling savings are more than offset by higher humidification costs).

The outside air and return air dampers should be modulated in sequence (the outside air damper fully opens before the return air damper begins to close) based on the cooling requirement when the economizer cycle is enabled and based on the minimum

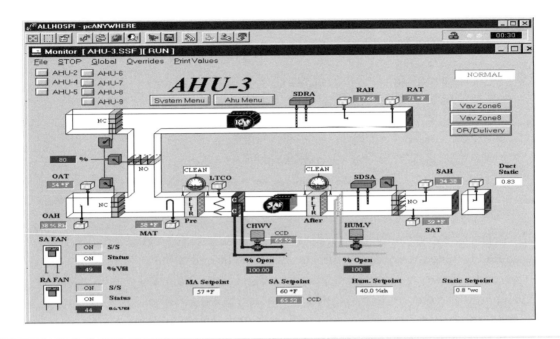

Figure 6-60: Typical SDVAV System

outdoor air requirement when the economizer cycle is disabled. Damper sequencing in this manner reduces the combined damper pressure drop, which reduces fan energy requirements. This method of damper sequencing also minimizes the potential for backward airflow through the relief damper, which can occur with air-side economizer cycles.

Heating and cooling equipment (e.g., preheat control valve, economizer dampers, and chilled water control valve) should be controlled by a single proportional-integral control loop with individual table statements for each device. The table statements are structured to prevent heating and cooling functions from overlapping. A sample set of table statements is provided below:

> **Preheat control valve:** Normally open valve modulates closed when control loop output increases from 0 to 25 percent.

> **Outside air damper:** Normally closed damper modulates open when economizer cycle is enabled and control loop output increases from 25 to 50 percent.

> **Return air damper:** Normally open damper modulates closed when economizer cycle is enabled and control loop output increases from 51 to 75 percent.

Chilled water control valve: Normally closed valve modulates open when control loop output increases from 76 to 100 percent.

The supply air temperature setpoints should be automatically reset according to terminal cooling requirements, outdoor air temperature, and/or occupancy schedule. The most efficient setpoint reset method is based on terminal cooling requirements. A separate proportional-integral control loop resets the supply air temperature setpoint between reasonable limits that are based on the highest terminal cooling requirement (cooling loopout) and a target maximum terminal cooling requirement (e.g., 95 percent). The upper and lower setpoint limits are based on the design heating and cooling conditions.

Resetting the supply air temperature setpoint according to the outdoor air temperature is less complex and easier for O&M staff to understand. As a result, it may provide more sustainable results. A sample supply air temperature setpoint reset schedule based on outdoor air temperature (OAT) is illustrated below:

Supply air setpoint: 61° F if OAT <= 50° F, 55° F if OAT >= 90° F and reset between 61° F and 55° F if OAT is between 50° F and 90° F

The supply air temperature setpoint reset strategy should include a maximum return air (or space) humidity override as previously described.

(d) **Multi-zone (MZ) systems.** MZ systems, which are similar to double-duct systems, are rarely used in health care facilities. The principal difference between MZ and double-duct systems is that the mixing dampers in an MZ system (referred to as "zone dampers") are located at the air-handling unit; there are no air terminals. MZ systems have the same inherent advantages and disadvantages as double-duct systems. Potential energy-conserving sequence strategies for MZ systems are the same as those previously indicated for double-duct systems.

The MZ zone dampers should be controlled in a manner that minimizes mixing. This can be accomplished by removing a section of the damper actuator rod between the hot deck and cold deck zone dampers and installing separate hot deck and cold deck damper actuators. The normally open hot deck zone dampers are controlled by direct-acting proportional-integral control loops according to the zone temperatures and the zone heating setpoints. The normally closed cold deck zone dampers are controlled by direct-acting proportional-integral control loops according to the zone temperatures and the zone cooling setpoints. The zone heating and cooling setpoints are separated by a reasonable deadband.

(e) **Single-zone (SZ) systems.** Single-zone systems include small air-handling units and fan coil units that sequence heating and cooling functions to maintain room temperature. Some SZ systems are also equipped for dehumidification (this requires the heating coil to be downstream of the cooling coil). Potential energy-conserving sequence modifications for SZ systems include converting to variable volume using a variable frequency drive, converting to variable volume using a multi-speed fan motor, and increasing the deadband between the heating and cooling functions.

(25) Establish revised air-handling unit outside airflow setpoints.

The RVS indicates minimum outside airflow setpoints for each air-handling unit. The air-handling unit minimum outside airflow setpoints should be determined using the individual space ventilation requirements indicated in ASHRAE Standard 170 and system efficiency factors calculated using the multiple space formula found in Appendix A of ASHRAE Standard 62.1-2010. The minimum outside airflow quantity must sufficiently offset the total exhaust (to maintain the desired building pressure at the entry level) and must also satisfy the minimum outside air change requirements for each room served. In taller buildings, where building pressure is more difficult to maintain, AHU minimum outdoor air quantities are automatically reset according to the building pressure relationship. The retrocommissioning team adjusts the minimum outdoor airflow settings on each air-handling unit to match the new setpoints.

(26) Establish revised exhaust fan airflow requirements.

The retrocommissioning team rebalances the health facility exhaust systems to match the quantities indicated on the RVS. The team also verifies that the exhaust fan airflows are equal to the sum of the room exhausts plus a reasonable allowance for duct leakage. If there is a significant discrepancy between the sum of the room exhausts and the fan exhaust airflow (indicating excessive leakage), the retrocommissioning team and the O&M staff work to identify and repair the leaks. Eliminating unnecessary exhaust is an important key to optimum building performance.

(27) Establish revised chilled water and heating water system sequences of operation for optimum energy efficiency (temperature setpoint reset, differential pressure setpoint reset, pump speed control and sequencing, etc.).

The retrocommissioning team implements selected modifications to the chilled water and heating water systems and conducts functional performance testing to assure the modifications work as intended. Potential energy-conserving sequence modifications for chilled water systems include conversions to variable primary operation, conversions to low-flow/high delta T operation, chilled water temperature setpoint reset, chilled water differential pressure reset, tower water temperature setpoint reset, use of hydronic free cooling, use of variable speed tower fans, most efficient pump sequencing, and optimal dispatch of chillers and cooling towers.

(28) Establish weekly occupied/unoccupied or on/off schedules for air terminals and fan coil units. Establish unoccupied heating and cooling setpoints.

The retrocommissioning team implements weekly schedules for air terminals and fan coil units serving intermittently occupied areas. An air terminal weekly schedule automatically changes the airflow setpoints and the thermostat heating and cooling setpoints based on day of the week and time of day. A fan coil unit weekly schedule automatically turns the unit on and off and adjusts heating and cooling setpoints based on day and time. Pushbuttons located at the thermostat allow occupants to override the weekly schedule to accommodate an unscheduled occupancy. When an override pushbutton is pressed, the equipment operates in the occupied mode for a preset period (typically 1 to 4 hours).

(29) Establish revised air terminal sequences of operation for optimum energy efficiency.

The retrocommissioning team implements selected modifications to the air terminal sequences of operation and conducts functional performance testing to assure the modifications work as intended. Potential energy-conserving sequence modifications for air terminals include use of weekly schedules, night setback/setup, unoccupied/occupied airflow settings, and minimum and maximum thermostat setpoints; reduced minimum airflow setpoints where allowed; and increased deadbands.

(30) Establish revised fan coil unit sequences of operation for optimum energy efficiency.

The retrocommissioning team implements selected modifications to the fan coil unit sequences of operation and conducts functional performance testing to assure the modifications work as intended. Potential energy-conserving sequence modifications for fan coil units include reduced fan speed; increased deadbands; and use of weekly schedules, night setback/setup, and minimum and maximum thermostat setpoints.

Reducing the fan speed during cooling operation will reduce the discharge air temperature and yield a lower room relative humidity. The reduction in relative humidity allows a 1 to 4° F increase in space temperature without diminishing occupant comfort. A reduction in relative humidity also reduces the potential for mold and mildew growth.

(31) Establish revised terminal airflow setpoints (eight settings).

The retrocommissioning team adjusts the terminal airflow setpoints (8 settings as described in the *Health Facility Commissioning Guidelines*) to the quantities indicated on the RVS. The team also verifies that each air terminal has the correct setup parameters (i.e., terminal size, calibration constant, etc.) and is programmed for automatic and regular calibration.

(32) Establish minimum and maximum limits for thermostat setpoints.

The EMS can restrict occupant thermostat control to a reasonable range for the room function. The EMS can also override the thermostat during unoccupied periods by establishing a lower heating setpoint (night setback) and a higher cooling setpoint (night setup).

The retrocommissioning team adjusts the occupied minimum and maximum limits for air terminal and fan coil unit thermostats. The limits permit occupant control of environmental conditions within a reasonable range of temperatures. The team should set the limits according to occupant comfort and criteria established by ASHRAE Standard 170.

Occupant comfort is determined by a number of factors, including room temperature, room surface temperature, clothing level, activity level, and relative humidity. The average of the room temperature and the room surface temperature (average of the wall, glass, and ceiling temperatures) is commonly referred to as the operative temperature. Summer and winter comfort zones as a function of operative temperature and dewpoint temperature are illustrated in Figure 6-61.

As indicated in the figure, occupant comfort requires a controlled dewpoint temperature (or relative humidity) between upper and lower limits. As a result, the HVAC system should be equipped

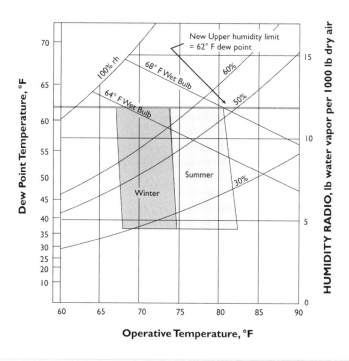

Figure 6-61: Occupant Comfort Zone

with dehumidification and humidification capability. Variable volume reheat HVAC systems with supply air temperature reset and maximum humidity override are energy efficient and provide inherent dehumidification. Humidification capability can also be provided by installing a humidifier, which should be located immediately upstream of the cooling coil. This location minimizes the potential for water carryover problems (the cooling coil is an effective mist eliminator). The humidifier introduces steam (water vapor) into the air stream. The steam source may be the central steam system (assuming the chemical treatment program is appropriate for this function) or an independent steam generator.

Space relative humidity generally increases with higher outdoor temperatures and drops with lower outdoor temperatures. Dehumidification requires simultaneous heating and cooling, and humidification increases heating fuel and water consumption. Striving for both occupant comfort and minimal operating cost encourages a higher maximum humidity level in the summer and a lower minimum humidity level in the winter.

ASHE has recently worked with ASHRAE to establish new recommendations for humidity levels in patient treatment areas, including operating rooms. Addendum d to ANSI/ASHRAE/ASHE Standard 170-2008: *Ventilation of Health Care Facilities* reduces the lower limit of acceptable humidity levels from 30 to 20 percent. An excerpt from the addendum appears in Figure 6-62.

TABLE 7-1 Design Parameters

Function of Space	Pressure Relationship to Adjacent Areas (n)	Minimum Outdoor ach	Minimum Total ach	All Room Air Exhausted Directly to Outdoors (j)	Air Recirculated by Means of Room Units (a)	RH (k), %	Design Temperature (l), °F/°C
SURGERY AND CRITICAL CARE							
Class B and C operating rooms, (m), (n), (o)	Positive	4	20	N/R	No	~~30~~20–60	68–75/20–24
Operating/surgical cystoscopic rooms, (m), (n), (o)	Positive	4	20	N/R	No	~~30~~20–60	68–75/20–24
Delivery room (Caesarean) (m), (n), (o)	Positive	4	20	N/R	No	~~30~~20–60	68–75/20–24
Treatment room (p)	N/R	2	6	N/R	N/R	~~30~~20–60	70–75/21–24
Trauma room (crisis or shock) (c)	Positive	3	15	N/R	No	~~30~~20–60	70–75/21–24
Laser eye room	Positive	3	15	N/R	No	~~30~~20–60	70–75/21–24
Class A Operating/Procedure room (o), (d)	Positive	3	15	N/R	No	~~30~~20–60	70–75/21–24
DIAGNOSTIC AND TREATMENT							
Gastrointestinal endoscopy procedure room	Positive	2	6	N/R	No	~~30~~20–60	68–73/20–23

Figure 6-62: ANSI/ASHRAE/ASHE Standard 170-2008, Addendum d

The retrocommissioning team also establishes night setback/setup room temperature setpoints for unoccupied periods where applicable. Room occupancy can be established by a weekly schedule, an occupancy sensor, a relay interlocked with the lights, or a simple wall switch or pushbutton. Setback/setup settings are generally not used to regulate temperatures in operating rooms and other critical areas because of infection control issues and concerns about warm-up and cool-down. However, administrative areas and other support areas not typically occupied at night or on weekends are good candidates for night setback and setup. For this strategy to be successful, it must be transparent to the occupants (i.e., the occupants should be unaware that a setback/setup strategy is in effect).

During the energy crunch of the 1970s, automatic temperature control systems were not as robust as current direct digital control (DDC) systems. Energy conservation efforts generally consisted of turning equipment off at designated times. Morning startup times were determined by subtracting the estimated time for warm-up and cool-down from the occupancy start time. Early energy conservation pioneers discovered, however, that actual warm-up and cool-down times vary throughout the year according to outdoor air temperature, sun position, cloud cover, length of time the space has been unoccupied, and building mass. The variance in warm-up and cool-down times and the lag between the outside air temperature and the temperature of the building surfaces and furnishings (commonly referred to as a "thermal flywheel") resulted in occupant discomfort and complaints. Temperatures in some rooms were not within an acceptable range when occupants arrived in the morning. The EMS manufacturers reacted to this situation by developing optimal start/stop programs that could learn from experience and automatically vary the start and stop times as needed to assure room temperatures remained within established limits during occupied periods.

Suggested minimum and maximum thermostat limits for occupied periods and night setback and setup temperature setpoints for typical health facility room functions are provided in Table 6-9.

Room Function	Unoccupied Heating Setpoint (°F)	Occupied Minimum Setpoint (°F)	Occupied Maximum Setpoint (°F)	Unoccupied Cooling Setpoint (°F)
Operating rooms	N/A	62	78	N/A
Cath labs	N/A	65	76	N/A
Recovery rooms	N/A	68	75	N/A
LDRP rooms	65	68	75	75
Radiology	65	68	75	75
Laboratory	65	68	75	75
Patient rooms	62	68	75	78
Waiting rooms	60	68	75	80
Dining room	60	68	75	80
Offices	60	68	75	80
Conference rooms	60	68	75	80
Kitchen	60	70	78	85

Table 6-9: Recommended Room Setpoints

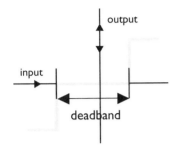

Figure 6-63: Control Loop Deadband

(33) Establish revised deadband settings for space heating and cooling setpoints.

A control loop deadband is a range of inputs for which there is no change in output. An optimum deadband setting takes into account the dynamic nature of space loads, allows reasonable overshooting of the control response, and reduces the potential for simultaneous heating and cooling. The relationship of control system input and output to the deadband setting is illustrated in Figure 6-63.

The retrocommissioning team sets the width of the deadband (deadband setpoint) for each room according to the specific room's function. Rooms housing critical functions (e.g., operating rooms and

Room Function	Recommended Deadband (°F)
Operating rooms	1.0
Cath labs	1.0
Recovery rooms	2.0
LDRP rooms	2.0
Radiology	2.0
Laboratory	2.0
Patient rooms	3.0
Waiting rooms	3.0
Dining room	3.0
Offices	4.0
Conference rooms	4.0
Kitchen	4.0

Table 6-10: Recommended Deadband Settings

intensive care units) require more precise temperature and humidity control than rooms housing less critical functions (e.g., offices and conference rooms). Recommended deadband settings for typical health facility room functions are indicated in Table 6-10.

(34) Document the work in a written report.

The retrocommissioning team documents the methodology, conclusions, recommendations, actions, and results of the retrocommissioning effort in a draft report. The retrocommissioning report includes the following sections:

1. Executive summary

2. Facility description

3. Retrocommissioning team member list

4. Baseline Energy Star rating

5. Target Energy Star rating and intermediate goals

6. Potential energy cost savings

7. Construction documents review

8. Facility survey

9. Control systems review

10. Supply-side energy cost reduction measures

11. Demand-side energy cost reduction measures

12. Retrocommissioning plan

13. Energy scorecard

14. Equipment test results

15. Trend data

16. Room ventilation schedule

17. Weekly schedules for air-handling units, exhaust fans, air terminals, fan coil units, and other equipment

18. Revised air-handling unit sequences of operation and airflow setpoints

19. Exhaust system balancing

20. Revised chilled water system sequences of operation

21. Revised heating water system sequences of operation

22. Revised air terminal sequences of operation and airflow setpoints

23. Revised fan coil unit sequences of operation

24. Revised thermostat setpoints and deadbands

25. Conclusions

26. Recommendations

27. Appendices

Appendices to the report should include floor plans, diagrams, utility rates, calculations, trends, and other documents generated by the retrocommissioning effort.

The RTL reviews the draft report with the O&M staff. The retrocommissioning team then modifies the draft report as needed and issues the final retrocommissioning report.

When the retrocommissioning work has been complete for one year, the retrocommissioning team should issue an addendum to the final report. This should include the following information:

1. Actual energy consumption and costs as compared to target levels

2. Current Energy Star rating

3. Unresolved performance issues

4. Equipment and system test results

5. Equipment and system trend data

6. Recommended changes in O&M procedures

7. Recommended O&M staff training.

6.1.3 Striving for Continuous Commissioning®

Use of an electronic commissioning tool that interfaces with the automatic temperature control system can significantly expedite the retrocommissioning effort. The tool uses a standard communication protocol to query a massive database and quickly identify previously undetected problem areas. After the retrocommissioning effort has been completed, O&M staff can use the tool to continuously identify problems and dispatch maintenance personnel to respond to them. The retrocommissioning effort should encourage the implementation of a continuous commissioning effort that is appropriate for the specific health care facility.

Absent a transition to continuous commissioning in which O&M staff diligently maintain the building systems at maximum efficiency, system performance will slowly degrade from the initial retrocommissioning results back to their original inefficient state. Continuous commissioning requires measurement and verification of actual results (instant feedback on changes in operating conditions), dashboards, and continuous staff training and retraining as previously described in Chapter 4.

6.2 RETROCOMMISSIONING CASE STUDIES

Retrocommissioning health care facilities can significantly reduce annual energy costs. The case studies presented in the *Health Facility Commissioning Guidelines* provide proven and verifiable evidence of the benefits of retrocommissioning. Case studies such as these can help health facility managers demonstrate the benefits of retrocommissioning to the C-suite.

For example, the retrocommissioning of an acute care hospital in Nashville yielded more than $1.2 million in annual energy cost savings and an increase in the facility's Energy Star rating from 36 to 56. The natural gas consumption at this hospital for each day of a typical month before (baseline) and after the retrocommissioning effort is compared in Figure 6-64.

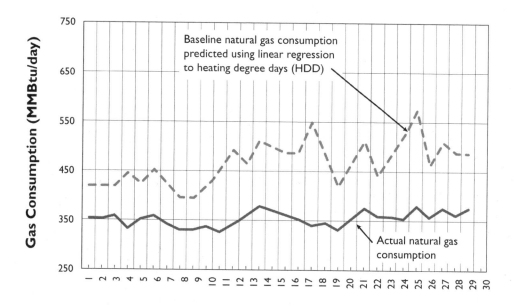

Figure 6-64: Hospital Natural Gas Consumption Before and After Retrocommissioning

APPENDICES

Sample HFCx Business Plan

EXECUTIVE SUMMARY

The Organization proposes to modify the equipment in the Central Energy Plant (CEP) and install an electric heat pump chiller to reduce dependence on natural gas by capturing heat recovered from chilled water production and using it for hydronic heating water production. The use of steam for heating will be replaced with hot water systems fueled from the production of chilled water. The technology for simultaneous production of heating and cooling water has continued to improve since installation of this type of equipment in the West Central Energy Plant (WCEP), and more companies are manufacturing heat pump chillers. These developments have fostered better competition in the marketplace and development of more design options.

The project efficiencies are such that, when properly commissioned, the project will generate $3.2 million in savings that can be directed to support the growth of the Organization's patient care, education, and research missions. The savings will be used to service the debt from bonds sold to pay for the CEP expansion; add 60 beds to the ninth floor of the hospital; remodel the second floor surgery, PACU, and pre-OP space; build out the 26,000 sq. ft. eighth floor in the Cancer Institute; and purchase 6.7 acres for the construction of 600 additional parking spaces as well as allowing 5 percent savings in reserve to manage the growth of future operational expenses.

Assuring the project is properly commissioned will optimize the value derived from developing the West Energy Plant by facilitating achievement of the most benefits at the best project delivery cost. The health facility commissioning authority (HFCxA) will document the value by measurement and verification of the outcomes to assure they meet or exceed the owner's project requirements.

CURRENT PLAN

The eastern portion of the Organization's campus is currently served by the Central Energy Plant (CEP), a traditional plant that incorporates chilled water production for use in cooling and utilizes natural gas to produce steam for heating. The plant serves 15 buildings and a total of 1.8 million square feet of occupied space. The chillers operate on a large general service (LGS) time-of-use rate plan that rewards customers for off-peak demand production, which is not consistent with the hours of operation of the facility. The CEP has equipment that is in various stages of its productive life cycle and does not require total replacement at this time. Various pieces of equipment in production are inefficient and would offer a good return on investment (ROI) if retired early and replaced with newer, high-efficiency equipment. In general, the operations of the plant are sound and do not represent operational risks associated with poor performance and low reliability. Nonetheless, there is a substantial need to upgrade equipment and keep the plant properly capitalized to prolong its useful life.

The Organization's deferred maintenance program has identified equipment in the CEP that is either at or near its useful life or represents a potential ROI with high net present value (NPV) and simple payback of less than seven years. Current funding levels can accommodate only about 60 percent of the projected need for replacement equipment, resulting in a continuing deferred maintenance agenda. To properly fund the replacement activities would require approximately $4 million per year for the next 10 years to control the deferred maintenance account and $2.5 million per year to manage replacements in perpetuity, discounting the future cost of money.

The CEP capacity is constrained and represents limited opportunities to expand services. The buildings served by the plant range from eight to 50 years old and have consistently increased in energy intensity and demand. Heat loading from newer diagnostic and therapeutic equipment; more, higher output computers; and higher density occupancies have created significant demand. The opportunities to meet this demand with current equipment are limited and inefficient because of the CEP design.

In 2006 the Organization began development of the WCEP to provide district power, cooling, and heating water to support the expansion of the campus. The project included participation from the State Hospital and the State Department of Health, which the new plant would serve along with the new properties in the campus expansion. The solutions included installation of an electric heat pump chiller to reduce dependence on natural gas and utilize the heat generated in the production of chilled water to produce hot water for heating. The simultaneous production of heating and cooling water from a single source was intended to dramatically reduce the production cost of the facility. The technology has delivered above expectations and has resulted in savings from the dramatic reduction of natural gas used in the facility.

Operation of the WCEP has resulted in dramatic savings for the district collaborative and the outcome for the Organization has been a carbon impact of almost zero despite the addition of more than a million square feet of new construction. Energy intensity reductions on the campus resulted in reductions in excess of 20 percent, earning an EPA Energy Star of 91 for one new building and the E²C award for the campus as a whole.

The east portion of the campus continues to operate using the older technologies in place prior to development of the WCEP. The Central Energy Plant (CEP) provides chilled water for cooling and steam for heating 15 buildings serving more than 1.8 million square feet of conditioned space.

The success of the WCEP design in generating savings by capturing heating water from the production of chilled water has resulted in significant savings. Chilled water production is required year-round; however, in the winter months much less is required. The full demand for heating water is much less than the demand for chilled water even during the peak heating season. By operating a smaller heat pump chiller in the cooler months, the demand for both cooling water and heating water can be met by capturing the heat created from the production of chilled water.

SWOT ANALYSIS

This analysis spells out the strengths and weaknesses of the current CEP, the opportunities presented if it is replaced, and the economic threats if no action is taken.

Strengths: The CEP has a proven track record of constantly and consistently providing safe and reliable operation. The technicians are competent in their management of the plant and are uniquely qualified to own and operate the equipment. Their track record for uptime in the plant is excellent and with the assistance of the contract engineering team has been able to support the Organization's missions. The CEP supports buildings used for patient care (both inpatient and outpatient), education, research, and administration. Many of these facilities present unique cooling and refrigeration requirements for the preservation of tissue and animals as well as critical patient care. The plant has proven its worth over time and has been the heart of the institution for more than 50 years.

Weaknesses: Much of the equipment in the CEP has been replaced over time as the Organization has worked to continuously upgrade efficiencies and safety. However, the controls process for managing the plant and its monitoring systems is antiquated and outdated. Many of the remote enunciators managed by the monitoring team are equally old and outdated. The control room is now a hodgepodge of system front end computers, remote enunciators, and alarm systems that can easily be misread or misinterpreted by monitoring technicians. Controls and alarms are especially problematic, and constant and diligent attention is required to assure the numerous alarms are sorted through for those that are critical to operations. The fact that the system generates steam for use in occupancy heating creates a critical safety factor and introduces significant maintenance issues to assure the steam traps are working properly. Although these systems are safe, by design they are neither the safest available nor the most cost efficient to operate.

Opportunities: Installing an electric heat pump chiller and running it off the WCEP's electrical grid would provide cost savings because the chiller can be used to generate heat as it produces chilled water. The chiller can be powered from the WCEP electrical distribution grid and generate further savings from the lower rates offered in the OIS rate structure applied to the WCEP. The savings generated could be redirected to service the debt from bonds sold to support $53 million in construction projects that will benefit the Organization's core missions of patient care, education, and research. A 5 percent reserve from the savings can be applied to cover the indirect costs associated with operating the new spaces. The improved efficiency of operations at the CEP that would result from installation of an electric heat pump chiller would offer an outstanding opportunity to redirect monies spent on utilities to growing mission activities. This project would build new reserves for the campus through expansion of revenues from additional patient beds, improved throughput in the ORs, and consolidation of translational research facilities.

Threats: The micro- and macroeconomic model traditionally applied to health care delivery is not aligned with current legislative mandates and reimbursement models. If health institutions will be charged to care for all citizens, regardless of ability to pay, and reimbursement continues to be reduced for the care provided, the delivery model will require major overhaul. This level of change will certainly impact the built environment, the business models currently used for campus operations, and the industry resources available to support them.

PROJECT GOALS

The primary objective of this proposal is to support growth of the Organization's mission departments with savings acquired through installation of new technologies and upgrades in the CEP. The savings will be used to service the debt from the sale of bonds in the amount of $53 million to fund expansion of inpatient beds, remodeling of the pre- and post-operative suites and five of the older OR suites. The bonds will also pay to relocate the Translational Research Center to the Cancer Institute and to purchase acreage and build additional parking.

The role of the health facility commissioning authority (HFCxA) is to assure the most cost-efficient systems are specified by the design team, installed by the construction team, and can be owned and operated by the maintenance team. An important responsibility of the HFCxA is to provide measurement and verification of the outcomes associated with operation of the facility. Although an excellent architect, engineer, and general contractor will be used, the HFCxA is necessary to assure high-quality outcomes and the project meets the owner's project requirements. In keeping with [state] Act X, additional requirements for independent measurement and verification (M&V) are required to meet state energy code requirements. The HFCxA is uniquely qualified to complete and document M&V and to assure the owner meets the requirements of the act.

The project teams will determine the facility's baseline energy consumption using the EPA's Energy Star Portfolio Manager and then keep the tool updated until the one-year warranty walkthrough, when operating costs can be validated. The requirements of Act X require energy performance at a level 10 percent better than required in the 2007 edition of ASHRAE 90.1: *Energy Standard for Buildings Except Low-Rise Residential Buildings*. It is through outstanding teamwork gained in the integrated project delivery model and third-party commissioning from a qualified health facility commissioning authority that this standard will be met and the savings documented.

BUSINESS STRATEGY

Undertaking proper design, construction, and commissioning activities for this project will assure savings from improved energy efficiency in the CEP sufficient to fund the next campus expansion to support the Organization's missions of patient care, education, and research. This project will include:

- **Use of the ASHE health facility commissioning process:** As outlined in the *Health Facility Commissioning Guidelines* (*HFCx Guidelines*), the process begins with selecting a qualified independent health facility commissioning authority (HFCxA) at the same time the design team and contractor are selected.

- **Central energy plant upgrades:** Install an electric heat pump chiller and related equipment.

- **Expanded patient care:** Add 60 beds for the hospital and improve throughput in the surgery department by doubling the size of pre-op holding and post-op holding areas.

    ◆ **Improved clinical care and education:** Improve the connectivity between the Cancer Institute and Multiple Myeloma Treatment facility by relocating the latter into a new floor of the Cancer Institute.

    ◆ **Expanded research capabilities:** Consolidate the Transitional Research Institute by co-locating the various components in the space previously occupied by MIRT.

The Organization will sell bonds to support the cost of the accumulated projects. The bonds will be serviced from the savings obtained by more energy-efficient generation of heating water.

Project Scope

The Organization proposes to replace an inefficient steam heating system with a new, high-efficiency hydronic heating system that utilizes a heat pump chiller/heater (HPCH) as the primary source of heating energy. The hydronic system will provide space heating and service water heating for 15 campus buildings that house education facilities, medical research laboratories, outpatient clinics, and an acute care hospital. The project's total cost will be $21,888,236.

The project's primary objective is to reduce energy usage, and it will also improve the efficiency and reliability of utilities service on the campus. The project will reduce the Organization's energy consumption (primarily natural gas usage) and is estimated to reduce energy costs by more than $3.6 million per year.

The project will include (1) installation of the HPCH, steam-fired heating water converters for supplemental and standby heating capacity, and related support equipment in an addition to the existing Main Central Energy Plant (MCEP); (2) installation of main heating water piping from the MCEP expansion to the campus buildings; (3) heat exchangers in individual buildings for service water heating; and (4) connections to existing building space heating and service water heating systems. The HPCH will be able to produce 1,800 tons of chilled water and 939 horsepower (1 HP = 34, 500 Btu/hour) of heating water simultaneously. The new central heating water system and the building systems will be controlled automatically by a direct digital control (DDC) system that is connected to the campus energy management system.

The project will incorporate other state-of-the art design features, including distributed pumping (no wasted pumping energy), individual building metering (providing a management tool needed for effective energy conservation), and dynamic sequencing of the HPCH and the supplemental steam-fired converters based on real-time natural gas and electricity rates.

The HPCH will produce useful heat six times more efficiently than the existing steam boilers. By recovering heating energy from the chilled water system instead of generating heating energy through combustion of fossil fuels, the HPCH will operate with a heating coefficient of performance (COP) of 5.0 compared to a COP of 0.78 for the existing natural gas-fired steam boilers.

The project team will include the Organization, XYZ Consulting Engineers, ABC Contractors, JKL Industrial Hygienist, and PQR Environmental Protection Consultants. The Organization will provide construction management and purchase the major equipment (HPCH and cooling tower). The XYZ Consulting Engineers will develop the final project drawings and specifications, review pricing, and review shop drawings and submittal data. XYZ will also provide hydraulic modeling, construction administration, and MV services. JKL Industrial Hygienist will prepare specifications for ACM abatement and provide on-site monitoring services. PQR Environmental Protection Consultants will provide ACM abatement and temporary insulation. ABC Contractors will purchase materials, purchase small equipment, and construct the project.

NEW SERVICE PROGRAMS

The Organization is installing a heat pump chiller/heater (HPCH) that can be operated in either heat pump mode or chiller mode. Typically, the unit will operate in heat pump mode. The only time it will operate in chiller mode is in the event of a standard chiller failure. When in heat pump mode, the unit will use approximately 3.5 MW of electricity to simultaneously produce 2,000 tons of cooling and 1,000 HP of heating (155 to 170 deg. F heating water). The heating water it produces will be used for space heating, dehumidification (reheat), and service water heating. The net heating coefficient of performance is approximately 5.6 as compared to 0.70 for the existing fossil fuel-fired steam boilers. The HPCH electricity source will come from the campus West Energy Plant, which is served by the Utility Company under an interruptible electricity rate structure (approximately 30 percent lower unit cost than the standard rate). The HPCH will produce approximately 50 percent of the annual cooling and approximately 85 percent of the annual heating requirements of the campus buildings it serves.

The plan is to issue a request for proposals (RFP) for the HPCH to multiple manufacturers. The team will accept proposals for a single unit as well as multiple units with the equivalent aggregate capacity.

The net savings of undertaking this project will be approximately $3.6 million per year:

1. The annual electricity cost of the 2,000 ton HPCH using current WEP OIS rates is $1.258 million per year.

2. Operating the HPCH will reduce the main plant chiller electricity

costs by $946,081 per year (on standard rates) and reduce the main plant boiler natural gas costs by $3,851,296 per year.

FINANCIAL PROJECTIONS

Total Project Cost: $21,888,236
CEP HPCH Energy and Cost Savings Calculations

Savings Calculations		
Item	**Units**	**HP Chiller** **2,000 ton with 155°F**
Design HP chiller cooling capacity	tons	2,000
HPCH annual hours of operation	hours/year	8,500
Average HPCH cooling load	% of capacity	92.8
Annual cooling heat transfer	ton-hours	15,781,687
Leaving chilled water temperature	deg. F	42.0
Leaving heating water temperature	deg. F	155.0
Heat pump chiller heater temperature lift	deg. F	113
HPCH efficacy	kW/ton	1.52
HPCH power consumption	kWh	23,988,164
HPCH chilled water pump power consumption	kWh	535,539
HPCH heating water pump power consumption	kWh	767,060
Additional WCEP electricity consumption	kWh	25,290,763
WCEP average electricity unit cost	cents/kWh	4.98
Annual HPCH electricity cost	$/year	1,258,238
Standard water chiller efficacy	kW/ton	0.70
Avoided standard water chiller power consumption	kWh	11,047,181
HPCH chilled water pump indirect power consumption	kWh	117,659
Net MCEP electricity savings	kWh	10,929,521
MCEP average electricity unit cost	cents/kWh	8.66
Annual standard chiller electricity cost savings	$/year	946,081
Net electricity consumption	kWh	14,361,242
Annual HPCH heating heat transfer	MMBtu	271,252
Annual heating water pump heat transfer	MMBtu	2,409
Total heating heat transfer	MMBtu	273,660
HPCH heating COP	N/A	3.3
Effective HPCH heating COP	N/A	5.6
Average natural gas cost	$/MMBtu	9.85
Steam boiler efficiency	$/MMBtu	70
Annual natural gas savings	MMBtu/year	391,084
Annual natural gas cost savings	$/year	3,851,296
Net annual energy cost savings	$/year	**3,539,139**
Net annual site energy savings	MMBtu/year	**342,069**

Energy Summary

Item	Units	Value
Current campus floor area	SF	4,013,244
Proposed energy costs	$	9,611,103
Proposed energy costs	$/SF	2.39
Reduction in energy costs	%	**26.9**
Proposed site energy consumption	MMBtu/year	665,867
Proposed site energy consumption	Btu/year/SF	165,917
Reduction in site energy consumption	%	**33.9**
Proposed source energy consumption	MMBtu/year	1,975,228
Proposed source energy consumption	Btu/year/SF	492,177
Reduction in source energy consumption	%	**10.3**

Energy Conversion Factors

Item	Site
Electricity	3,413
Natural gas	1,000,000

PROJECT LIFE CYCLE COST ANALYSIS

Assumptions

Item	Units	Value
Energy cost escalation rate	%	1.7
Maintenance cost escalation rate	%	2.0

Results

Item	Units	Value
Life cycle cost savings	$	91,205,035
Net present value of savings	$	**35,058,211**
Internal rate of return	%	**21.01%**

QUALITY CONTROLS

To assure the success of the project, the following controls should be implemented:

+ Monthly reports from each member of the HFCx team and subsequent managers

+ Roll-up report from the HFCxA responsible for the project

+ Financial updates (at least monthly) as budget projections improve

+ Evaluation at critical project milestones, including SD, DD, and CD phases of design and 25%, 50%, 75%, and final construction completion. M&V at annual warranty walkthrough by the HFCxA

+ Chief Facility Officer oversight and privilege to expunge the project at any time during design phase if projections do not meet owner's project requirements, HFCx team is not productive, or project deliverables and outcomes are poor.

Health Facility Commissioning Glossary

AHJ (authority having jurisdiction): A government agency or office that regulates a health facility.

Airborne infection isolation: Institution of a set of procedures and building design features intended to reduce risk from the spread of airborne infectious agents.

Airborne infection isolation (AII) room: A single-occupancy patient care room specifically designed and constructed to isolate patients who are infected with diseases that can be spread by airborne droplet nuclei.

Airflow offset: A difference in the flow of air between adjacent spaces that is intended to create a pressure differential between the spaces.

Air-side economizer cycle: Increasing the flow of outside air above the minimum required for ventilation when outside air conditions can reduce the need for mechanical cooling.

Alkalinity: A measure used to estimate the capacity of water to neutralize acids or caustic wastes. Note: Alkalinity does not refer to pH, but rather to the ability of water to resist changes in pH.

AHJ: *See* Authority having jurisdiction.

AIIR: *See* Airborne infection isolation room.

AMCA: *See* Automated meting and cost allocation.

Apparent power: The product of the root-mean-square voltage and the root-mean-square current delivered in an alternating current circuit, with no account taken of the power factor (i.e., the phase difference between voltage and current).

Approach temperature: The difference between the leaving temperatures of fluids in a heat exchanger.

Automated metering and cost allocation (AMCA): Software that automatically allocates utility production costs to individual consumers based on metered consumption and demands.

BAS: *See* Building automation system.

Basis of design (BOD): The design team's documentation of the primary thought processes and assumptions behind design decisions that are intended to meet the owner's project requirements. The BOD describes the assumptions used for sizing and selection of systems (e.g., codes, standards, operating conditions, design conditions, weather data, interior environmental criteria, and other pertinent design assumptions).

Best practice: A technique, method, process, activity, or incentive that informed judgment regards as more effective at delivering a particular outcome than any other when applied to a particular condition or circumstance.

Bias: *See* Deadband.

Blowdown rate: The rate at which water is periodically discharged from a boiler or cooling tower system to reduce the buildup of suspended and total dissolved solids.

Building automation system (BAS): A control system designed to automatically control and monitor building systems.

Building information modeling (BIM): The process of generating and managing building data during the life cycle of a building using three-dimensional, real-time, dynamic building modeling software to increase productivity in building design and construction. The process produces a building information model, which encompasses building geometry, spatial relationships, geographic information, and quantities and properties of building components. This model can be used to support operations and maintenance once the building is occupied.

Building maintenance program (BMP): A structured approach to managing preventive maintenance of building equipment and systems to assure their reliable performance.

Cash-in/cash-out: A process used by natural gas utilities to reconcile differences between the amount of gas used by a customer and the amount of gas purchased by the customer for a given period. Typically applies to customers that purchase natural gas in an unbundled manner.

Combined billing: Consolidation of data from multiple meters prior to application of rates, also known as electronic master metering.

Combined heating and power (CHP): A process for deriving electricity and heat from a single fuel source.

Commissioning: The process of assuring that all building systems and their components perform in accordance with design intent, that the design intent is consistent with the owner's project requirements, and that operations and maintenance staff are adequately prepared to operate and maintain the facility.

Commissioning conference: A meeting organized by the health facility commissioning authority in which representatives of the design team, owner, contractor, subcontractors, and operations and maintenance staff review the commissioning process.

Commissioning plan: A comprehensive plan that establishes the scope, structure, and schedule for commissioning activities.

Commissioning specifications: A document that defines the roles, requirements, responsibilities, and scope of work of all members of the project team. Note: This document is a component of the contract documents.

Computerized maintenance management system (CMMS): Software that enables facility managers and operations and maintenance (O&M) staff to track the status of maintenance work and associated costs.

Condensing boiler: A boiler designed to recover latent energy from the boiler stack to preheat cold water.

Conductivity: The measure of the ease with which an electric charge or heat can pass through a material.

Constant-volume system: A system that provides a fluid (air or water) at a fixed volume per unit of time.

Contract documents: Documents that establish the obligations of the design team, the health facility commissioning authority, contractor, and other parties involved in a specific project. The documents may include general conditions, specifications, change orders, and drawings. Typically, "contract documents" refers to the project drawings and specifications.

Control loop hunting: Excessive oscillation of a control damper, valve, or other device as a result of unstable control.

Cooling tower: A device for heat removal that uses water evaporation to transfer process-waste heat into the atmosphere.

C-suite: Widely used term for the senior executives of a corporation. Note: The term is derived from the "c" with which the executives' titles begin (e.g., chief executive officer, chief financial officer, and the like).

Cycle of concentration: The number of times the solids in a particular volume of water in a boiler or cooling tower are concentrated.

Dashboard: A software tool used to monitor or check the functioning of a system or piece of equipment and to display leading indicators of critical operations and performance.

Daylighting: The controlled admission of natural light into occupied space that is used to reduce or eliminate the need for electric lighting.

DCV: *See* Demand-controlled ventilation.

Deadband (also known as "bias"): An area of a signal range or band where no action occurs (i.e., the actuators hold their current positions). Deadbands are used to allow slight variation in the measured condition to reduce energy costs.

Deaerator: A device to remove air and other dissolved gases from boiler feedwater.

Decoupling: A closed loop water distribution system design feature that allows water to bypass system distribution and then return to the source equipment to reduce required pumping horsepower.

Delta temperature (Delta T): Shorthand for the difference in two comparative temperatures.

Demand-controlled ventilation (DCV): Adjustment of outside ventilation air according to the number of occupants and the ventilation demands those occupants create. DCV is part of the ventilation system control strategy for a building and can be used to reduce the total outdoor air supply during periods of reduced occupancy.

Demand limiting: A process of monitoring total electrical power consumption and reducing or offsetting loads to avoid exceeding a preset level that would trigger excessive utility demand charges.

Demand side energy cost reduction measures: Steps taken on the customer's side of the power meter (as opposed to the utility's side of the meter) that will reduce consumption and cost.

Desiccant: A substance or agent that chemically absorbs water and is used to remove moisture from an airstream.

Design intent: The original thoughts, concepts, and purpose behind a proposed solution to a project and its components, usually expressed through plans, narratives, and specifications.

Design-build: A project delivery system in which the owner signs a single contract that covers both the design and construction disciplines for the project.

Distributed generation: A concept whereby a facility can self-generate 100 percent of its total power demand and agrees to operate off the utility grid during periods of high demand in exchange for negotiating a lower rate structure with the utility.

Distributed pumping: An arrangement of pumps in a central distribution system in which the pumps are located in the buildings close to the load and sized to match specific building flow/head needs rather than pumping solely from the central source.

Diversion meter: A device used to measure the flow of water from outside connections that does not discharge into the sanitary sewer system. These devices are typically used to avoid sanitary sewer charges related to cooling tower or boiler makeup water.

Dual-duct system: An air-conditioning system in which conditioned air is supplied via parallel hot and cold ducts. Mixing terminals control space temperature by regulating the two airstreams based on room-mounted thermostats.

E²C: *See* Energy efficiency commitment.

Effective room leakage area: The measure of air leakage in or out of a particular space through wall violations, door undercuts, and other passageways other than HVAC supply, return, or exhaust ducts.

Energy efficiency commitment (E²C): An ASHE program for sharing of fundamental concepts, real data, proven strategies, financial tools, and local success stories by ASHE members. The program promotes sharing of expert knowledge of where to find the energy savings inherent in a building design. The program includes awards and other incentives for marginal improvements in source energy use intensity.

Energy efficiency scorecard: A means of monitoring and tracking energy use efficiency and intensity for a specific facility. The scorecard identifies daily, monthly, and annual energy cost savings resulting from energy conservation efforts.

Energy management system: A general term sometimes used interchangeably with building automation system (BAS), computerized maintenance management system (CMMS), HVAC controls system, or other facility operational systems.

Energy model: A computer-based tool that simulates energy consumption of a building over a period based on building design, operational schedule, climate, and other factors.

Engineer of Record (EOR): The registered Professional Engineer responsible for the design of his or her particular portion of a project, signified by stamping and signing contract documents for AHJ review and to serve as contract documents.

Enthalpy wheel: A type of energy recovery heat exchanger that transfers thermal and latent energy between supply and exhaust airstreams in an air-handling system.

EPA Energy Star: A joint program of the U.S. Environmental Protection Agency and the U.S. Department of Energy that provides a method for facilities of various types to benchmark energy consumption and compare their performance to a control group of peer facilities. An Energy Star rating is derived from a statistical ranking with respect to comparable facilities in the database.

Essential electrical power system: A system for providing power in the event of normal power failure to feed the critical, life safety, and equipment branches in a health facility.

Exfiltration: The flow of conditioned air out of the building through the building envelope, doors, or other passageways, typically the result of having an overall positive pressure relationship. The opposite of infiltration.

Face velocity: The average velocity of air measured across the area of an opening, device, or element through which air is passing.

Fan heat gain: The increase of temperature within a given airstream as a result of fan and motor energy.

FGI *Guidelines*: Recommendations published by the Facility Guidelines Institute (FGI) for minimum program, space, engineered system, and equipment needs for various health care facilities. Adopted in whole or in part by a number of states to serve as licensing standards.

Final filter: A high-efficiency filter bank typically located downstream of any heating or cooling coils, fans, humidifiers, and other components.

Final commissioning report: A document developed at the conclusion of the commissioning process to document that final equipment and system functional testing processes verified compliance with the OPR, BOD, and contract documents and to outline/detail any remaining issues to be monitored or resolved.

Functional performance test (FPT): Test of dynamic function and operation that is conducted for components, equipment, systems, and integrated systems. Systems are tested under various modes (e.g., design loads, part loads, component failures, unoccupied periods, varying outside air temperatures, life safety conditions, power failure, etc.). Systems are run through all specified operational sequences. Components are verified to be responding in accordance with the contract documents. Functional performance tests are executed after pre-functional checklists, equipment start-ups, and contractor testing, adjusting, and balancing (TAB) are complete.

Gray water: Non-potable waste water that has been treated to varying degrees and made available for reuse for irrigation, cooling tower makeup, and other non-potable purposes.

Guaranteed maximum price (GMP): A definition of project construction cost based on intermediate design documents at which a construction manager or other entity is willing to contractually commit that the project can be delivered at or below that price.

Head: The difference between pump discharge and suction pressures expressed in units of elevation (e.g., feet).

Health facility commissioning authority (HFCxA): The individual or entity responsible for managing, coordinating, executing, and documenting commissioning activities.

HFCx: Health facility commissioning.

HFCxA: *See* Health facility commissioning authority.

Hybrid boiler plant: A hydronic heating plant that combines condensing boilers and non-condensing boilers in a single system. It may also refer to a heating system with multiple fuel choices (e.g., diesel fuel, electricity, natural gas, etc.).

Hydronic free cooling system: A system that produces chilled water without mechanical refrigeration by using a heat exchanger to transfer heat directly from the chilled water system to the condenser water system.

Infiltration: The flow of unconditioned outside air into the building through the building envelope, doors, or other passageways, typically the result of having an overall negative building pressure. The opposite of exfiltration.

Inlet vane: An optional component on a fan that modulates the fan capacity and energy consumption by pre-swirling and restricting the air before it enters the fan wheel inlet.

Integrated project delivery: A project delivery approach in which the design and construction forces work in a close partnership from project inception through final commissioning, often using a common contract that is signed by all project parties.

Internal rate of return (IRR): A calculation done in capital budgeting to predict the return on invested capital. Specifically, the IRR of an investment is the interest rate at which the net present value of costs of the investment (negative cash flows) equals the net present value of the benefits of the investment (positive cash flows). Although technically incorrect, sometimes used interchangeably with return on investment.

Interoperability: The degree to which separate systems and components are able to function together (interoperate) to provide satisfactory overall facility performance.

LDC bypass: The practice of connecting directly to a major natural gas distribution main pipeline rather than taking service through the local distribution company (LDC).

Life cycle cost: The sum of all recurring and one-time costs over the specified life span of a good, service, structure, or system. The life cycle cost includes purchase price, installation cost, operating costs, maintenance and upgrade costs, and remaining (residual and salvage) value at the end of ownership or of its useful life.

Life safety plan: A document, usually a floor plan, that designates required occupancy separation, fire-rated partitions, smoke-tight barriers, corridor walls, and suite barriers to demonstrate compliance with the applicable version of the *Life Safety Code.*

Lighting efficiency: The ratio of the amount of light produced by a lamp measured in lumens to the amount of power consumed to produce it measured in watts. Note: Lighting efficiency is typically expressed in lumens per watt.

Master metering: A process of arranging electric power or natural gas meters so that a service for multiple buildings is taken through a single meter. Note: With master metering, each individual building may or may not have an individual meter.

Maximum daily quantity: Volume of natural gas consumption that cannot be exceeded in a given 24-hour period.

Measurement and verification: A process and arrangement of instrumentation that will allow accurate and real-time documentation of actual system performance and energy consumption.

MODBUS: A serial communications protocol that allows communication between multiple devices. Typically used to connect different manufacturer devices to a common network.

Multi-zone system: An HVAC system that uses zone dampers located at the air handler to mix heated air and chilled air to regulate the temperature of a space or zone.

Net present value (NPV): Total value of future cash flows discounted back to the current date.

Night setback/setup: An HVAC system control strategy whereby setpoints are relaxed during unoccupied periods for the purpose of reducing energy consumption.

Normal power: Primary source of electrical power supplied to a facility from a utility grid.

Occupancy sensor: Motion sensor used to automatically control electric lighting and other loads based on detection of occupants in the monitored area.

Ongoing commissioning: A process designed to assure that buildings and systems are maintained at optimum performance levels.

Operations and maintenance (O&M) manuals: Documents that indicate actual installation and configuration options, preventive maintenance and repairs, operational sequences, replacement parts and instructions, warranty information for the equipment, and contact information for key personnel and support staff. Typically developed by the installing contractor and given to the owner at the completion of a project.

Owner's project requirements (OPR): For a commissioning project, documentation that defines the functional requirements of a facility and the expectations of the owner as they relate to the systems to be commissioned. At a minimum, the OPR should establish the facility purpose, expected life, expected project cost, energy efficiency and sustainability goals, outdoor design conditions, and indoor environmental conditions.

Parallelling switchgear: A system of electrical equipment and controls that allows multiple engine-driven generators to be phase synchronized to feed a common load.

Performance contract: A model of financing energy-saving measures (design fees, installation, and incentives) with a share of future anticipated savings.

PFC: *See* Pre-functional checklist.

PI: *See* Proportional-integration.

PID: *See* Proportional-integral-derivative (PID) loop.

Power factor: The ratio of real power in kW to apparent power in kVA. Typically calculated as the cosine of the phase angle between the voltage and current waveforms.

Pre-filter: The initial barrier in an air-handling system that provides gross filtration of airborne particulates to protect heating and cooling coils and final filter beds.

Pre-functional checklist (PFC): A list of static inspections and elementary component tests that verify proper installation of equipment (e.g., installation and arrangement of associated services such as ductwork, piping, hydronic specialties, sensor locations, dampers, belt tension, oil levels, labels affixed, gauges in place, sensors calibrated, etc.).

Pressure-independent air terminal: A variable and constant volume air terminal that can maintain constant or required air volume (within a defined range) regardless of changes in inlet air pressure.

Project scope: Definition of the goals, objectives, departments, size, schedule, and cost of a project.

Proportional-integral (PI) loop: A generic control loop feedback mechanism that is a commonly used feedback controller in building control systems. The loop calculates an output based on the difference between the input value and the control setpoint (proportional component) and the length of time the difference has occurred (integral component).

Proportional-integral-derivative (PID) loop: A generic control loop feedback mechanism that is a commonly used feedback controller in building control systems. The loop calculates an output based on the difference between the input value and the control setpoint (proportional component), the length of time the difference has occurred (integral component), and the rate of change of the input (derivative component).

Real-time pricing: A type of utility tariff where the unit price varies throughout the day in response to the actual cost of service and demand.

Recommissioning: Repeating the commissioning process on a previously commissioned facility or systems with the goal of achieving optimum performance.

Retrocommissioning: Commissioning an existing building that has not previously been commissioned with the goal of achieving optimum performance.

Return on investment (ROI): The measured benefits received from an investment based on its actual economic performance. Although technically incorrect, sometimes used interchangeably with internal rate of return (IRR).

Room ventilation schedule: A schedule indicating the proper supply, return, and exhaust airflows for each zone in a health care facility based on heating and cooling loads and code requirements.

R-value: A measure of thermal resistance to the flow of heat used in the building and construction industry. Greater R-values indicate a higher level of thermal resistance and better insulating properties. The R-value is the inverse of the U-value.

Stack effect: The difference in the pressure relationship between the inside of a building and the exterior of a building caused by the buoyancy of warmer air and changes in elevation within the building. The stack effect causes taller buildings to experience negative building pressure relationships at lower levels in the winter and positive building pressure relationships at lower levels in the summer.

Start-up plan: A written plan for activities and tasks to be completed prior to initiating operation of any equipment or system component and for testing and verification purposes during initial operation.

Submittal documents: Drawings, data, samples, and so on that are submitted for review, evaluation, and approval prior to their inclusion in a project.

Synthetic natural gas: An artificial version of natural gas produced by mixing propane and air.

Systems manual: A manual focused on operating systems. At a minimum, it should include the final version of the OPR and the BOD, system single-line drawings, as-built sequences of operation, control shop drawings, original control setpoints, operating instructions for integrated systems, recommended retesting schedules and blank test forms, and sensor and actuator recalibration schedules. One of the manual's most important functions is provision of a condensed troubleshooting guide for O&M personnel at the system level.

Testing, adjusting, and balancing (TAB): A process by which the contractor tests, adjusts, and balances the air and hydronic systems. The contractor completes the TAB work prior to functional performance testing.

Thermal storage: Use of various equipment arrangements, controls, and related technologies to store thermal energy during off-peak or low-utility-cost hours for use during high-demand, high-cost periods. Typically used in reference to chilled water storage tanks or ice tanks.

Time-of-use electricity rate: Electricity pricing that varies with demand according to the time of day and week. Time-of-use rates are designed to provide a financial incentive to transfer electricity consumption from peak demand periods to off-peak periods.

Utility management plan (UMP): A document required by the Joint Commission that establishes policies and procedures related to safe and effective operation and failure response of a health care facility's utility systems.

U-value: A measure of the rate at which heat transfers through a building element over a given area under standardized conditions. It is the inverse of the R-value.

Value engineering (VE): When used properly, value engineering is an organized process of identifying and evaluating methods of improving project value by either reducing cost or increasing performance (efficiency, longevity, etc.). Sometimes called value analysis.

Variable frequency drive (VFD): A component that controls the rotational speed of an alternating current (AC) electric motor by controlling the frequency of the electrical power supplied to the motor.

Variable-volume system: A system that provides a fluid (air or water) at a varying volume per unit of time in response to varying loads or occupancy.

Health Facility Commissioning Crosswalk

This health facility commissioning (HFCx) crosswalk is a tool intended to help clarify the differences between the various commissioning processes promoted in the marketplace. The crosswalk compares the steps defined by the ASHE health facility commissioning process with those of several other approaches to commissioning. The tabular format of the comparison highlights the similarities and differences in all the approaches and provides a relatively thorough review of the commissioning process prescribed by each approach.

To create the crosswalk, a master list was compiled of the commissioning tasks in all the publications reviewed; this list was then sorted by project phase: predesign, design, construction, transition to operational sustainability, postoccupancy and warranty, and retrocommissioning. The resulting tabular lists provide a thorough overview of the commissioning activities deemed important by each approach to commissioning.

The publications included in the crosswalk represent widely known credible voices in the building construction and facility management industries. Of all these commissioning approaches, however, only the ASHE *Health Facility Commissioning Guidelines* specifically addresses commissioning from the perspective unique to health care facilities.

COMMISSIONING SOURCES INCLUDED IN THE CROSSWALK

ACG: AABC Commissioning Group. *ACG Commissioning Guideline for Building Owners, Design Professionals and Commissioning Service Providers.* Washington: Associated Air Balance Council Commissioning Group, 2005. http://www.commissioning.org/Commissioningguideline/ACGCommissioningGuideline.pdf (accessed Jan. 1, 2011).

The *ACG Commissioning Guideline* has been used as reference for candidates taking the AABC commissioning certification examination. It focuses on HVAC commissioning and was written by industry professionals experienced in the testing of HVAC systems. *Environmental Building News* refers to it as "one of the clearest descriptions of the commissioning process."

APPA: Heinz, J. A., and R. B. Casault. *The Building Commissioning Handbook*. Alexandria, Va.: APPA, 2004.

The Building Commissioning Handbook is a useful resource that describes in detail the roles of the building owner, design professionals, contractor, testing contractor, commissioning authority, subcontractors, vendors, sub-consultants, and testing, adjusting, and balancing firms in addition to the owner's operations staff, all of whom have a stake in the total effort. The book discusses the commissioning process, equipment testing, systems functional performance testing, intersystem functional performance testing, scheduling, documentation, training costs, and advertising for and selecting a commissioning authority. APPA's goal for building commissioning is to assist in the construction of a facility that will operate as intended. APPA recommends commissioning every new facility, and recommends commissioning static and dynamic building systems as well as health and life safety systems.

ASHE: American Society for Healthcare Engineering (ASHE). *Health Facility Commissioning Guidelines*. Chicago: ASHE of the American Hospital Association, 2010.

ASHE's *Health Facility Commissioning Guidelines* presents a commissioning process specifically designed for the complexities entailed in commissioning a health care facility. The ASHE commissioning process, referred to as health facility commissioning (HFCx), is cost-effective and efficient and fosters delivery of the desired return on investment. It makes the entire project team, including the commissioning authority, accountable for actual building performance. ASHE's collaborative approach delivers a health care physical environment that meets the goals of the health care organization and the needs of its community. The *HFCx Guidelines* text covers initial commissioning collaboration, continuing commissioning procedures, and retrocommissioning tactics.

ASHRAE: American Society of Heating, Refrigerating and Air-Conditioning Engineers. Guideline 0-2005: *The Commissioning Process*. Atlanta: ASHRAE, 2005.

ASHRAE Guideline 0-2005 reads like a code text and covers the entire process for all phases of project delivery in less than 60 pages. The ASHRAE process is driven by the owner's project requirements—29 criteria that "help the project team to properly plan, design, construct, operate and maintain systems and assemblies" (p. 6). The document thoroughly covers commissioning activities from predesign to warranty but does not address the practice of retrocommissioning. ASHRAE 0-2005 applies directly to commissioning mechanical systems; however, the outlined steps are defined well enough that other types of systems can be added to the commissioning scope as well.

GSA: U.S. General Services Administration Public Buildings Service. *The Building Commissioning Guide*. Washington, D.C.: U.S. General Services Administration, 2005. http://www.wbdg.org/ccb/GSAMAN/buildingcommissioningguide.pdf (accessed May 2011) or http://www.gsa.gov/portal/category/21595 (an HTML publication, accessed May 2011)

The Building Commissioning Guide published by the GSA is organized in three parts:

1. The first part reviews the philosophy of building commissioning, including the GSA's definition of and expectations for commissioning.

2. The second part outlines the building commissioning process then discusses the GSA project processes for the planning, design, construction, and post-construction stages. A matrix of commissioning activities that identifies who is responsible for each is provided, along with more detailed discussion of these steps. .

3. The appendices include a sample scope for commissioning services, a commissioning systems selection matrix, glossary, etc.

LEED: U.S. Green Building Council. *LEED Reference Guide for Green Building Design and Construction*. Washington: U.S. Green Building Council, 2010.

The U.S. Green Building Council developed this LEED reference guide, which focuses on design, construction, and renovation of commercial and institutional buildings, for building owners and project teams who want to apply for LEED certification. Commissioning is a requirement for certification, and the publication lists a series of tasks that should be included in the commissioning process.

NEBB: National Environmental Balancing Bureau. *Design Phase Commissioning Handbook*. Gaithersburg, Md.: NEBB, 2005.

National Environmental Balancing Bureau. *Procedural Standards for Retro-Commissioning of Existing Buildings*. Gaithersburg, Md.: NEBB, 2009.

National Environmental Balancing Bureau. *Procedural Standards for Whole Building Systems Commissioning of New Construction*, 3rd ed. Gaithersburg, Md.: NEBB, 2009.

NEBB's three volumes on commissioning were developed to provide a uniform and systematic set of criteria to assure optimum commissioning of buildings and systems. They are intended for use by commissioning authorities, building owners, and facility maintenance personnel and cover the commissioning of both new and existing facilities, but do not include information related to health care facilities.

PECI: Energy Design Resources. *Building Commissioning Guidelines: A Source Book on Building Systems Performance*. Prepared for Pacific Gas and Electric Company by Portland Energy Conservation (PECI) for the statewide Energy Design Resources program, 2001. http://www.energydesignresources.com/ DirectDownload.htm?media/2296/EDR_CommissioningHandbookComplete.pdf (accessed April 1, 2011).

PECI wrote the *Building Commissioning Guidelines* for building owners and designers. Part 1 of the document provides clear arguments and case studies to help owners select a suitable commissioning provider and discusses the role of the owner throughout the commissioning process. Part 2 is written for designers. Stressing the importance of commissioning new construction, techniques and materials used in green design, and restating LEED requirements for commissioning, the *Guidelines* makes the case for designers to support the process and describes how they also benefit from commissioning. This section also presents a more detailed commissioning process focused on design-build projects, including sample documentation in the appendices. In both Parts 1 and 2, a strong case is made for using an "independent third party under contract to the owner" for commissioning services as a best practice. The document is very thorough, but does not address building types and therefore does not mention health care facilities.

HEALTH FACILITY COMMISSIONING CROSSWALK

Predesign Phase

Master List	Commissioning Process Sources							
Commissioning Activity	ACG	GSA	ASHRAE	LEED	APPA	NEBB	PECI	ASHE
Decide to commission	X		X					**X**
Send out request for qualifications/proposal (RFQ/RFP) to commissioning authority (CxA) candidates	X						X	**X**
Interview CxA candidates					X		X[1]	**X**
Select a CxA	X			X	X		X[2]	**X**
Develop CxA agreement					X[3]		X	**X**
Identify Cx team		X	X			X	X	**X**
Develop Cx team structure	X	X	X			X	X	**X**
Define Cx scope	X		X			X	X	**X**[4]
Develop preliminary Cx plan	X	X	X		X	X	X	**X**
Establish Cx budget	X	X	X		X	X		**X**
Negotiate the HFCxA fee and contract								**X**
Perform commissioning cost-benefit analysis	X	X[5]						**X**
Create and document Cx team communication plan			X		X			
Review design intent document	X[6]						X[7]	**X**
Define roles and responsibilities in predesign (15 items)			X[8]					**X**
Create/develop owner's project requirements (OPR) (29 criteria)		X	X[9]	x	X	X	X	**X**
Review lessons learned from previous projects			X					**X**
Verify that Cx activities are clearly stated in all scopes of work			X					**X**
Review predesign documents for compliance with OPR (9-step process)			X			X[10]		**X**
Prepare Cx process progress reports			X					**X**
Establish issues log procedures (11 criteria)			X[11]			X		**X**
Create issues log			X			X		**X**
Determine the documents that will make up the systems manual						X[12]		**X**
Review/update OPR						X	X	**X**
Accept OPR, Cx plan, and issues log procedures	X		X			X	X	**X**
Prepare predesign phase documentation			X[13]			X		
Select design professional					X[14]			
Provide design professional agreement					X[15]			
Identify preliminary Cx time requirements for each project phase	X[16]							
Owner formally accepts predesign phase requirements			X				X	

Note: The footnoted material in the tables identifies material in a publication that provides significant explanation of a subject *or* an activity defined or described differently by that commissioning approach. Footnoted material of the latter type is followed by an asterisk.

[1] Interviews of CxA candidates—PECI (p. 54). "To properly plan, schedule and execute a successful commissioning project, the chosen provider should have broad experience working as a team member in other commissioning projects." This statement is followed by a list of recommended minimum qualifications and a list of optional qualifications.

[2] Select a commissioning authority—PECI (p. 56). The author emphasizes throughout the handbook that the commissioning provider (CP) should be an "independent third party under contract to the owner." *

[3] Owner provides commissioning authority agreement—APPA (p.43). The agreement is a simple two-page document that can be changed to suit the contracting details for each project. The agreement consists of Attachments A, B and C, which are the Conditions of Agreement, Rate Guidelines for Time and Expense Agreements, and Scope of Services.

[4] Define Cx scope—ASHE (pp. 23–25). The first step in establishing the scope for a commissioning project is to identify the systems to be commissioned. The comprehensive commissioning scope for health care facilities should consider building envelope, life safety, HVAC systems, HVAC system controls, plumbing systems, medical gas systems, electrical systems, fire alarm system, information technology, fire protection system, exterior lighting, refrigeration, vertical transport, and materials and pharmaceutical handling.

[5] Commissioning cost-benefit analysis—GSA (p. 19). As part of the initial budget for Cx this publication proposes a cost-benefit analysis during predesign. "Beyond operating efficiency, successful building commissioning has been linked to reduced occupant complaints and increased occupant productivity."

[6] CxA reviews design intent document—ACG (p. 26). The design intent document defines the technical design criteria required to satisfy the building's intended use and occupancy needs.

[7] CxA reviews design intent document (DID)—PECI (p. 59). This publication emphasizes the design intent document more than most. "Design Intent Documentation forms the foundation of the commissioning process . . . this design intent documentation includes owner's requirements for the project, design intent acceptance criteria for each requirement, and references to the portions of the design basis and design narrative that relate to each requirement." *

[8] Roles and responsibilities in predesign—ASHRAE (p. 6). For the list of 15 items, refer to Section 5.2.1.6. in ASHRAE Guidelines 0.

[9] Create/develop owner project requirements (OPR)—ASHRAE (p. 6). For the list of 29 criteria, refer to Section 5.2.2.4. in ASHRAE Guidelines 0.

[10] Review predesign documents for compliance with OPR—APPA (p. 40)

- Project description
- Objectives
- Functional uses

- Occupancy requirements
- Indoor environmental quality requirements
- Performance criteria
- Quality of materials
- Construction considerations
- Budget considerations and limitations

[11] Establish issue log procedures—ASHRAE (p. 8). For the list of 11 criteria, refer to Section 5.2.5.2.

[12] Determine the documents that will make up the systems manual—NEBB (p. 55). The final systems manual may include the following and should be provided in electronic format:

- Summary
- Final approved submittals and shop drawings
- Final OPR
- Final BOD
- Final contract documents (record drawings/as-builts)
- Final operations and maintenance manuals
- Final commissioning report
- Operator training materials
- Recommended standard operating procedures
- TAB report

[13] Predesign phase documentation—ASHRAE (p. 8). For the list of documents required, refer to Section 5.4.1. This list includes "commissioning process progress reports." *

[14] Select design professional—APPA (p. 44). This publication suggests this may happen before, during, or after the predesign phase. *

[15] Owner provides design professional agreement—APPA (p. 44). The owner must clearly identify the design professional's responsibilities in developing construction documents and in participating in the commissioning process.

[16] Preliminary Cx time requirements for each project phase—ACG (p. 27). This publication suggests outlining Cx time requirements by phase and inserting them into the project schedule. *

Design Phase

Master List	Commissioning Process Sources							
Commissioning Activity	ACG	GSA	ASHRAE	LEED	APPA	NEBB	PECI	ASHE
Organize and attend predesign conference					X			X
Cx scoping meeting							X	
Set project energy efficiency goals								X[1]
Design meetings	X	X	X			X	X	
Design review (6-step process)	X	X	X	X	X[2]		X	
Develop OPR								X
Develop BOD (8 criteria) or design narrative		X	X[3]	X	X	X	X[4]	X
Review OPR		X		X			X	X
Review BOD or design narrative		X		X	X		X	X
Review schematic design documents	X			X	X	X		X
Develop Cx plan								X[5]
Develop Cx specifications	X	X	X	X	X		X	X[6]
Retain CxA		X[7]						
CxA interviews facility manager							X[8]	
Define roles and responsibilities in design phase (18 criteria items)		X	X[9]		X		X	X
Review design development (DD) documents/verify that BOD follows OPR			X			X		X
Define equipment and systems			X				X	
Establish communication protocols			X		X			
Review HVAC control system sequences of operation								X
Include Cx process requirements in construction documents		X	X		X	X	X	X[10]
Update Cx plan		X	X		X	X	X	X
Update Cx specifications								X
Develop construction checklists			X				X	
Establish system manuals	X	X	X[11]				X	
Establish training requirements (7 criteria)	X	X	X[12]			X	X	
Review submittals	X	X	X				X	
Team accepts design phase Cx process	X	X	X					
Update issues log		X	X			X	X	
Update OPR		X	X			X		
Conduct functional performance tests	X[13]							X
Use system verification checklists	X							
Develop utility management plan (UMP)								X[14]
Attend pre-bidding conference					X	X	X	X
Evaluate shop drawings						X		
Owner formally accepts design phase requirements			X				X	

[1] Set project energy efficiency goals—ASHE (pp. 31–32). The HFCxA should work with the owner, design team, and contractor to establish an aggressive yet attainable and fiscally responsible energy efficiency goal. This goal can be set using the EPA Energy Star Target Finder tool, which can be accessed at www.energystar.gov.

[2] Design review steps—APPA (pp. 54–56). General design reviews include these:

  + Basis of design review

  + Discipline-specific design review

  + Discipline coordination drawing review

  + Specification review

  + Calculations review

[3] Develop basis of design (BOD)—ASHRAE (pp. 9–10). For the list of eight criteria, refer to Section 6.2.2.1.

[4] Develop basis of design/design narrative—PECI (p. 62). This publication introduces the term "design narrative": "The designer compiles the design concepts and design basis into a design narrative document that the commissioning provider reviews for clarity, completeness and compliance with the owner's project requirements." *

[5] Develop Cx plan—ASHE (pp. 37–39). The health facility commissioning agent (HFCxA) develops a HFCx plan for the commissioning team to follow. Refer to Section 2.7.2 for the list of 12 components.

[6] Develop Cx specifications—ASHE (p. 39). Refer to Section 2.8.2 for commissioning specification elements.

[7] Retain commissioning agent—GSA (pp. 26–27). The commissioning agent should be chosen primarily on the basis of qualifications and not solely on the basis of price. It is recommended that the commissioning agent be contracted using a two-phase fee negotiation process: (1) design stage responsibilities and (2) construction and post-construction activities.*

[8] CxA interviews facility manager—PECI (p. 24). The purpose of the interview is to determine the ability and availability of the O&M staff to operate and maintain building equipment and systems.

[9] Define roles and responsibilities in design phase—ASHRAE (p. 9). For the list of 18 criteria, refer to Section 6.2.1.3.

[10] Include commissioning process requirements in construction documents—ASHE (pp. 41–42). The HFCxA reviews the construction documents with health facility O&M staff and documents their comments and concerns. Refer to Section 2.11.2 for the list of 10 objectives.

[11] Establish system manuals—ASHRAE (pp. 11–12). For the list of 10 criteria, refer to Section 6.2.6.4.

[12] Establish training requirements—ASHRAE (p. 12). For the list of 7 criteria, refer to Section 6.2.7.7.

[13] Conduct functional performance tests (FPTs)—ACG (p. 31). The tests are needed to demonstrate correct operation under all modes of operation and include applicable pass/fail criteria. The commissioning authority must witness all FPTs to verify results.

[14] Develop utility management plan—ASHE (pp. 42–44). The Joint Commission and similar organizations accredit many health care facilities. One requirement in the Joint Commission's accreditation manual is the development of a comprehensive utility management plan (UMP). Refer to ASHE 2.13.3 for the components included in an UMP.

Construction Phase

Master List	Commissioning Process Sources							
Commissioning Activity	*ACG*	*GSA*	*ASHRAE*	*LEED*	*APPA*	*NEBB*	*PECI*	**ASHE**
Select and approve testing contractor (TC)					X[1]			
Hold pre-construction Cx conference	X		X		X	X	X	**X**
Participate in pre-bid conference			X[2]					
Coordinate participation of owner's representatives			X					
Identify specialists for specific systems and assemblies			X			X	X	
Update OPR to reflect owner-directed and construction process changes			X			X		
Update Cx plan	X		X[3]	X	X	X	X	
Develop issues log								**X**
Update issues log							X	
Review submittals	X	X	X	X	X	X	X	**X**
Review shop drawings								**X**
Prepare O&M manuals	X	X		X	X			**X⁴**
Review O&M manuals								**X**
Coordinate drawing review							X	
Review change orders							X	
Schedule Cx activities	X		X[5]		X	X	X	
Develop and document test procedures		X	X[6]	X	X	X	X	
Conduct Cx team meetings	X	X	X	X	X	X	X	**X**
Attend selected project meetings								**X**
Conduct periodic site visits (OPR compliance)	X		X	X	X	X	X	
Lead O&M staff tours								**X**
Complete pre-functional checklists and inspections								**X**

Construction Phase *(continued)*

Master List								Commissioning Process Sources
Commissioning Activity	ACG	GSA	ASHRAE	LEED	APPA	NEBB	PECI	ASHE
Review HVAC control system programming								**X**
Verify completion of construction checklist items	X	X	X	X	X		X[7]	
Witness and document equipment start-up	X	X	X			X		**X**
Confirm TAB completion and documentation	X	X						**X**
Conduct functional performance testing	X	X	X	X	X	X	X[8]	**X**
Verify training (OPR compliance)	X	X	X	X	X		X	
Write and review Cx process progress reports	X	X	X	X	X	X	X	
Verify updates to BOD			X	X			X	
Verify updates to system manuals/construction phase documentation		X	X	X	X	X	X	
Prepare final Cx report							X	
Conduct systems verification checks (SVCs)	X[9]							
Conduct controls point-to-point checks	X[10]							
Correct problems and retest	X							
Facilitate pressure testing								**X[11]**
Review training plans							X	
Review record drawings								**X[12]**
Owner formally accepts construction phase requirements			X				X	

[1.] Select and approve testing contractor (TC)—APPA (p. 79). For large, complex projects, the specifications must require the prime contractor to engage a TC and include a subsection that defines the TC's qualifications and responsibilities. The TC must be selected and approved prior to the preconstruction commissioning conference. *

[2.] Participate in pre-bid conference—ASHRAE (p. 14). Time should be allotted during the pre-bid conference for the commissioning team to alert bidders to commissioning process requirements they may be unfamiliar to them.

[3.] Update commissioning plan—ASHRAE (p. 14). For the list of 5 criteria, refer to Section 7.2.5.1.

[4.] Prepare O&M manuals —ASHE (pp. 46–47). Contractors must submit O&M manuals for approval as soon as possible after their shop drawings have been approved. The HFCxA then reviews the manuals to assure proper content and format. The manuals should be available to operations personnel prior to and during training. *

[5] Schedule commissioning activities—ASHRAE (p. 15). For the list of 9 criteria, refer to Section 7.2.8.3.

[6] Develop and document test procedures—ASHRAE (pp. 15–16). For the list of criteria, refer to sections 7.2.9.1 and 7.2.10.1.

[7] Verify completion of construction checklist items—PECI (p. 25). This publication suggests including the facility maintenance staff in this process as much as possible.*

[8] Conduct functional performance testing—PECI (p. 25). This publication suggests including the facility maintenance staff in this process as much as possible. *

[9] Conduct systems verification checks (SVCs)—ACG (p. 34). The purpose of these tests is to assure that systems have been installed properly, conform to the specifications, and are ready for safe start-up.

[10] Conduct controls point-to-point checks—ACG (p. 35). These checks confirm that all control-point wiring has been correctly installed and terminated, sensors have been calibrated, and field devices operate correctly. These are physical observations carried out by the automatic temperature controls (ATC) contractor.

[11] Facilitate pressure testing—ASHE (pp. 49–52). Refer to sections 3.13.1 through 3.13.4 for code requirements, steps for positive pressure rooms, steps for testing negative pressure rooms, and steps for testing the building envelope.

[12] Review record drawings—ASHE (p. 52). The HFCxA should review the record drawings with O&M personnel and identify known discrepancies between these documents and as-installed conditions. A list of discrepancies should then be forwarded to the owner, contractor, and design teams for incorporation into the record documents.

Transition to Operational Sustainability

Master List	Commissioning Process Sources							
Commissioning Activity	ACG	GSA	ASHRAE	LEED	APPA	NEBB	PECI	**ASHE**
Facilitate development of operating and maintenance dashboards								**X**[1]
Coordinate contractor callbacks			X					
Convene lessons-learned workshop		X	X					
Update OPR, BOD and Cx plan			X		X	X		
Update schedules						X		
Facilitate maintenance staff training								**X**
Document HVAC controls installation	X							
Facilitate implementation of HVAC control system trends								**X**[2]
Verify preliminary TAB report	X[3]							
Conduct functional performance tests	X					X		
Correct problems and retest	X					X[4]		
Verify completion of deferred testing						X[5]		
Produce system manuals			X			X		**X**
Facilitate development of the maintenance budget								**X**[6]
Facilitate fire and smoke damper inspections and testing								**X**
Facilitate completion of the statement of conditions								**X**
Facilitate development and implementation of the building maintenance program								**X**[7]
Prepare final Cx report	X	X	X	X		X		
Provide acceptance phase documentation						X[8]		
Train owner's O&M staff	X		X			X		
Owner formally accepts occupancy and operations phase requirements			X					

[1] Facilitate development of O&M dashboards—ASHE (pp. 53–55). Many health care facilities have had significantly reduced maintenance staffing levels and budgets in recent years. Dynamic O&M dashboards created for the automatic temperature control system are well-suited to meet the resulting need. Refer to Section 4.1.2 for the 13 system requirements for dashboards.

[2] Facilitate implementation of HVAC control system trends—ASHE (pp. 57–59). The contract design scope should require creation of various trends to help the O&M staff monitor the operation of key equipment and systems in the facility. Often the design documents require the HVAC control system to be capable of trending the systems but do not specify what trends are acceptable. In such cases,

the HFCxA should assist the O&M staff in identifying and tracking key trends. Refer to sections 4.3.1 and 4.3.2 for information on trending and the four trends to consider developing.

[3] Verify preliminary TAB report—ACG (p. 38). The TAB agency completes and submits the preliminary TAB report to the designer. The designer requests TAB report verification by the commissioning authority that TAB was based on the commissioning specifications and conducted with TAB agency equipment and personnel assistance. The TAB agency performs services to address inconsistencies identified during verification or designer comments and resubmits the final TAB report to the designer for approval.

[4] Correct problems and retest—NEBB (p. 47). After corrective action, retests are performed to verify conformance in accordance with the commissioning plan.

[5] Verify completion of deferred testing—NEBB (p. 47). Some testing must be deferred for budgetary issues, seasonal requirements, etc. The commissioning agent verifies and documents that these deferred tests are performed by the responsible member of the commissioning team.

[6] Facilitate development of the maintenance budget—ASHE (covered in Chapter 4). The HFCxA works with the health facility manager to use ASHE and ASHE/IFMA tools to predict annual maintenance and energy costs and develop budgets.

[7] Facilitate development and implementation of the building management program—ASHE (covered in Chapter 4). The HFCxA works with the health facility manager to develop the utility management plan (UMP).

[8] Provide acceptance phase documentation—NEBB (p. 49). Required documents should include:

- Commissioning meeting minutes
- Functional performance test reports
- Training documentation
- Updated issue log with noted corrections
- Updated commissioning plan
- Updated OPR
- Updated BOD from the design professionals
- Final commissioning report

Postoccupancy and Warranty Phase

Master List	Commissioning Process Sources							
Commissioning Activity	*ACG*	*GSA*	*ASHRAE*	*LEED*	*APPA*	*NEBB*	*PECI*	***ASHE***
Review trend data								**X**[1]
Conduct acceptance phase commissioning follow-up						X		
Conduct construction phase commissioning follow-up						X		**X**
Hold warranty phase commissioning review meeting						X		**X**
Prepare periodic Cx process reports			X					
Maintain OPR and BOD			X					**X**
Periodically evaluate OPR			X					**X**
Maintain systems manual			X					**X**
Conduct ongoing training of O&M staff			X				X	**X**
Monitor and analyze performance data			X		X		X	**X**
Perform deferred and seasonal testing	X	X	X		X	X	X	**X**
Estimate energy savings and implementation costs							X	**X**
Reinspect/review performance before end of warranty period		X	X	X	X		X	**X**
Benchmark energy performance								**X**[2]
Conduct final satisfaction review with customer agency		X[3]						**X**
Correct problems and retest	X						X	**X**
Hold lessons learned workshop			X			X		**X**
Complete final commissioning report	X	X						**X**
Provide warranty phase documentation						X[4]		**X**
Recommission at appropriate intervals		X			X		X[5]	**X**

[1] Review of trend data—ASHE (pp. 65–68). When a facility is occupied and the systems are subjected to actual load conditions, trends provide the facility manager with critical data that allow him or her to optimize system operations for both building comfort and energy management. Refer to sections 5.1.1 through 5.1.5 for information on trending for terminal boxes, heating hot water system, air-handling units, chilled water systems, and other equipment.

[2] Benchmark energy performance—ASHE (p. 70). After the building has been in service for a year, its actual energy efficiency is benchmarked by the owner or the HFCxA. The benchmarking process is based on actual energy and water consumption and costs as compared to the EPA target.

[3] Conduct final satisfaction review with customer agency—GSA (p. 51). A review should occur one year after occupancy between the commissioning team and selected customer agency representatives. The purpose of this review is to obtain honest, objective, and constructive feedback on what worked well throughout the

commissioning process and what the commissioning team could have done better.

[4] Provide warranty phase documentation—NEBB (p. 51). Required documents should include:

  • Final commissioning report warranty addenda

  • Updated issue log if appropriate

  • Retesting forms with deferred testing results, if appropriate

  • Lessons learned workshop report

[5] Recommission every three to five years—PECI (p. 28). This publication suggests recommissioning in two to three years.*

Retrocommissioning

Master List		Retrocommissioning Process Sources						
Retrocommissioning Activity	*ACG*	*GSA*	*ASHRAE*	*LEED*	*APPA*	*NEBB*	*PECI*	*ASHE*
Establish an Energy Star Portfolio Manager account								**X**
Obtain 24 months of utility bills and enter data into Portfolio Manager								**X**
Obtain baseline Energy Star rating								**X**
Establish Energy Star target								**X**
Identify potential savings to reach target level								**X**
Identify current facility HVAC commissioning requirements	X					X[1]	X	
Analyze energy cost benefits	X							**X**[2]
Select a retrocommissioning team	X					X		**X**
Develop a retrocommissioning proposal						X		**X**
Conduct documentation and site reviews	X					X		**X**[3]
Obtain original TAB reports control diagrams								**X**
Assess TAB services	X							**X**
Document and verify TAB results	X							**X**
Develop a scorecard to track actual energy cost savings								**X**
Conduct functional performance tests	X							**X**[4]
Review O&M practices	X							**X**
Review O&M instruction and documentation	X					X		**X**
Complete retrocommissioning report	X							**X**
Identify and solve comfort and operational problems							X	**X**
Assess retrocommissioning project scope					X		X	
Develop retrocommissioning plan					X		X	**X**
Develop retrocommissioning cost estimate					X		X	**X**
Identify OPR					X			
Identify O&M staff who will participate in retrocommissioning					X			**X**
Interview management staff						X		**X**
Interview O&M staff					X	X		**X**

(continued on next page)

Retrocommissioning *(contuinued)*

Retrocommissioning Activity	ACG	GSA	ASHRAE	LEED	APPA	NEBB	PECI	ASHE
Perform walkthrough of all spaces					X			**X**
Interview selected occupants					X	X		
Identify retrocommissioning interference and impact					X			
Develop assessment of performance goals vs. system capacities					X			**X**[5]
Evaluate remaining life of equipment					X			
Develop a retrocommissioning plan outline					X	X		
Gain owner's approval of scope, plan, and cost					X	X		
Formalize professional services agreement					X			**X**
Analyze existing documentation					X	X		**X**[6]
Update and enhance system documentation					X			**X**
Analyze existing physical conditions					X	X		**X**[7]
Review operational records						X		**X**
Analyze historical energy consumption data					X	X		**X**
Develop component verification test procedures					X			
Mitigate potential risks associated with component testing					X			
Establish and review trends for key equipment operating parameters								**X**
Advise occupants of effect of testing					X			
Perform component verification tests					X	X		
Review test results					X	X		
Record corrective actions already taken					X			**X**
Recommended problem resolution						X		**X**
Set performance goals					X			**X**
Develop room ventilation schedule								**X**
Develop weekly occupied/unoccupied schedules for AHU								**X**
Develop and revise AHU sequence of operation and setpoints								**X**
Establish outside airflow setpoints and exhaust airflow requirements								**X**
Establish revised chilled water and heating water sequences of operation								**X**
Establish weekly occupied/unoccupied schedules for air terminal units and fan coils								**X**
Establish revised air terminal and fan coil unit sequences of operation								**X**
Establish air terminal airflow setpoints (8 settings)								**X**
Establish minimum and maximum limits for thermostat setpoints								**X**
Establish revised deadband settings for space heating and cooling setpoints								**X**

(continued on next page)

Retrocommissioning *(contuinued)*

Master List	Retrocommissioning Process Sources							
Retrocommissioning Activity	ACG	GSA	ASHRAE	LEED	APPA	NEBB	PECI	**ASHE**
Determine goals that are compatible with existing system capacities						X	X	
Develop plan and cost for replacing dysfunctional components						X		**X**
Review additional considerations						X8		
Prepare corrective action report							X9	**X**
Revise project plan and schedule						X		**X**
Obtain owners approval for cost of replacement						X	X	**X**
Develop contracts for repair of systems						X10		
Document energy and demand goals for equipment						X		**X**
Update retrocommissioning plan and schedule						X		**X**
Develop functional performance test procedures for systems to be retrocommissioned						X	X	
Coordinate participation of owner's staff in systems performance testing						X		**X**
Provide appropriate training for staff						X		**X**
Advise occupants of timetable and impacts of testing						X		
Correct easily fixable deficiencies						X	X	**X**
Assess the results of retrocommissioning programs						X		X	**X**
Prepare the report to owner						X	X	**X**
Establish operational stability						X		**X**
Conduct site investigations							X	**X**
Confirm use of site datalogger							X11	**X**
Perform design calculations/studies							X12	
Conduct a lessons learned workshop							X	**X**

[1] Identify and assess current facility HVAC commissioning requirements (CFR)—NEBB Retro (p. 32). The retrocommissioning agent (RCxA) must update the original OPR to create a current CFR. If no OPR exists, the RCxA should create a CFR for a retrocommissioning of existing buildings (RCx-EB) project. The CFR will be updated and expanded as the project proceeds to completion.

[2] Analyze energy cost benefits—ASHE (p.72). Identify and evaluate potential supply-side and demand-side energy cost reduction opportunities to reduce energy expenditures.

[3] Conduct documentation and site reviews—ASHE (p. 71). ASHE identifies the need for a review of the construction drawings and specifications developed for the original construction and any renovations to the facility.

[4] Conduct functional performance tests—ASHE (p. 72). ASHE recommends detailed testing of water and air systems in order to record and measure data that determine power consumption and electrical demand.

[5] Develop assessment of performance goals vs. system capacities—ASHE (p. 72). ASHE recommends comparing the actual performance of the equipment to the manufacturers' rated performance data to identify discrepancies.

[6] Analyze existing documentation—ASHE (p. 71). ASHE recommends obtaining and reviewing the major equipment submittal data from the original construction and any renovations.

[7] Analyze existing physical conditions—ASHE (p. 72). ASHE recommends conducting a detailed survey of the facility, focusing on the mechanical and electrical rooms as well as any energy-consuming equipment and systems. Also, review in detail the automatic temperature control systems and identify existing sequences of operation.

[8] Review additional considerations—APPA (p. 130). Additional considerations include the need to clean ductwork and rebalance systems. One of the common goals of retrocommissioning is to maximize the capability of the ventilation systems because the function of old, tired systems has slowly degraded over the years.

[9] Prepare corrective action report—NEBB Retro (p. 37). The RCxA meets with the owner to present the findings and recommendations from the retrocommissioning process. Specifically, the meeting should identify how the recommended solutions improve the building performance issues based on the identified CFR.

[10] Develop contracts for repair of systems—APPA (p. 131). To prepare the contract for rebalancing the HVAC systems, the CxA will need to provide a set of systems drawings that clearly identify the layout of the systems and the new air distribution quantities for every supply air outlet diffuser or grille and exhaust air inlet grille and provide the total air volumes for the fans serving the systems. Duct cleaning and rebalancing of systems should be performed if needed.

[11] Confirm use of site data loggers—NEBB Retro (p. 34). During the early stages of the site investigation phase, the RCxA should have launched data loggers throughout the facility to establish existing operating parameters such as temperature, humidity, lighting levels, air pressure, timed events, etc. If the control system has been calibrated, it can be used instead of the data loggers to obtain data trends.

[12] Perform design calculations/studies—NEBB Retro (p. 34). The building may require design calculations where site investigations have determined that significant changes from the intent of previous designs have occurred. These studies/calculations may include fire and life safety calculations, energy load calculations, electrical power and lighting calculations, domestic water usage and sanitary/storm drainage calculations, etc. The studies/calculations may be performed by any member of the RCx-EB team qualified to do so. If performed by an RCx-EB team member other than the RCxA, the RCxA should review the calculations. This information will be used to determine changes required to improve existing building systems.

Sample Commissioning Request for Qualifications

SOLICITATION FOR COMMISSIONING SERVICES

(Owner)
(Project Name)
(Location)

(Date)

BACKGROUND

(**Owner**) is seeking the services of a qualified Health Facility Commissioning Authority (HFCxA) for a new health care construction project. The project is a (**Project description, including current status and schedule**).

The project is presently in the design phase. Construction is anticipated to begin in (**Month-year**) and to be completed in (**Month-year**).

The design of the project is by (**Architect and/or Engineer**). (**Construction Manager Firm Name**) is the Construction Manager. The HFCxA will report to the Owner. The Owner's Representative is:

(Owner's Rep Name)
(Title-if applicable)
(Company)
(Address)
(City, ST ZIP)

SCOPE OF WORK

The primary role of the HFCxA is to ensure that the Owner's Project Requirements (OPR) are developed during the planning phase and are achieved through the design, construction, and operation of the facility.

The following is a summary of the commissioning process the Owner intends to have implemented on this project. This process is as defined in the ASHE *Health Facility Commissioning Guidelines*. For this proposal, the following process will be followed.

I. COMMISSIONING PROCESS

A. Commissioning Process during Design

   1) Meetings

   a) Predesign conference—The HFCxA will organize and attend a predesign conference at the beginning of the Design Phase. The HFCxA will prepare an agenda for the meeting that addresses the project goals, scope, team member responsibilities, delivery process, project budget, schedule, and performance expectations.

   b) Design review meetings—The HFCxA will be required to attend the design review meetings at the end of each design phase (SD, DD, CD). The meetings will be held at the (Architect's *complete as appropriate*) office in (City, State).

   2) Owner's project requirements (OPR)—The HFCxA will facilitate development of the OPR. The Owner, design team, and HFCxA will work collaboratively to develop the OPR.

   a) The HFCxA will work with the Owner, design team, and contractor or third-party project manager hired by the Owner to establish an aggressive yet attainable and fiscally responsible energy efficiency goal.

   b) The HFCxA will chair an OPR charrette and prepare an agenda for the charrette that covers all elements of the OPR as defined in the ASHE *Health Facility Commissioning Guidelines*.

   c) The HFCxA will prepare a draft of the OPR from the minutes of the OPR charrette for for final review and comment by the participants. The HFCxA will prepare a final OPR based on the draft review comments. The HFCxA will modify the OPR as the project progresses through the design and construction phases.

   3) Commissioning specifications

   a) The HFCxA will develop full commissioning specifications based on the OPR.

   b) The HFCxA will coordinate with the design team to integrate the commissioning specifications into the project specifications prepared by the project architect and engineers.

c) The commissioning specifications will include the elements defined in the ASHE *Health Facility Commissioning Guidelines*, including a detailed description of the responsibilities of all the parties, details of the commissioning process, reporting and documentation requirements (including formats), deficiency resolution, pre-functional checklist requirements, functional testing requirements, test and balancing requirements, training, O&M manuals, record document requirements, and retesting responsibilities.

4) Design documents—The HFCxA will review the design documents with a focus on commissionability, design completeness, cost-effectiveness, coordination of trades, and energy efficiency. The HFCxA will include the hospital O&M staff in this review. For each review, the HFCxA will prepare a written list of comments for the Owner and design team. The HFCxA will conduct the following reviews:

a) Basis of design (BOD)—Review the BOD to verify compliance with the OPR. The design engineer is to provide the BOD documentation for use during this review.

b) Plan reviews—Perform reviews at 100% completion of schematic design documents (SDs), design development documents (DDs), and construction documents (CDs).

c) HVAC control system sequences of operation—Review these sequences carefully to make certain they contain adequate detail and incorporate energy-efficient processes (e.g., static pressure setpoint reset, supply air temperature setpoint reset, occupancy sensors, unoccupied/occupied air changes rates, weekly scheduling with optimal start/stop, etc.).

4) Utility management plan (UMP)—The HFCxA will facilitate the development of the UMP. The HFCxA will work with the facility manager, design team, and contractor to facilitate development of the plan prior to completion of the final design. The UMP will include all the components as outlined in the ASHE *Health Facility Commissioning Guidelines*.

6) Commissioning plan—The HFCxA will develop a commissioning plan that encompasses the design, construction, and occupancy and operations phases. In the design phase, the HFCxA will develop the initial commissioning plan, including the following:

a) A project-specific description of equipment to be commissioned

b) A description of the roles of the HFCx team, including the responsibilities of the Owner, A/E, contractors, and HFCxA

    c) Sample prototypical pre-functional checklists (PFCs) for each piece of equipment in the commissioning scope

    d) Sample prototypical functional performance tests (FPTs) that define acceptable results of the tests to be performed

B. Commissioning Process During Construction and Acceptance Phases

  1) Meetings

    a) Kick-off meeting—The HFCxA will plan and conduct a pre-construction commissioning meeting within 60 days of contract award.

    b) Commissioning meetings—The HFCxA will coordinate and direct the commissioning activities in conjunction with the contractor and/or construction manager in a logical, sequential, and efficient manner using consistent protocols, clear and regular communications and consultations with all necessary parties, frequently updated timelines and schedules, and technical expertise. Meetings will be held as necessary to coordinate the commissioning process. At minimum, the HFCxA will conduct "milestone meetings" at the beginning of each phase of commissioning, including the following:

        i. Shop drawing submission
        ii. Equipment installation
        iii. Creation of pre-functional checklists
        iv. Equipment start-up
        v. Functional performance testing
        vi. Submission of operating and maintenance manuals
        vii. Owner training
        viii. Seasonal testing
        ix. One-year warranty testing

    c) Project meetings—The HFCxA will review the minutes of the regular project meetings and attend selected project meetings as needed to resolve issues and concerns and coordinate the commissioning process.

  2) Construction phase commissioning plan—The HFCxA will revise the commissioning plan developed during design, including scope and schedule, as necessary.

    a) The HFCxA will prepare project-specific pre-functional checklists (PFCs) for each piece of equipment in the commissioning scope and include these in the commissioning plan. Generic PFCs or equipment start-up checklists are not acceptable.

b) Prepare project-specific functional performance test (FPT) procedures that define acceptable results of the tests to be performed and include these in the commissioning plan. Generic FPTs are not acceptable.

3) Reviews

a) Shop drawings—The HFCxA will review contractor submittals applicable to systems being commissioned to ensure compliance with the commissioning plan, commissioning specifications, and OPR. The HFCxA also reviews these documents with facility O&M personnel. The HFCxA will forward comments and concerns in writing to the design team and the Owner. Reviews must be concurrent with A/E reviews, must be conducted in a timely manner, and must not affect the construction schedule of the contractor.

b) O&M manuals—The HFCxA will review the manuals to ensure proper content and format.

c) Start-up plan—The HFCxA will review the start-up plan to ensure operational parameters outlined in the OPR will be met. The review will include start-up training procedures for maintenance personnel who will be operating the equipment after occupancy.

d) HVAC control system programming—The HFCxA will review the programs before implementation and again after implementation to ensure proper performance of the HVAC system.

e) Training program—The HFCxA will review training procedures for all equipment included in the commissioning plan to ensure an appropriate transition to operational sustainability by maintenance personnel. These training procedures should be specific to the unique parameters the O&M staff will need to manage to ensure the equipment performs at the desired efficiencies outlined in the OPR. These training procedures are in addition to standard training in systems operation normally associated with turnover/takeover activities at the end of a project.

f) TAB report—The HFCxA will review the testing, adjusting, and balancing (TAB) report prepared by the contractor and prepare a written response. The HFCxA will also spot-check a representative sample of airflow and water flow readings as documented in the TAB report. The duration of the sampling will be two eight-hour days.

g) Record drawings—The HFCxA will review the record drawings with O&M personnel and identify known discrepancies between these documents and as-installed conditions. The HFCxA will forward a list of these discrepancies to the Owner, contractor, and design team for incorporation into the record documents.

4) Scheduling—The HFCxA will coordinate the commissioning tasks with the general contractor (GC) and construction manager (CM) to ensure that commissioning activities are included in their master schedule. The HFCxA will develop a testing plan for all equipment, systems, and integrated systems.

5) O&M staff construction site tours—The HFCxA will lead facility O&M personnel on regular tours of the construction site, discussing the equipment, systems, OPR, BOD, scheduled maintenance requirements, sequences of operation, and so on. The HFCxA maintains a list of O&M staff comments and concerns and works with the contractor and design team to respond to these.

6) Pre-functional inspections and checklists—The HFCxA will execute the PFCs in phases (e.g., equipment installation, piping rough-in, electrical rough-in, controls rough-in, feeder and load side termination for electrical systems, etc.) as the work progresses. The purpose of this process is to document that installation occurs per the contract documents as the work is installed rather than waiting until all installation is complete. Resolution of deficiencies is documented on subsequent site visits. All elements of equipment and system installation and all PFCs must be complete prior to functional testing.

7) Equipment and systems start-up—The HFCxA reviews equipment start-up procedures, witnesses the start-up of critical systems, and reviews the completed start-up documentation.

8) Functional performance tests—The HFCxA will direct execution of the functional performance tests by the responsible subcontractors. The FPTs are conducted at design full load, part load, and emergency conditions. The tests proceed from tests of simple system to tests of complex system to tests of integrated systems. The HFCxA invites O&M personnel to attend and witness testing. The HFCxA documents test results and recommends systems for acceptance.

a) Facilitate pressure testing—Per ASHE *Health Facility Commissioning Guidelines* requirements, pressure testing will be conducted on isolation rooms and associated anterooms, operating rooms, procedure rooms, airborne infection isolation (AII) rooms, and protective environment (PE) rooms.

b) Fire and smoke damper testing—The HFCxA will verify that all dampers have been tested per the ASHE *Health Facility Commissioning Guidelines* and provide a report (as defined in those guidelines) that lists each damper number, damper location, date of inspection, and damper inspection results.

c) The HFCxA will functionally test O&M dashboards and document the accuracy of the data they report.

d) The HFCxA will document that specified trends are implemented and operational as required by the commissioning specifications.

9) Site visits—The HFCxA will perform site visits, as necessary, to observe component and system installations.

a) Maintain a master issues log and separate testing record. The log will include a definition of each issue, the date it was identified, a proposed corrective plan, the responsible party, the date of anticipated resolution, and its current status.

b) Provide the Owner with written progress reports and test results with recommended actions.

10) Training

a) The HFCxA will monitor scheduling and execution of the training process to ensure it is conducted as specified and as planned in the training program. The HFCxA will also monitor recordings made of the training process to ensure their quality is acceptable according to specifications.

b) The HFCxA will develop testing to assess the O&M staff's knowledge.

11) Final commissioning report and systems manual—The HFCxA will complete the commissioning report and a systems manual for turnover/takeover at the completion of the construction phase. These documents will conform to the requirements of the ASHE *Health Facility Commissioning Guidelines*.

C. Commissioning During the Occupancy and Operation Phases

1) Maintenance budget—The HFCxA will facilitate development of the facility's maintenance budget. The recommended staffing level and maintenance budget for the facility should be determined using

benchmarking tools such as those defined in the ASHE *Health Facility Commissioning Guidelines*.

2) Maintenance program—The HFCxA will facilitate development of the facility's maintenance program. The scope of the HFCxA's involvement in the development and implementation of the maintenance management program will be as recommended in the ASHE *Health Facility Commissioning Guidelines*.

3) Testing—Coordinate required seasonal or deferred testing and deficiency corrections and provide final testing documentation for the commissioning record and O&M manuals.

4) Postoccupancy visits—The HFCxA will return to the site 10 months into the 12-month warranty period and review with facility staff the current building operation and the condition of outstanding issues related to the original and seasonal commissioning. Also interview facility staff and identify problems or concerns they have with operating the building as originally intended.

5) Documents to address continuing problems—The HFCxA will assist facility staff in developing reports and documents and requests for services to remedy outstanding problems.

6) Lessons learned meeting—The HFCxA will accomplish a meeting with the Owner, contractors, designers, operators, and occupants one year after occupancy to identify lessons learned.

7) Measurement and verification (M&V)

   a) The HFCxA will work with the facility manager to establish a Portfolio Manager account on the EPA Energy Star website.

   b) The HFCxA will help the facility manager enter actual electricity, heating fuel, and water consumption and costs into the Portfolio Manager account.

   c) The HFCxA will assist the facility manager with development of an energy efficiency scorecard and assist the facility manager in publishing the scorecard each month.

   d) If the actual Energy Star rating is less than the target Energy Star rating, the HFCxA will work with the facility manager, design team, and contractor to identify the cause of the disparity and implement corrective action (provide a 40 man-hour contingency for the investigation into why the ES rating is less than the target).

2. WHAT THE COMMISSIONING AUTHORITY IS NOT RESPONSIBLE FOR

The HFCxA is not responsible for design concept, design criteria, compliance with codes, design or general construction scheduling, cost estimating, or construction management. The HFCxA may assist with problem-solving or resolving non-conformance or deficiencies, but ultimately that responsibility resides with the architect and the general contractor.

3. SYSTEMS AND ASSEMBLIES TO BE COMMISSIONED

A. The following systems are to be commissioned:

1) Building Envelope

    a) Insulation

    b) Glazing

    c) Vapor barriers

    d) All elements of the building exterior wall

    e) Roof

    f) Building pressure testing

2) Life Safety

    a) Fire-resistive ratings

    b) Smoke barriers

    c) Smoke-tight partitions

    d) Stair pressurization system

    e) Fire command center

3) HVAC Systems

    a) Air terminals

    b) Induction units

    c) Fan coil units

    d) Unit heaters

    e) Air-handling units

    f) Energy recovery units

    g) Exhaust system

    h) Chilled water system

    i) Heating water system

    j) Steam system

    k) Humidifiers

    l) Fire and smoke dampers

    m) Special applications

        • Operating rooms (anesthetizing locations)

        • Airborne infection isolation (AII) rooms

        • Protective environment (PE) rooms

        • Data center

        • Pharmacy

        • Imaging

4) Controls

    a) Workstations

    b) System graphics and dashboards

    c) Networks

    d) Controllers

    e) Sensors

    f) Actuators

    g) Meters

5) Plumbing Systems

    a) Domestic cold water

        • Meter

        • Backflow preventers

        • Booster pump

- ◆ Water softener
- b) Domestic hot water
  - ◆ Water heater
  - ◆ Recirculation system
- c) Sump pumps
- d) Natural gas
- e) Fuel oil
- f) Propane or synthetic natural gas
- g) Disinfection systems
- h) Rainwater harvesting
- i) Process cooling

6) Medical Gas Systems

- a) Oxygen
- b) Bulk oxygen system
- c) Remote oxygen supply connection
- d) Nitrogen
- e) Nitrous oxide
- f) Medical vacuum
- g) Waste anesthesia gas disposal
- h) Instrument air
- i) Medical air
- j) Manifold rooms
- k) Master and area alarms
- l) Valves
  - ◆ Source
  - ◆ Future
  - ◆ Riser
  - ◆ Service
  - ◆ Zone

7) Electrical Systems

- a) Meter
- b) Primary transformers
- c) Main switchgear
- d) Panelboards
- e) Isolated power systems
- f) Power conditioners
- g) Power factor correction equipment
- h) Uninterruptible power supplies
- i) Step-down transformers
- j) Generators
- k) Paralleling switchgear
- l) Automatic transfer switches
- m) Lightning protection systems
- n) Grounding systems

8) Fire Alarm System

- a) Workstations
- b) Controllers
- c) Sensing devices
- d) Interface with life safety systems
- e) Interface with fire protection system
- f) Interface with HVAC system
- g) Interface with elevators

9) Information Technology

- a) Telephone
- b) Data
- c) Intercom
- d) Paging
- e) Doctor's dictation
- f) Telemetry
- g) Security
- h) Master clock
- i) Dedicated antenna
- j) Television
- k) Nurse call

l) Infant abduction

m) Wireless access points

n) Cellular phone repeaters

10) Fire Protection System

a) Backflow preventer

b) Fire pump/jockey pump

c) Drains

d) Tamper and flow switches

e) Valves

f) Fire department connections

g) Standpipes

h) Sprinkler heads

i) Pre-action systems

j) Clean agent systems

11) Interior Lighting

a) Occupancy sensors

b) Controls

12) Exterior Lighting

a) Controls

b) Illumination levels

13) Refrigeration

a) Food services refrigerators

b) Food services freezers

c) Clinical refrigerators and freezers

d) Blood banks

14) Vertical Transport

a) Elevators

b) Escalators

c) Dumbwaiters

15) Materials and Pharmaceutical Handling

a) Pneumatic tube

b) Linen and trash conveyance

c) Electronic transportation vehicles (ETVs)

4. DESIRED QUALIFICATIONS

A. Principal HFCxA

It is desired that the person designated as the principal HFCxA satisfy the following requirements:

1) Has acted as the principal HFCxA for at least three projects of equivalent or larger size during the past three years.

2) Is experienced in the quality process.

3) Has extensive experience in the operation and troubleshooting of HVAC systems, energy management control systems, and lighting controls systems. Extensive field experience is required. A minimum of five full years in this type of work is required.

4) Is knowledgeable in building operation and maintenance and O&M training.

5) Is knowledgeable in test and balance of both air and water systems.

6) Is experienced in energy-efficient equipment design and control strategy optimization.

7) Has direct experience in monitoring and analyzing system operation using energy management control system trending and stand-alone data logging equipment.

8) Has excellent verbal and written communication skills. Highly organized and able to work with both management and trade contractors.

9) Has a bachelor's degree in Mechanical Engineering and PE certification.

B. HFCxA Team Members

The HFCxA firm will demonstrate depth of experienced personnel and capability to sustain loss of assigned personnel without compromising quality and timeliness of performance.

4. INSTRUCTIONS TO PROPOSERS

A proposer must include execution of all phases of commissioning in a single proposal. The proposal must be signed by an officer of your firm with the authority to commit the firm.

A. Provide a summary description of your firm's commissioning experience within the past five years.

B. Provide a detailed project organizational chart indicating names of dedicated project staff and their specific duties and responsibilities. Provide an organizational chart of your firm.

C. List the key individual who will serve as the principal HFCxA for this contract and describe his or her relevant qualifications and experience. This information is required in addition to any detailed resumes the proposer submits. The contract will require that this individual be committed to the project for its duration.

D. Provide project and professional references and experience for three to five commissioning projects for which the proposer was the principal HFCxA in the last three years. Include a description of each project, identify when the proposer came into the project, and describe the involvement of each individual on the proposer's team in the project. For each project, attach a sheet that includes the name and telephone number of the Owner's project manager.

E. Describe your proposed approach to managing the project expertly and efficiently, including your team participation. Describe what approach you will take to integrate commissioning into the normal design and construction process. Describe what you will do to foster teamwork and cooperation from contractors and designers.

F. As an attachment, provide the following work products written by members of the proposer's team:

1) Commissioning plan that was executed

2) Commissioning specifications

3) An actual Functional Test Procedure that was executed

5. ADDITIONAL CONDITIONS

Owner is not obligated to request clarifications or additional information but may do so at its discretion. Owner reserves the right to extend the deadline for submittals.

Award, if made, shall be to the responsible HFCxA whose proposal is determined in writing to be the most advantageous for the Owner, taking into account all of the evaluation factors set forth in this RFP. No other factors or criteria shall be used in the evaluation. The Owner reserves the right to reject any and all proposals submitted in response to this RFP.

Confidentiality of documents: Upon receipt of a proposal by Owner, the proposal shall become the property of the Owner without compensation to the submitting firm.

6. RESPONSES ARE DUE (DATE)

Please provide (**xx**) paper copies or one electronic copy (e-mail, CD, or thumb drive media is acceptable).

Sample RFQ
Evaluation Form

Proposal submitted by: _____ Date: _____

Proposal reviewed by: _____ Date: _____

#	Factor	Rating (1-5)[1]	Weight (1 to y)[2]	Total Points[3]	Comment
	Example	*4*	*3*	*12*	
1	Size of firm				
2	% of work that is commissioning				
3	Evaluated qualifications				
4	Fee				
5	Location (proximity to site)				
6	Rated expertise area #1 (List)				
7	Rated expertise area #2 (List)				
8	Rated expertise area #3 (List)				
9	Commissioning methodology				
10	Completeness of RFQ answers				
11	Overall impression				
	TOTAL				

[1] The health facility commissioning authority is rated for each factor on a scale of 1 to 5, with 5 being the highest and 1 the lowest.

[2] For each project, assign a weight to the factors based on their importance in choosing a health facility commissioning authority. Use a scale from 1 to y (the total number of factors to be evaluated, 11 in the example given) in which 1 is the most important and y is the least important factor.

[3] The total score for each factor is calculated using this formula: Rating x Weight = Total Points.

Sample HFCxA Interview Evaluation Form

Proposal submitted by: _____ Date: _____

Proposal reviewed by: _____ Date: _____

#	Item	Rating (1 to 5)[1]	Weight (1 to y)[2]	Total Points[3]	Comment
	Example	*4*	*3*	*12*	
1	Presentation effectiveness				
2	Ability to stay on project focus				
3	Team experience				
4	Discussion of methodology				
5	Complete presentation within time				
6	Overall impression				
	TOTAL				

[1] The health facility commissioning authority is rated for each factor on a scale of 1 to 5, with 5 being the highest and 1 the lowest.

[2] For each project, assign a weight to the factors based on their importance in choosing a health facility commissioning authority. Use a scale from 1 to **y** (the total number of factors to be evaluated, 6 in the example given) in which 1 is the most important and **y** is the least important factor.

[3] The total score for each factor is calculated using this formula: Rating × Weight = Total Points.

Sample HFCxA
Selection Form

Proposal submitted by: _____ Date: _____

Proposal reviewed by: _____ Date: _____

#	Item	RFQ Points	Interview Points	Total Points	Comment
	Example	54	27	81	
1	Company A				
2	Company B				
3	Company C				
	Final Selection is:				

Note: The total points are calculated by adding together the RFQ points and the interview points.

Sample Predesign Phase HFCx Responsibilities and Tasks Matrix

Task	Predesign Phase Health Facility Commissioning (HFCx) Responsibilities and Tasks		HFCx Design Team Members						
			Owner's representative	Facility manager	Team member	Team member	Team member	Team member	HFCx authority
1	Overall coordination of Cx during predesign	Lead							*
	a. Plan and schedule meetings.								*
	b. Distribute meeting minutes.								*
	c. See that all tasks are completed.								*
2	Develop documentation of owner's project requirements (OPR).	Lead	*						
	a. Assist in the development of the OPR.		*	*	*	*	*	*	*
	b. Review and comment on development of the OPR.		*	*	*	*	*	*	*
	c. Distribute final document.		*						
3	Develop commissioning plan (CP).	Lead							*
	a. Review and comment on development of CP.		*	*	*	*	*	*	*
	b. Distribute final document.								*
	c. Maintain CP.								*
4	Identify commissioning team communications.	Lead							*
	a. Identify the means and methods of communications for the commissioning team.		*						*
	b. Encourage and expedite communications between team members.								*
5	Provide and maintain commissioning deficiency log for predesign phase commissioning tasks.	Lead							*
	a. Develop and distribute deficiency log.								*
	b. Review log and respond appropriately.		*	*	*	*	*	*	*
5	Develop predesign schedule.	Lead							*
	a. Participate in the development of the predesign phase commissioning schedule.		*	*	*	*	*	*	*
	b. Distribute and maintain predesign commissioning schedule.								*

Sample Matrix for Preparing a Utility Management Plan (UMP)

[Facility] Utility Management Plan Required Environment of Care Compliance Documentation

[Company] Project #/Name:

Category	TEST TYPE or Documentation Required	Initial Testing of Inspection Required	TJC EC # or other	CODE REF
EC Mgt + Risk	EC Utility Systems Management Plan		01.01.01 EP8, 04.01.01 EP15	NA
EC Mgt + Risk	PRA for project area		02.06.05 EP2 EP3	NA
Safety Security	Identify EC safety risks. Risks are identified from internal sources such as ongoing monitoring of the environment, results of root cause analyses, results of annual proactive risk assessments of high-risk processes and from credible external sources such as SEAS.	Yes	02.01.01 EP1, 04.01.01 EP14, LD.04.0405 EP7, EP8, EP10	NA; these are safety risks other than those handled by specific codes (mentioned below).
Safety Security	The hospital takes action to minimize or eliminate identified safety risks in the physical environment.		02.01.01 EP3	NA
EC Mgt + Risk	Leaders identify an individual(s) to manage risk, coordinate risk reduction activities in the physical environment, collect deficiency information (including injuries, problems, or use errors), and disseminate summaries of actions and results.		01.01.01 EP1, 04.01.01 EP1	NA
EC Mgt + Risk	Leaders identify an individual(s) to intervene whenever environmental conditions immediately threaten life or health or threaten to damage equipment or buildings.		01.01.01 EP2, LD.04.04.05 EP5	NA
EC Mgt + Risk	EC Safety Management Plan		01.01.01 EP3, 04.01.01 EP15	NA
EC Mgt + Risk	EC Security Management Plan		01.01.01 EP4, 04.01.01 EP15, 02.01.01	NA
EC Mgt + Risk	EC Hazardous Materials and Waste Management Plan		01.01.01 EP5, 04.01.01 EP15	NA
EC Mgt + Risk	EC Fire Safety Management Plan		01.01.01 EP6, 04.01.01 EP15	NA

RESP	START DATE	GC Responsibility				Owner Responsibility				Verified Exists (Y/NA)	Reviewed (Y/NA)	Detailed Status	Detailed Status	COMPANY CONFIDENITAL	Ongoing	NEW HOSPITAL Order #
		# of DAYS	Tickler Date	Due Date	RECEIVED	# of DAYS	Tickler Date	Due Date	RECEIVED					COMMENTS or N/A for this project		
Owner														Verify signed-off Utility Systems Management Plan includes project area	A	7
Owner											NA			Verify PRA was done for all areas covered by the project. Verify documentation of action taken as a result of PRA.	Yes	NA because no patients
Owner											NA			Verify safety risk assessments were done. Safety Management Plan should identify processes (EC tours proactivity, external sources) for risk assessments.		NA because no patients
Owner											NA			Safety Management Plan should include this process. Establish schedule and personnel for safety rounds with management processes.		7
Owner											NA			Signed appointment letter, position description	A	3
Owner											NA			Signed appointment letter, position description	A	I
Owner														Verify signed-off Safety Management Plan includes project area.	A	7
Owner														Verify signed-off Security Management Plan includes project area.	A	7
Owner														Verify signed-off Hazardous Materials and Waste Management Plan includes project area.	A	7
Owner														Verify signed-off Fire Safety Management Plan includes project area.	A	7

Sample Commissioning Conference Agenda

I. Introductions and sign-in

II. Commissioning goal

   A. Team approach to documenting completion of project per construction documents

   B. Commissioning to be done in accordance with the project specifications

III. Equipment and systems to be commissioned *(see master equipment list)*

   A. HVAC systems

   B. Domestic hot water systems

   C. Water softener, R.O. system, elevator sump pump, fire protection pump

   D. Normal electrical power distribution systems

   E. Emergency power/automatic transfer switches

   F. Nurse call system

   G. Security system

IV. Commissioning tasks *(responsibilities)*

Issue commissioning plan updates. (HFCxA).

   A. Integrate activation of building systems in the project schedule. (contractor).

     1) The contractor should include activation of the following on the overall project schedule:

       a) Natural gas service

       b) Water service

    c) Electrical service

  2) The schedule should include, at minimum, each element listed below in Section VII (Milestones and project phases) for each system to be commissioned.

    a) Review submittals and shop drawings. (HFCxA)

    b) Complete startup plan and forward to HFCxA. (contractors).

    c) Complete initial training plan and forward to HFCxA. (contractors)

    d) Complete prefunctional checklists. (HFCxA)

    e) Perform fire and fire/smoke damper testing. (HFCxA)

    f) Conduct O&M staff tours. (HFCxA)

    g) Review control system programming. (HFCxA)

    h) Complete startup and compile documentation, including duct and pipe pressure testing and pipe flushing reports, and forward to the HFCxA. (contractors)

    i) Review testing and balancing report. (HFCxA)

    j) Conduct demonstration of systems (contractors); direct and document demonstration/performance. (HFCxA)

    k) Perform pressure testing. (contractors and HFCxA)

    l) Review O&M manual and record drawings. (HFCxA)

    m) Compile/prepare data for systems manual. (contractors and HFCxA)

    n) Review contractor-provided training. (HFCxA)

V. COMMISSIONING DOCUMENTATION (CONTRACTORS)

  A. The contractor should forward the following to the HFCxA:

    1) Shop drawings

    2) Record drawings

    3) Duct and pipe pressure testing reports

    4) Cleaning and flushing procedures and records

    5) Startup plan and records

    6) Training plan and records

    7) Testing and balancing report

    8) Certifications

a) Fire alarm system

b) Medical gas system

9) O&M and systems manual data

B. The HFCxA will review and provide comments on the above and distribute comments to the project team. The project team should review the comments and address them in writing to the HFCxA.

VI. Milestones and project phase discussion

A. Shop drawing phase

B. Site visits by the HFCxA

1) Installation documentation (pre-functional checklist execution)

2) O&M staff tours during construction

C. Permanent services (power, natural gas, water)

D. Startup of systems, including the use and maintenance of building systems for temporary heating and cooling (if planned)

E. Owner training

F. HVAC testing and balancing

G. HVAC control system calibration and point-to-point verification

H. Functional testing

I. Integrated systems testing

J. Project turnover

1) Final report

2) O&M manuals

3) Systems manual

4) Dashboards

5) HVAC trends

6) Measurement and verification (M&V)

K. Opposite season testing

L. End-of-warranty period review and meetings

VII. Commissioning deliverables (HFCxA)

A. Reviews defined above

B. Meeting minutes

C. Site visit reports, including current issues log

D. Testing plan

E. Functional performance testing and integrated systems testing documentation

F. Commissioning progress reports

G. Final report

H. Systems manual

VIII. Communications

A. Commissioning team meetings—These will be held as needed throughout construction, including one meeting to be held prior to functional testing.

B. Commissioning deliverables—Most of the deliverables (see item VII just above) will be shared with all or part of the commissioning team to communicate progress, issues that require attention, or schedule. Some clients may desire to review deliverables before distribution to the entire project commissioning team, so the HFCxA will coordinate distribution procedures with the client.

C. Resolution of items noted in the issues log—Items noted in the issues log will be addressed by the responsible party. This party will notify the HFCxA in writing when the item has been corrected/addressed and the HFCxA will back-check the item as corrected/addressed then close out the item on the issues log.

IX. OPEN DISCUSSION/QUESTIONS AND COMMENTS

Sample Issues Log

Note: This sample is an excerpt from a project issues log.

Expansion of ABC Hospital

As of: _____ (Date)

Item #	Equip-ment	Room Number	Obser-vation Date	Description	Refer-ence	Notes	Category	Date Cx Verified
1	CT-3, 4, 5	Roof	1/21/09	LPS connection to steam basin heater does not comply with piping detail on H605: no strainer is installed, isolation valve is not installed on downstream of the control valve, and pressure gauge is not installed.	H605 Detail	11/12/09 – Corrections complete. Item closed.	Pre-Functional	HFCxA 11/12/09
2	RF-6	Mechanical 5M00M01	9/22/09	Access to bolted access door on unit casing is impeded by motor housing on adjacent fan. This door appears to be the only way to service the fan bearings.	Access/ Service Require-ment	12/15/09 – Accepted by owner, as un-necessary for maintenance.	Pre-Functional	HFCxA 12/15/09
3	AHU-6	Level 5	9/22/09	Factory-provided coil piping in interior of unit – plugs for flow control valves were oriented so that there was only 3-½-in. of clearance between the top of the plugs and rigid obstructions in the units. Our concern is that the balancer will not be able to insert flow meter tips without the valves being rotated. This will most likely be a typical comment for all units.	15500-3.16G4	1/18/10 – TAB contractor has stated the clear-ance is sufficient as is. Item closed.	Pre-Functional	HFCxA 1/18/10
4	TB-142	Greeter RN1 112	9/22/09	Coil HHW return piping and domestic water piping are run in close contact, which will prevent the specified thick-ness of insulation from being applied to both. Specification 15500-2.33U requires a minimum ½-in. space from finished covering and adjacent work.	15500-2.33U		Pre-Functional	
5	Exhaust Air Valves (Typical)	Various Locations	9/22/09	H707 Detail requires air valves to be in-dependently supported. None of the air valves installed on the 3rd Floor this far are provided with independent support.	H707 Exhaust Air Valve Detail	12/15/09 – Cor-rection in prog-ress. 1/13/10 – Additional locations noted: EV-605; EV-704; EV-705; and EV-706.	Pre-Functional	

(continued)

SAMPLE ISSUES LOG *(continued)*

Item #	Equip-ment	Room Number	Obser-vation Date	Description	Refer-ence	Notes	Category	Date Cx Verified
6	Interim CHWS FPT	Control Room (Pent-house)	11/12/09	When the refrigerant differential pressure is at its minimum and the con-denser water differential pressure is at its minimum, the CW setpoint will reset to 70 degrees as required, but the bypass valve will not operate to allow the CW to meet the setpoint.	Chilled Water Sequence of Opera-tions	Informational note for owner on existing sys-tem – Not part of B3C project scope.	Functional Performance Test	
7	Interim CHWS FPT	Control Room (Pent-house)	11/12/09	The second cooling tower in the free cooling mode would not stage up prop-erly. BCM added the second cooling tower to the program to maintain the condenser water temperature during the free cooling mode.	Chilled Water Sequence of Opera-tions	11/12/09 – BCM corrected the issue and the second tower is staging up cor-rectly.	Functional Performance Test	SRM 11/12/09
8	CT-2	Roof	11/12/09	The isolation valve for CT-2 did not close when the cooling tower shut down. BCM controls corrected the program on-site.	Chilled Water Sequence of Opera-tions	11/12/09 – BCM corrected the program to allow the isolation valve to close.	Functional Performance Test	SRM 11/12/09
9	Interim CHWS FPT	Control Room (Pent-house)	11/12/09	The BAS controls graphics will not indicate when the condenser water set-point resets to 46 degrees F in the free cooling mode, and does indicate that the system is in free cooling mode.	Chilled Water Sequence of Opera-tions	Informational note for owner on existing sys-tem – Not part of XYZ project scope.	Functional Performance Test	
10	Interim CHWS FPT	Control Room (Pent-house)	11/12/09	The condenser water temperature sen-sor is located before the bypass valve, but the sensor needs to be located after the bypass valve. The sensor needs to be relocated to allow the low con-denser water temperature sequence in mechanical cooling to operate correctly, and also when the system is transferring from free cooling to mechanical cooling.	Chilled Water Sequence of Opera-tions	Informational note for owner on existing sys-tem – Not part of XYZ project scope.	Functional Performance Test	
11	FCU-4; CT-3, 4, 5	Mechani-cal Room	11/12/09	Valve tags have not been installed as specified on valves serving this equip-ment.	15500-3.7E1		Pre-Functional	
12	CT-3, 4, 5	Roof	11/12/09	Specifications require new CW, LPS, and LPC piping aluminum insulation jacketing to be secured by 1-in. bands on 12-in. centers. We noted that small diameter piping was not banded, but secured by what appeared to be rivet-type connec-tors.	15500-2.310	12/16/09 – Corrected.	Pre-Functional	HFCxA 12/16/09
13	Waste Piping Hangers	Ortho OR 5 (Space 305)	12/1/09	Hangers on waste piping near return duct in northwest corner of Ortho OR 5 (Space 305) extend outside of wall. Recommend hangers are relocated or recommend use of a different type of pedestal hanger at this location.	Con-struction Standard	Please advise of corrective action to be taken.	Pre-Functional	

Sample Commissioning Milestone Meeting Agenda

I. Status of shop drawings

The following shop drawings have not been received:

A. Domestic hot water booster pump

B. Occupancy sensors

II. Status of pre-functional checklists

Contractor should forward completed PFCs as they are completed:

A. MEP – ongoing

B. Domestic hot water – received except for tankless systems

C. Lighting controls – partially completed, but contractor has indicated they will complete as the installation takes place

III. Review of equipment/system startup schedule

IV. Review of test and balance schedule

V. Review of functional testing schedule

The following functional testing should be scheduled within the next two months:

A. FCUs 1, 2

B. Chiller plant control sequence

C. Dishwasher hoods

D. Fire alarm sequences w/AHUs

E. Emergency power blacksite test

F. Lighting controls – 1st floor

VI. Review of training plan and O&M manual

As per the commissioning coordination meeting held on July 1, the following should be forwarded to the HFCxA for review:

A. The contractor's training plan

B. The O&M manual

Sample Air-Handling Unit Pre-Functional Checklist

Note: The example provided is an excerpt from an AHU pre-functional checklist.

(Facility Name)

Date:
Unit #: AHU-DT-10-01
Area Served: Diagnostic & Treatment Area – Level B, 1, 3, 4, 8, 9
Location: Mechanical 10320U

Model Verification			
Manufacturer	2		1 = Specified
Model	2		2 = Installed
Serial #	2		* = Submittal
Airflow, SP	1	CFM = 45,000 ; Min OA = 16,000	Change
CHW Coil	1	EAT (db/wb) = 83.6/70.4°F ; LAT (db/wb) = 50/49°F ; CFM = 45,000 ; P.D. = 1.0 in. w.c. ; MBH = 2,740; EWT/LWT = 43/ °F ; GPM = 370 ; Max P.D. = 20 ft.	
HW Coil	1	EAT = -15 °F ; LAT = 55 °F ; CFM = 45,000; MBH = 3,410; EWT/LWT = 180/ °F ; GPM = 175 ; Max P.D. = 15 ft.	
Pre-Filter	1	2" Panel Type MERV 8; 35% Efficient	
	2		
Final Filters	1	12" Cartridge Type MERV 14; 90-95% Efficient	
	2		

(continued)

SAMPLE AIR-HANDLING UNIT PRE-FUNCTIONAL CHECKLIST *(continued)*

	36633384		

Reference	Equipment Installation/General	Comp. Y/N
23 7328 2.2 A	Unit base is constructed of structural steel.	
Detail 1 M8.20	Unit arrangement is per section detail:	
23 7328 3.1 B	Unit is installed a proper height for condensate trap depth.	
23 7328 2.6 A	Access doors are hinged and flush-mounted. Access doors are sufficient size for service and no less than 16-in. wide.	
Construction Standard	Inspection and access doors are operable.	
23 7328 2.21 A	Fluorescent lights installed in all access sections. Single switch with pilot light is provided near middle of unit.	
Construction Standard	All shipping bolts and brackets removed.	
20 0000 3.11 A	Equipment has been cleaned and finish touched up if necessary.	
23 7328 2.6 A	Access sections have a minimum of 30 in. between other equipment.	
23 7328 2.18 A	24" section provided a minimum of 15 in. downstream of CHW coil drain pan for future UV section.	
Detail 1 M8.20	Sound attenuators are installed per section detail.	
Detail 1 M8.20	Air blenders are installed per section detail.	

(continued)

SAMPLE AIR-HANDLING UNIT PRE-FUNCTIONAL CHECKLIST *(continued)*

Reference	Humidifier Section	Comp. Y/N
Detail 2 M8.06	Supports are provided for humidifier.	
Detail 2 M8.06	Humidifier piping is installed per detail 2 on M8.06 (attached for reference)	
23 2120 2.2 B	Steam condensate thermometer is 9-in. scale cast aluminum-type with clear acrylic window. Adjustable stem angle with permanently stabilized glass tube. Range = 30 to 300°F with 2°F increment.	
23 8413 2.1 D	Dispersion tubes discharge up and down perpendicular to airflow.	
23 8413 3.2 B	Minimum of 3 elbows for steam and condensate line expansion/contraction.	

Reference	Chilled Water Coil	Comp. Y/N
Construction Standard	Coils are clean and any damage to coil tubing or fins has been repaired.	
23 7328 2.10 D	Coil piping and flange arrangement provided pull access from one side of the unit.	
Construction Standard	Water flow through cooling coil is piped for counterflow (coolest water to coolest air).	
23 7328 2.10 B	Chilled water piping supported independently of coils.	
Construction Standard	Chilled water control valves properly installed with shaft above horizontal and correct flow direction.	
Detail 3 M8.05	Chilled water piping is piped per detail 3, M8.05 - (attached for reference)	
Detail 3 M8.05	Cooling coil control valve is two-way valve and is functional.	
Detail 3 M8.05	Chilled water coil air vents and drains and valves are installed per detail:	
Detail 3 M8.05	Piping offset provided with flanges for ease of coil removal.	
Detail 3 M8.05	Dirt legs with drain valves and caps are provided at the bottom CHWS and CHWR main lines.	
23 7328 2.10 E	Drain pan is minimum 2-in. stainless steel between 4 and 12 in. downstream of coil, sloped in direction of airflow and sloped to prevent standing water. Drain pan may be recessed, integral with unit floor.	
23 2120 2.2 B	Chilled water thermometer is 9-in. scale cast aluminum type with clear acrylic window. Adjustable stem angle with permanently stabilized glass tube. Range = 0 to 100°F with 1°F increment.	
23 2120 2.4 B,C,D,E	Chilled water pressure gauges are 4½-in. diameter, dial type. Range 0–200 psi. Operating pressure at gauge midpoint. Gauge accuracy is 1% of full scale.	

Reference	Condensate Drain Piping	Comp. Y/N
	Condensate drainage piped per detail:	
Detail 4 M8.04	Top of trap to drain connection is 5 in.	
Detail 4 M8.04	Trap is 3 in. deep.	
Detail 4 M8.04	Total height is 8 in.	

(continued)

SAMPLE AIR-HANDLING UNIT PRE-FUNCTIONAL CHECKLIST *(continued)*

Reference	Pre-Heat Hot Water Coil	Comp.Y/N
Construction Standard	Coils are clean and any damage to coil tubing or fins has been repaired.	
23 7328 2.9 D	Coils are removable though access door or removable access panel.	
23 7328 2.9 B	Heating hot water piping is supported independently of coils.	
Detail 2 M8.05	Hot water piping is piped per detail 2, M8.05 (attached for reference).	
Controls M7.26	Manual air vent provided per control diagram	
Controls M7.26	Temperature transmitter provided per control diagram	
Detail 2 M8.05	Heating coil vents and drains and valves are installed.	
23 7328 2.3 E 2 & 3	Drain pan is stainless steel, sloped in direction of airflow, and sloped to prevent standing water.	
Detail 2 M8.05	Piping offset with flanges is provided for ease of coil removal.	
23 2120 2.2 B	Heating hot water thermometer is 9-in. scale cast aluminum type with clear acrylic window. Adjustable stem angle with permanently stabilized glass tube. Range = 30 to 240°F with 2°F increment.	
23 2120 2.4 B,C,D,E	Heating hot water pressure gauges are 4½-in. diameter, dial type. Range 0–200 psi. Operating pressure at gauge midpoint. Gauge accuracy is 1% of full scale.	
Reference	HHW Recirculation Pump	Comp.Y/N
23 2123 2.3 E	Pump is directly hung from motor shaft without flexible couplings.	
23 2123 3.2 C	Pump and motor are lubricated.	
23 2123 2.3 H	Pump has regreaseable bearings or oil-lubricated sleeve bearings.	
23 2123 2.3 C	Casing is tapped and plugged for vent, drain, and suction and discharge gauges.	
Construction Standard	Pipe fittings are complete.	
Detail 2 M8.05	Recirculation pump and bypass is piped per details 2 and 6 on sheet M8.05 (attached for reference).	
Controls M7.26	Spring-loaded check valve, balancing valve, flanges, increaser provided per controls diagram on sheet M7.26	
23 0550 2.16 A Chart	Piping supported w/spring isolators to 100 pipe diameters or 50 ft. from the pump, whichever is greater.	
Detail 6 M8.05	Pressure gauge installed across pump and strainer with shutoff valves.	
23 2120 2.4 B,C,D,E	Heating hot water pressure gauges are 4½-in. diameter, dial type. Range 0–200 psi. Operating pressure at gauge midpoint. Gauge accuracy is 1% of full scale.	
23 2123 3.1 F	Full line size spring-loaded check valve and balancing valve in pump discharge.	

(continued)

SAMPLE AIR-HANDLING UNIT PRE-FUNCTIONAL CHECKLIST *(continued)*

Reference	Duct and Plenum	Comp.Y/N
Construction Standard	Duct installation complete.	
20 0000 3.3 E	Access doors are provided at all automatic dampers, fire dampers, smoke dampers, smoke detectors, fan bearings, heating and cooling coils, reheat coils, humidifiers, filters, bird/insect screens, valves and control devices and turning vanes in ductwork.	
Construction Standard	Duct connections to unit allow for straight and smooth airflow.	
23 3314 3.7 A	Flexible connections are provided for ductwork that is connected to equipment containing rotating equipment.	
Controls M7.26	Dampers (outside air, return air, mixing, relief) are installed and functional.	
Construction Standard	Damper actuators and linkages are connected.	
23 3314 3.19 D	Smoke detectors are mounted and labeled with unique tag numbers on access doors.	

Reference	VFDs - SF-DT-10-01A and B	Comp.Y/N
	Variable frequency drive (VFD) provided with the following:	
20 0514 2.7 C	HOA switch	
20 0514 2.7 A	Door interlock	
20 0514 2.7 E	Power on indication	
20 0514 2.7 D	Manual speed control	
20 0514 2.7 F	Drive run indication	
20 0514 2.7 G	Drive fault indication with testable feature	
20 0514 2.7 O 1	Manual bypass	
20 0514 2.9 A 3 & 4	Integral disconnect: molded-case switch with rotary switch	
20 0514 2.5 A	BAS interfacing	
20 0514 2.7 1	Speed indication (meter or digital)	
20 000 3.3 B	Adequate working clearance is provided for VFD.	
20 0514 2.7 K	VFD screen display is functioning properly and is viewable.	
20 0553 3.4 A	VFD is labeled with plastic nameplate.	
Construction Standard	Power available to VFD.	
20 0514 3.3 H	Floor-mounted drives are mounted on a $3\frac{1}{2}$-in. concrete pad with a $\frac{3}{4}$-in. neoprene pad.	
Construction Standard	Drive is securely mounted.	

(continued)

SAMPLE AIR-HANDLING UNIT PRE-FUNCTIONAL CHECKLIST *(continued)*

Reference	Electrical and Controls	Comp.Y/N
Controls M7.26 - M7.38	Return inlet smoke/isolation damper installed before fan.	
Controls M7.26 - M7.38	Return smoke detector Installed.	
Controls M7.26 - M7.38	Return outlet isolation damper installed and actuator is connected.	
Controls M7.26 - M7.38	Return temperature sensor installed.	
Controls M7.26 - M7.38	Return humidity sensor installed.	
Controls M7.26 - M7.38	Static pressure sensor installed in return air duct before common plenum connection.	
Controls M7.26 - M7.38	Static pressure sensor installed at return fan before sound attenuator.	
Controls M7.26 - M7.38	Low static pressure switch installed across return fans.	
Controls M7.26 - M7.38	Return air damper correctly installed and actuator is connected.	
Controls M7.26 - M7.38	Outside air flow transmitter installed.	
Controls M7.26 - M7.38	Outside air damper correctly installed and actuator connected.	
Controls M7.26 - M7.38	Relief air damper correctly installed and actuator is connected.	
Controls M7.26 - M7.38	Static pressure sensor installed in relief air duct.	
Controls M7.26 - M7.38	Prefilter dirty filter transmitter installed and hooked up across prefilter.	
Controls M7.26 - M7.38	Mixed air temperature sensor installed before preheat coil.	
Controls M7.26 - M7.38	Mixed air static pressure sensor is installed.	
Controls M7.26 - M7.38	Preheat temperature sensor installed after the preheat coil.	
Controls M7.26 - M7.38	Preheat discharge water temperature sensor is installed.	

(continued)

SAMPLE AIR-HANDLING UNIT PRE-FUNCTIONAL CHECKLIST *(continued)*

Controls M7.26 - M7.38	Freezestat installed upstream of cooling coil.	
Controls M7.26 - M7.38	Chilled water return temperature sensor installed.	
Controls M7.26 - M7.38	95% Final filter dirty filter transmitter installed and hooked up across final filter.	
Controls M7.26 - M7.38	Supply duct smoke detector installed before smoke isolation damper.	
Controls M7.26 - M7.38	AHU inlet isolation damper correctly installed and actuator is connected.	
Controls M7.26 - M7.38	Supply discharge smoke/isolation damper is installed and connected.	
Controls M7.26 - M7.38	Discharge air temperature sensor installed before smoke/isolation damper.	
Controls M7.26 - M7.38	Discharge humidity sensor installed in supply duct.	
Controls M7.26 - M7.38	High static pressure switch installed in supply air duct prior to the smoke/isolation damper.	
Controls M7.26 - M7.38	Static pressure sensor installed before AHU outlet smoke/isolation damper.	
Reference	**Insulation**	**Comp. Y/N**
20 0700 3.1 A Chart	Concealed Supply Air Duct Insulation: Flexible Glass Fiber 1½" thick insulation with laminate jacket.	
20 0700 3.1 A Chart	Return Air Duct Insulation: Rigid Glass Fiber 1½" thick insulation with heavy duty jacket.	
20 0700 3.1 A Chart	Mixed Air Duct Insulation: Rigid Glass Fiber 1½" thick insulation with heavy duty jacket.	
20 0700 3.1 A Chart	Chilled Water piping is insulated with Rigid Foam Insulation using a heavy-duty jacket: Less than 8" Diameter Piping = 1" Thick Insulation; 8" and Greater Diameter Piping = 1½" Thick Insulation	
20 0700 3.1 A Chart	Heating Hot Water piping (141°F–200°F) is insulated with Rigid Glass Fiber using a heavy-duty jacket: 2" and Less Diameter Piping = 1" Thick Insulation; 2" and Greater Diameter Piping = 1½" Thick Insulation	
20 0700 3.1 A Chart	Low Pressure Steam and Condensate piping is insulated with Rigid Glass Fiber using a heavy-duty jacket: 1¼" and Less Diameter Piping = 1½" Thick Insulation; 1½" to 6" Diameter Piping = 2" Thick Insulation; 8" and Larger Diameter Piping = 3½" Thick Insulation	
Reference	**Filters**	**Comp. Y/N**
23 7328 2.8 B	Space provided downstream of pre-filter for future carbon filter.	
23 7328 2.8 C	Space provided downstream of final-filter for future HEPA filter.	
23 4114 2.10 A	Filter holding frames incorporate gaskets and clips for no air bypass.	
23 4114 2.12 B	Filter gauge installed: Prefilter Range – 0–1.0 in. w.c.; Final Filter Range – 0–2.0 in. w.c.	
23 4114 3.1 B	Clearance provided to service filters.	

(continued)

SAMPLE AIR-HANDLING UNIT PRE-FUNCTIONAL CHECKLIST *(continued)*

Reference	**Operational Checks** (These augment mfr's list. This is not the functional performance testing.)	**Comp.Y/N**
	VFD has been set up per the manufacturer's recommendations	
	The HOA switch properly activates and deactivates the unit	
	Manual bypass starts the unit across the line	
	Operation is vibration free, with no unusual noises.	
	There is no leaking apparent around joints and fittings.	
	Specified sequences of operation and operating schedules have been implemented.	

Notes

Date:		MDL/ Verified
Present Were:		
Note 1		
Note 2		
Note 3		
Note 4		
Note 5		
Note 6		
Note 7		
Note 8		
Note 9		
Note 10		
Details		

(continued)

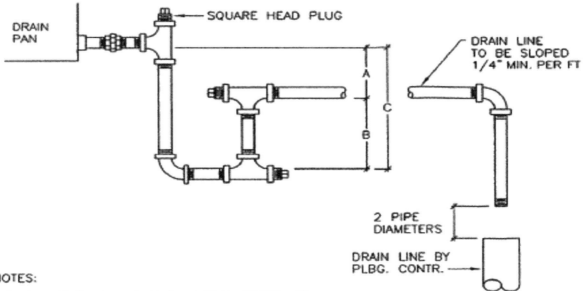

NOTES:

(1) FILL TRAP MANUALLY ON INITIAL START-UP.

(2) TRAP EACH COMPONENT DRAIN CONNECTION.

(3) PIPE SIZE SHALL BE 3/4" OR DRAIN PAN
    CONNECTION SIZE, WHICHEVER IS LARGER.

(4) DRAW-THRU UNITS   BLOW-THRU UNITS
    A = SP + 1"   A = 1/2"
    B = 1/2 SP + 1/2"   B = SP + 1/2"
    C = 1-1/2 SP + 1-1/2"   C = SP + 1"

    SP TO BE MAXIMUM STATIC PRESSURE (SP) ON
    DRAIN PAN INCLUDING MAXIMUM FILTER
    PRESSURE DROP AND PRESSURE DROP OF
    FUTURE COMPONENTS OF UNIT IF APPLICABLE.

(5) RAISE COIL SECTION OR ENTIRE AIR HANDLING UNIT
    WITH STRUCTURAL MEMBERS OR STANDS TO PROVIDE
    PROPER TRAP HEIGHT.

UNIT	A	B	C
AHU-DT, SUG, ED, LAB, MS, ICU, KT, HM	5	3	8
AHU-SG, CHW	4.5	2.75	7.25
PAHU	3	1.5	4.5
HRU-LAB	4	2.5	6.5

COOLING COIL AND HEAT RECOVERY COIL
CONDENSATE DRAIN TRAP PIPING

4 / M8.04 SCALE: NONE

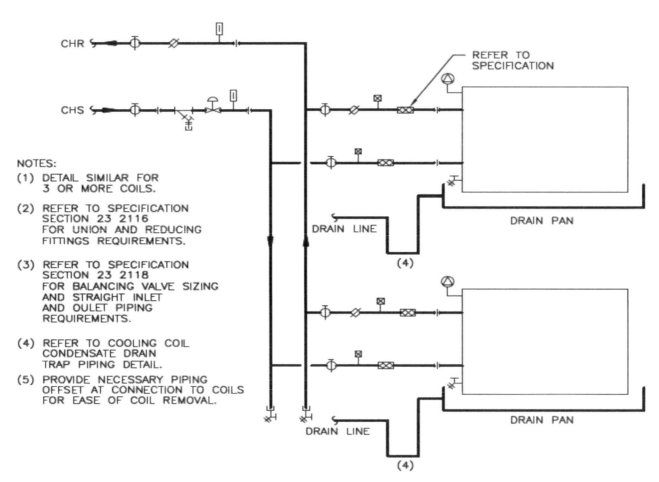

NOTES:

(1) DETAIL SIMILAR FOR
3 OR MORE COILS.

(2) REFER TO SPECIFICATION
SECTION 23 2116
FOR UNION AND REDUCING
FITTINGS REQUIREMENTS.

(3) REFER TO SPECIFICATION
SECTION 23 2118
FOR BALANCING VALVE SIZING
AND STRAIGHT INLET
AND OULET PIPING
REQUIREMENTS.

(4) REFER TO COOLING COIL
CONDENSATE DRAIN
TRAP PIPING DETAIL.

(5) PROVIDE NECESSARY PIPING
OFFSET AT CONNECTION TO COILS
FOR EASE OF COIL REMOVAL.

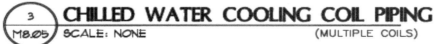

CHILLED WATER COOLING COIL PIPING

3 / M8.05   SCALE: NONE   (MULTIPLE COILS)

Sample Equipment/System Start-Up Plan

STEAM BOILER/HEATING HOT WATER LOOP START-UP PLAN

Multiple contractors are involved with the steam boiler/heating hot water loop start-up process, and all parties are required to complete their work and prepare for the system to provide hot water. The construction team (HFCxA, mechanical contractor, and equipment manufacturer) must complete the items on the manufacturer's checklist as well as those on the pre-functional checklist from the health facility commissioning agent (HFCxA). The boiler manufacturer prepares the system for start-up. After all parties of the construction team and state and local authorities agree the boilers are ready for start-up, the boiler manufacturer and electricians apply power to the boiler.

Step 1: Pump alignment must be completed before the pumps are started. This takes place after piping is complete and data sheets have been obtained for start-up records.

Step 2: Before the pipes are flushed, the steam and hot water piping systems are to be pressure-tested in accordance with specifications. The HFCxA or the CM/general contractor should witness this process.

Step 3: The power supply is applied to the hot water pumps with start-up personnel assisting the electricians to verify phasing and proper voltages. The pumps are started before the boilers and are utilized to flush the piping system.

Step 4: The local water authority should be consulted about the type of chemical to be used and whether and in what concentration it is safe to dump into the sanitary sewer. How much can be drained within a certain period will need to be determined (e.g., 5 to 10 GPM continuous to sanitary drain for 24/48 hours).

Step 5: Generally, the design documents require the piping system to be flushed for 48 hours. Chemical treatment must be applied to the system as specified in the design. The flush will need to circulate through main piping but not through equipment, so there must be means of bypassing equipment at each device. The steam heat exchanger(s) are bypassed as well. No flow stations or sensors sensitive to chemicals should be installed in piping during the flushing process.

Once the flush has circulated and maintained the required minimum velocity for the time specified, the system should continue to circulate while dumping the flush chemicals to the drain. The flow rate should be confirmed either by available flow meters or by calculation based on pressure differential in the system. The makeup flow must be adequate to offset the discharge (dumped) flow throughout the discharge period to maintain constant velocity in the piping system.

Once the system has been determined to be clean, a water sample should be taken and tested to confirm proper PPM values before rust inhibitors are introduced. Start-up screens should not be removed until the last piece of equipment has been connected and circulated. Copies of the flush used should be given to the general contractor for record-keeping.

Heating Water Pump Start-up/Flushing Checklist

1. Verify all piping is complete, with high-point vents and temporary flush lines to each device.

2. Confirm all pumps have been laser-aligned and documented.

3. Confirm piping has been tested and verified by the general contractor.

4. Confirm proper values of flush additive have been provided for pipe volume.

5. Confirm all pumps are properly lubricated.

6. Confirm temporary spool-piece bypass lines are in place where check valves have been installed on each AHU.

7. Confirm VFDs for pumps are wired and properly programmed.

8. Fill system with water and bleed air from all high-point vents.

9. Enable pump to operate and circulate.

10. Confirm proper GPM flows by differential on pump.

11. Install flush chemicals into system and circulate according to proper timeline (chemically treated assist).

12. Monitor loop temperature to verify it does not exceed maximum temperature recommendations for chemicals.

13. Drain system slowly to maintain proper loop inlet pressures with bypass/makeup water.

14. After it is clean of soap, test the system to determine proper PPM for pure water.

15. Introduce rust inhibitor in one-shot feeder.

16. Verify rust inhibitor is adequate when the final system has been installed and placed online.

17. Chemical treatment personnel test water and rust inhibitor quality.

18. Remove temporary spool-piece bypass lines and reinstall check valves on each AHU.

Step 6: Once all heating hot water piping has been properly flushed and inhibitors added, the temporary bypasses around equipment should be removed and connected to the various loads as designed.

Step 7: The steam control valves for the heat exchanger must be verified for proper 1/3 and 2/3 operation before steam is applied to the header.

Step 8: Condensate return piping and pumping stations should be flushed with clean water back to the boiler room until the water is observed to be thoroughly clean and dirt-free. This will require disconnecting the condensate piping system from the loop and temporarily piping the condensate system to floor drains for visual observation. It may be necessary to introduce water into each pumping station by pouring water into condensate receivers to allow water to return to the boiler room. Each condensate return station will need electricity applied for pumps to lift the condensate.

Step 9 (steam boiler start-up): The water feed system should be tested to confirm proper levels before introducing makeup water feed to the boiler(s). Gas pressure to the facility should be verified with the gas company and boiler manufacturer. The 1/3 and 2/3 steam-reducing stations should be adjusted to the hot water heat exchangers. The steam piping system is temporarily disconnected to provide a means of blowing steam at a target, at the end of the main, for 1 to 2 hours or until the target is observed to be slag-free. Once this has taken place, the system will blow steam at dirt-legs for the period and pressure noted in the specifications. It may be necessary to accommodate cooldowns for drains in the areas where steam is to drain to floor drains. The ability of makeup station feed water to prevent low water feed levels to the boiler will need to be assessed and tracked during this period.

Step 10: After all parties of the construction team and state and local authorities agree the boilers are ready for start-up, the boiler manufacturer and electricians apply power to the boiler.

Sample Functional Performance Testing Plan

Note: This sample is an excerpt of a functional performance testing plan for a seven-story facility.

Functional Performance Testing Plan for [Facility]

As of: (Date)

Area Served	Equipment	Start-up complete	Installation and PFC complete	TAB complete	HVAC controls calibration, pt to pt, programming complete	Fireman override panel interface complete	Contractor pretest complete	Functional test with HFCxA	Comments
	Air-Handling Units								
7th floor A & B (4th–6th floor similar)	AHU 7-1 (7)								
	EF-7-1								
	RF 7-1								
	RP 7-1					N/A			
4-7 Area A	EF ISO 1 & 2								
	EF ISO 1								
	EF ISO 2								
	Isolation Room Monitors			N/A		N/A			
3rd Floor C									
	AHU 3-2 (3C)								
	EF 3-2								
	RF 3-2								
	RP 3-2					N/A			
	Isolation Room Monitors			N/A		N/A			
3rd floor A									
	AHU 3-4 (3A)								
	EF-3-4								
	RF 3-4								
	RP 3-4					N/A			
	REF-3-4								
	Isolation Room Monitors			N/A		N/A			

(continued)

FUNCTIONAL PERFORMANCE TESTING PLAN *(continued)*

Area Served	Equipment	Start-up complete	Installation and PFC complete	TAB complete	HVAC controls calibration, pt to pt, programming complete	Fireman override panel interface complete	Contractor pretest complete	Functional test with HFCxA	Comments
Patient Tower	Heating Water System								
	HEX 3			N/A		N/A			
	HEX 4			N/A		N/A			
	HWP-4					N/A			
	HWP-5					N/A			
	HWP-6					N/A			
	CRU-2			N/A		N/A			
2nd floor C									
	AHU 2-6 (3B)								
	EF 2-6A								
	EF 2-6B								
	RF 2-6								
	RP 2-6					N/A			
	Isolation Room Monitors			N/A		N/A			
2nd floor A									
	AHU 2-1 (3A)								
	EF-2-1A								
	EF-2-1B								
	EF-2-1C								
	RF 2-1								
	RP 2-1					N/A			
	Isolation Room Monitors			N/A		N/A			
2nd floor B									
	AHU 2-2								
	EF 2-2A								
	EF 2-2B								
	EF 2-2C								
	RF 2-2								
	REF-2-2								
	RP 2-2					N/A			
	Isolation Room Monitors			N/A		N/A			
2nd floor D									
	AHU 2-3 (3C - NE)								
	AHU 2-4 (3C - NE)								
	AHU 2-5								
	MUAU 3 (3C - NE)								
	RP MUAU 3					N/A			
	EF 2-3A								
	Typ, list all EFs and RFs								
	Typ, list all coil pumps					N/A			

(continued)

FUNCTIONAL PERFORMANCE TESTING PLAN *(continued)*

Area Served	Equipment	Start-up complete	Installation and PFC complete	TAB complete	HVAC controls calibration, pt to pt, programming complete	Fireman override panel interface complete	Contractor pretest complete	Functional test with HFCxA	Comments
Floors 1 and 2	Heating Water System								
	HEX 1			N/A		N/A			
	HEX 2			N/A		N/A			
	HWP-1					N/A			
	HWP-2					N/A			
	HWP-3					N/A			
	CRU-1			N/A		N/A			
1st floor D									
	AHU 1-5								
	AHU 1-6								
	AHU 1-7								
	EF 1-5A								
	Typ, list all EFs and RFs								
	Typ, list all coil pumps					N/A			
1st floor B									
	AHU 1-4								
	EF 1-4A								
	Typ, list all EFs and RFs								
	Typ, list all coil pumps					N/A			
1st floor A									
	AHU 1-2								
	AHU 1-3								
	AHU 1-8								
	EF 1-2A								
	Typ, list all EFs and RFs								
	Typ, list all coil pumps					N/A			
1st floor C									
	AHU 1-9								
	MUAU 1								
	MUAU 2								
	RP MUAU 1					N/A			
	RP MUAU 2					N/A			
	EF 1-9								
	Typ, list all EFs and RFs								
	Typ, list all coil pumps					N/A			

(continued)

FUNCTIONAL PERFORMANCE TESTING PLAN *(continued)*

Area Served	Equipment	Start-up complete	Installation and PFC complete	TAB complete	HVAC controls calibration, pt to pt, programming complete	Fireman override panel interface complete	Contractor pretest complete	Functional test with HFCxA	Comments
All Areas	Chilled Water System								
	Chiller 1					N/A			
	Chiller 2					N/A			
	Chiller 3					N/A			
	Cooling Tower 1					N/A			
	Cooling Tower 2					N/A			
	Cooling Tower 3					N/A			
	VFPCHP-1					N/A			
	VFPCHP-2					N/A			
	VFPCHP-3					N/A			
	CWP-1					N/A			
	CWP-2					N/A			
	CWP-3					N/A			
	Refrig Exhaust/ Alarm								
	Sand Filter system			N/A		N/A			
All Areas	Steam Boiler/ Distribution System								
	Boiler 1			N/A		N/A			
	Boiler 2			N/A		N/A			
	Boiler 3			N/A		N/A			
	Deaerator			N/A		N/A			
	PRS 1 & 2			N/A		N/A			
	PRS 3			N/A		N/A			
	PRS 4			N/A		N/A			
Boilers	Fuel Oil Sytem			N/A	N/A	N/A			
	CRU-3			N/A		N/A			
	CRU-4			N/A		N/A			
All Areas	Medical Air Compressor			N/A	N/A	N/A			Alarm interface complete?
All Areas	Medical Vacuum Pump			N/A	N/A	N/A			Alarm interface complete?
All Areas	Lighting Control System			N/A	N/A	N/A			
All Areas	Nurse Call System			N/A	N/A	N/A			

(continued)

Sample Functional Performance Test Matrix for Equipment

[Facility Name]

Emergency Generator Functional Performance Test

Date:
Unit: Generator 1
Location:

Reference	Load Testing	Complete, Yes/No
NFPA 110	On-site (site-load) installation acceptance test:	
	From "cold start," primary power is disconnected to all ATSs.	
	Time delay on start is recorded.	
	Time taken to reach operating speed recorded.	
	Voltage and frequency overshoot recorded.	
	Time taken to achieve steady state condition recorded.	
	Load bank test results have been provided and comply with the following staged increments:	
	Load 25% - 10 minutes	
	Load 50% - 30 minutes	
	Load 75% - 30 minutes	
	Load 100% - 4 hours	
NFPA-110	At conclusion of site-load test, generator allowed to cool for 5 minutes and started individually and closed to 100% nameplate KW.	
	Generator cooldown and shutdown period recorded.	
	Oil pressure is recorded in 15-minute intervals during load test.	
	Water temperature is recorded in 15-minute intervals during load test.	
	Water pressure is recorded in 15-minute intervals during load test.	
	Oil pressure is recorded in 15-minute intervals during load test.	
	KW Output is recorded in 15-minute intervals during load test.	
NFPA-110	Cranking time until the prime mover starts and runs shall be recorded.	
NFPA-110	Time taken to reach operating speed recorded.	
NFPA-110	Voltage and frequency overshoot recorded.	
NFPA-110	Time taken to reach steady state recorded.	

(continued)

EMERGENCY GENERATOR FUNCTIONAL PERFORMANCE TEST *(continued)*

Reference	Crank Cycle Test	Complete, Yes/No
NFPA 110	Starting battery pack is tested to be capable of maintaining cranking speed per NFPA 110 (75-second cranking cycle; 15-sec crank, 15-sec rest, 15-sec crank, 15-sec rest, 15-sec crank).	

Reference	Generator Control Panel (Verify proper operation of each.)	Complete, Yes/No
	Monitoring gauge panel (dead front, vibration isolated) to include:	
	Mode select switch - RUN-OFF-AUTO-MANUAL	
	Emergency stop switch - red mushroom-head pushbutton	
	Reset switch - used to clear a fault and restart generator after fault condition shutdown	
	Panel lamp switch - used to light the entire panel with DC control power. Automatically switches off after 10 minutes, or after being depressed a second time.	
NFPA-110	Overcrank shutdown - red	
NFPA-110	Low coolant temperature alarm - red	
NFPA-110	High water temperature pre-alarm - amber	
NFPA-110	High water temperature shutdown - red	
NFPA-110	Low oil pressure pre-alarm - amber	
NFPA-110	Low oil pressure shutdown - red	
NFPA-110	Overspeed shutdown - red	
NFPA-110	Low fuel main tank	
NFPA-110	Low coolant level	
NFPA-110	EPS supplying load	
NFPA-110	Controls not in auto	
NFPA-110	High battery voltage	
NFPA-110	Low cranking voltage	
NFPA-110	Low battery voltage	
NFPA-110	Battery charger failure alarm	
	Ground fault alarm	
	Control system annunciates high alternator temperature as a fault condition via two embedded resistance temperature detectors.	

Reference	Generator Control Panel (Verify proper operation of each.)	Complete, Yes/No
NFPA-110	Lamp Test	
	Panel illumination lights with on/off switch	
NFPA-110	Contacts for local and remote common alarm	
	The following features have been installed and are operating properly:	
	Engine oil pressure	
	Engine coolant temperature	
	Engine oil temperature	
	Engine speed	
	Number of hours of operation	
	Number of start attempts	

(continued)

EMERGENCY GENERATOR FUNCTIONAL PERFORMANCE TEST *(continued)*

	Battery voltage	
	Generator Set AC Output Metering:	
	3-phase analog voltmeter, ammeter(3-phase), frequency meter, and kilowatt meter	
	Digital metering set for RMS voltage and current, frequency, output current, output KW, KW hours, and power factor. Voltage is available L-L, L-N, 3-phase.	
	Control Switches:	
	Mode select switch - RUN-OFF-AUTO-MANUAL	
	Emergency stop switch - red mushroom-head pushbutton	
	Reset switch - used to clear a fault and restart generator after fault condition shutdown	
	Panel lamp switch - used to light the entire panel with DC control power. Automatically switches off after 10 minutes, or after being depressed a second time.	
	Control Panel is shock-mounted on unit.	
263213.2.3.G.3.k	The following status reports are functional: Engine running, circuit breaker open, circuit breaker closed.	

Reference	Generator Control Panel (Verify proper operation of each.)	Complete, Yes/No
263213.2.3.G.3.h	The following control features are installed and operational:	
263213.2.3.G.3.h	Voltage level adjustment rheostat	
263213.2.3.G.3.h	Overspeed level adjustment	
263213.2.3.G.3.h	Overvoltage level adjustment	
263213.2.3.G.3.h	Undervoltage level adjustment	
263213.2.3.G.3.h	Overfrequency level adjustment	
263213.2.3.G.3.h	Underfrequency level adjustment	
263213.2.3.G.3.h	Automatic remote start capacity	

Reference	Remote Annunciator Panel	Complete, Yes/No
	Remote annunciator panel with battery power is provided and includes the following operational indications:	
	Panel illuminating lights for:	
NFPA-110	Overcrank shutdown	
NFPA-110	Low coolant temperature alarm	
NFPA-110	High water temperature pre-alarm	
NFPA-110	High water temperature shutdown	
NFPA-110	Low oil pressure pre-alarm	
NFPA-110	Low oil pressure shutdown	
NFPA-110	Overspeed shutdown	
NFPA-110	Low fuel main tank	
NFPA-110	Low coolant level	
NFPA-110	Controls not in auto	
NFPA-110	Low cranking voltage	
	Ground fault alarm	
	Lamp test switch	
	Alarm horn and silence switch	

(continued)

EMERGENCY GENERATOR FUNCTIONAL PERFORMANCE TEST *(continued)*

Reference	Alarm and Shutdown Settings	Complete, Yes/No
	At conclusion of alarm and shutdown testing/verification, document as-left setpoints for each:	
	Overcrank shutdown	
	Low coolant temperature alarm	
	High water temperature pre-alarm	
	High water temperature shutdown	
	Low oil pressure pre-alarm	
	Low oil pressure shutdown	
	Overspeed shutdown	
	Low coolant level	
	High battery voltage	
	Low battery voltage	
	Ground fault alarm	

Notes

Date Present Were		MDL/ VERIFIED
Note 1		
Note 2		
Note 3		
Note 4		
Note 5		
Note 6		
Note 7		
Note 8		
Note 9		
Note 10		

Sample Functional Performance Test Matrix for a System

[Facility Name]

Emergency Generator Functional Performance Test

Date:
Location:

Mode	Test Procedure		Comp. Y/N
Normal (Utility) Mode	Pre-test status	Verify by visual response that:	
		1. All ATSs are in the normal position.	
		2. All paralleling gear generator mains are open.	
		3. All paralleling gear feeder breakers are open.	
		4. The emergency power system is in automatic/standby mode.	
Emergency Mode (Enter)	Drop utility power to an ATS.	Verify by visual response that:	
		1. ATS(s) send system a run request.	
		2. All available generators are started.	
		3. First generator up to voltage and frequency closes to the bus.	
		4. Priority 1 and Priority 2 loads are powered in under 10 seconds. Inhibit relay prevents all ATSs not part of life safety and critical branches from transferring to emergency power.	
		5. The remaining generators are synchronized and paralleled onto their respective bus as they come up to voltage and frequency.	
		6. Bus optimization timer begins.	
		7. At conclusion of bus optimization timer, bus optimization step timer begins.	
		8. At conclusion of bus optimization step timer, if total bus KW plus the next priority (ATS) KW Level is below the bus loaded to capacity KW level, Priority 3 ATS is added to generator system.	
Removal of Inhibit Signals		9. Following addition of load, bus optimization step timer begins.	
		10. At conclusion of bus optimization step timer, if total bus KW plus the next priority (ATS) KW level is below the bus loaded to capacity KW level, Priority 4 ATS is added to generator system.	

(continued)

EMERGENCY POWER SYSTEM FUNCTIONAL PERFORMANCE TEST *(continued)*

Mode	Test Procedure		Comp. Y/N
Emergency Mode (Exit)	Restore utility power to an ATS.	Verify by visual response that:	
		1.ATS(s) sense the utility source is within acceptable operational tolerances.	
		2.As each ATS transfers back to utility power, it removes its run request from the generator plant.	
		3.When the last ATS has retransferred to the utility and all run requests have been removed from the generator plant, all generator circuit breakers are opened.	
		4.The generators are allowed to run for their programmed cooldown period.	
		5.The power system returns to normal mode.	
Load-Sensitive Load Shed (Remove)	Remove generators and add load from loadbank as necessary to perform load shed remove operations until only Priority 1 loads are connected to bus.	Verify by visual response that:	
		1.With total bus KW above bus loaded to capacity KW level, load shed timer begins.	
		2.At conclusion of load shed timer, if total bus KW has remained above bus loaded to capacity KW level, Priority 4 loads are removed from generator system.	
		3.With total bus KW above bus loaded to capacity KW level, load shed timer begins.	
		4.At conclusion of load shed timer, if total bus KW has remained above bus loaded to capacity KW level, Priority 3 loads are removed from generator system.	
Under-Frequency Load Shed (Remove) (not in spec)	1.With only one generator in auto, remove normal power from one of each priority level ATS.	Verify by visual response that:	
		1.All generators start and connect to bus. Following load shed operations, all priority level ATSs are connected to emergency power.	
	2. Manually create an under-frequency situation on the paralleling gear bus.	2.All non-Priority 1 ATSs are removed from the emergency power system.	
Generator Demand (Remove)	Place one ATS in emergency mode to create a minimal load on the system.	Verify by visual response that:	
		1.All generators start, connect to bus, and ATS transfers to emergency power.	
		2. Load demand start timer begins.	
		3. Following completion of load demand start timer, if total bus KW remains below generator demand dropout setpoint, one generator stops and begins cooldown.	
Generator Demand (Add)	Following completion of generator demand (remove) test, add load from ATSs and load bank as required.	Verify by visual response that:	
		1. If total bus KW is above generator demand pickup setpoint, start timer begins.	
		2. Following completion of engine start timer, if total bus KW remains above generator demand pickup setpoint, generator Priority 2 starts and connects to paralleling gear.	

Notes

Date Present Were		MDL/ VERIFIED
Note 1		
Note 2		
Note 3		
Note 4		
Note 5		
Note 6		
Note 7		
Note 8		
Note 9		
Note 10		

Sample Integrated Systems Test Procedure Matrix

[Facility Name]

Integrated Systems Testing Under Emergency Power –
Functional Performance Test

Note: A master list of systems on emergency power must be generated. Full system functionality per piece of equipment connected to the essential system must be confirmed on normal power prior to emergency power operation.

Date:

Equipment #:   Systems as noted under individual test sections

CHILLER PLANT

Mode	Test Procedure	Expected Response	Comp.Y/N
Transition to Emergency Power	Normal power feed to facility is shut down.	Verify by visual response that:	
		1. Chillers, cooling tower, chilled water pumps, and condenser water pumps are powered and operational.	
		2. Chillers stage to maintain CHWS temperature setpoint.	
		3. CHW pump VFDs modulate to maintain system DP setpoint.	
		4. Cooling towers stage and fan VFD speeds modulate to maintain condenser water return temperature setpoint.	
		5. Condenser water pumps operate to satisfy system flow requirements.	
		6. System operates at steady state in the maintenance of water temperature and system DP setpoints.	
		7. BAS control graphics update to reflect conditions.	

(continued)

INTEGRATED SYSTEMS TESTING UNDER EMERGENCY POWER – FUNCTIONAL PERFORMANCE TEST *(continued)*

AHUS – CHECK TYPICAL AHU SEQUENCE ON SAMPLING OF UNITS, CHECK UNIT START/STOP ON ALL AHUS ON EP

Mode	Test Procedure	Expected Response	Comp. Y/N
Transition to Emergency Power	Normal power feed to facility is shut down.	Verify by visual response that:	
		1. Outside air damper and discharge air damper are open.	
		2. Supply fan and return fan VFDs start at minimum speed.	
		3. After a 5-second delay, VFDs gradually begin to increase speed under static pressure control.	
		4. Once pressure on both sides of the supply isolation dampers is equal, supply isolation dampers open gradually as VFDs increase in speed.	
	Emergency power Sequence	5. Supply and return fans index to 50% speed (maximum).	
		6. All floor supply and return control and isolation dampers open.	
		7. Floor terminal boxes reset to 50% airflow conditions.	
	DAT control (not in economizer)	8. CHW coil and preheat coil control valves modulate in sequence to maintain discharge air temperature setpoint of ___ F (adj).	
	Humidification control	9. Humidifier control valves remain closed when OA temperature > DAT setpoints	
		10. When activated, steam humidifier control valves modulate to maintain return air RH of ___% (adj), subject to a supply RH high limit of 90% (adj).	
	CO2 control	11. CO2 sensor feedback modulates minimum outside air between 30% (fixed) and floor pressure sensor minimum targets (0.001" SP, adj) with respect to outside conditions	
		12. When CO2 sensor senses 800 PPM, minimum outside air reverts to 30%.	
		13. BAS control graphic updates to indicate condition.	

SMOKE MANAGEMENT SYSTEMS - ATRIUM (CHECK EA TYP SEQUENCE)

Mode	Test Procedure	Expected Response	Comp. Y/N
Transition to Emergency Power	Normal power feed to facility is shut down.	Verify by visual response that:	
		1. All HOA/VFD switches are in auto position.	
		2. System operates when emergency power is available.	
		3. System operates when utility power is restored.	

(continued)

INTEGRATED SYSTEMS TESTING UNDER EMERGENCY POWER –
FUNCTIONAL PERFORMANCE TEST *(continued)*

SMOKE MANAGEMENT SYSTEMS - STAIRWELL #1 PRESSURIZATION (CHECK EA STAIRWELL)

Mode	Test Procedure	Expected Response	Comp. Y/N
Transition to Emergency Power	Normal power feed to facility is shut down.	Verify by visual response that:	
		1. All HOA/VFD switches are in auto position.	
		2. System operates when emergency power is available.	
		3. System operates when utility power is restored.	

HEATING HOT WATER SYSTEM - CHECK EA SYSTEM

Mode	Test Procedure	Expected Response	Comp. Y/N
Transition to Emergency Power	Normal power feed to facility is shut down.	Verify by visual response that:	
		1. All HOA/VFD switches are in auto position.	
		2. System operates when emergency power is available.	
		3. System operates when utility power is restored.	

ISOLATION ROOM EXHAUST SYSTEMS – CHECK EA ISOLATION EF SYSTEM

Mode	Test Procedure	Expected Response	Comp. Y/N
Transition to Emergency Power	Normal power feed to facility is shut down.	Verify by visual response that:	
		1. Supply fan VFDs start at minimum speed.	
		2. Supply fan VFDs ramp until static pressure is equal on both sides of the isolation damper, then isolation dampers open.	
		3. VFD speed modulates to maintain static pressure setpoint in ductwork.	
		4. BAS control system and graphic update indicates condition.	

SUMP PUMP – CHECK EA SUMP PUMP

Mode	Test Procedure	Expected Response	Comp. Y/N
Transition to Emergency Power	Normal power feed to facility is shut down.	Verify by visual response that:	
		1. System operates when emergency power is available.	
		2. System operates when utility power is restored.	

DOMESTIC WATER BOOSTER PUMP – CHECK EA PUMP PACKAGE IF MORE THAN ONE

Mode	Test Procedure	Expected Response	Comp. Y/N
Transition to Emergency Power	Normal power feed to facility is shut down.	Verify by visual response that:	
		1. System operates when emergency power is available.	
		2. System operates when utility power is restored.	

(continued)

INTEGRATED SYSTEMS TESTING UNDER EMERGENCY POWER – FUNCTIONAL PERFORMANCE TEST *(continued)*

MEDICAL VACUUM PUMP

Mode	Test Procedure	Expected Response	Comp. Y/N
Transition to Emergency Power	Normal power feed to facility is shut down.	Verify by visual response that:	
		1. System operates when emergency power is available.	
		2. System operates when utility power is restored.	

MEDICAL AIR COMPRESSOR

Mode	Test Procedure	Expected Response	Comp. Y/N
Transition to Emergency Power	Normal power feed to facility is shut down.	Verify by visual response that:	
		1. System operates when emergency power is available.	
		2. System operates when utility power is restored.	

ALARM SWITCHES – FLOW SWITCH (FIRE ALARM ACTIVATION)

Mode	Test Procedure	Expected Response	Comp. Y/N
Transition to Emergency Power	Normal power feed to facility is shut down.	Verify by visual response that:	
		1. System alarm LED flashes.	
		2. Audible devive in FACP sounds distinctive signal.	
		3. LCD display indicates information associated with condition, including type of point and location.	
	Activate FP flow switch.	4. Printing and history storage equipment logs and prints the event information along with the time and date stamp.	
		5. System outputs for condition are activated.	
		6. System stays in alarm condition until reset.	

ALARM SWITCHES – TAMPER SWITCH (SUPERVISORY ACTIVATION)

Mode	Test Procedure	Expected Response	Comp. Y/N
Transition to Emergency Power	Normal power feed to facility is shut down.	Verify by visual response that:	
		1. System trouble LED flashes.	
		2. Audible devive in FACP sounds distinctive signal.	
		3. LCD display indicates information associated with condition, including type of point and location.	
	Activate FP tamper switch.	4. Printing and history storage equipment logs and prints the event information along with the time and date stamp.	
		5. System outputs for condition are activated.	
		6. System stays in alarm condition until reset.	

(continued)

INTEGRATED SYSTEMS TESTING UNDER EMERGENCY POWER – FUNCTIONAL PERFORMANCE TEST *(continued)*

ELEVATOR OPERATION UNDER EMERGENCY POWER

Mode	Test Procedure	Expected response	Comp. Y/N
Transition to Emergency Power	Normal power feed to facility is shut down.	Verify by visual response that:	
		1. All cars come to a complete stop when emergency power is lost.	
		2. Cars remain in operation when emergency power is energized subject to elevator emergency selector switch panel mounted in lobby.	
		3. No more than one elevator (per group) is in operation at a time.	
		4. "Elevator emergency power" signal is illuminated.	
	Normal power feed to facility is restored.	5. All cars come to a complete stop when normal power is restored.	
		6. Elevators continue typical operation under normal power.	

PNEUMATIC TUBE SYSTEM

Mode	Test Procedure	Expected Response	Comp. Y/N
Transition to Emergency Power	Normal power feed to facility is shut down.	Verify by visual response that:	
		1. Pneumatic trash/linen system is powered and continues to operate.	
		2. Fans and compressors are powered.	
		3. Update with sequence of operations provided by manufacturer.	

Notes

Date Present Were		MDL/ VERIFIED
Note 1		
Note 2		
Note 3		
Note 4		
Note 5		
Note 6		
Note 7		
Note 8		
Note 9		
Note 10		

ASHE-IFMA
Hospital Staffing Tool

Statistics have been gathered based on completed surveys indicating the number of workers employed in each hospital operation. The staffing has been split by trade. The data provided show the number of FTEs based on facility size, provision of labor, and ratio of space per position. Variations may be explained by cross-training of different trades.

Category	GSF/FTE	Recommended Number
Electricians	213,000	24.41
Plumbers	484,000	10.74
Controls	600,000	8.67
HVAC	283,000	18.37
Stationary Engineers	170,000	30.59
Carpenters	496,000	10.48
General Mechanics	124,000	41.94
Locksmiths	1,060,000	4.91
Painters	397,000	13.10
Supervisors	448,000	11.61
Managers	485,000	10.72
Help Desk	587,000	8.86
Administrative Assistants	600,000	8.67
Total	25,608	203.06
Floor Area (GSF)	5,200,000	

Input Floor Area (GSF)	5,200,000

CATEGORY				GSF/FTE	Recommended FTEs
Electricians				264,304	19.7
Facility Size (GSF)	N	# FTE	Actual # FTEs	GSF/FTE	
150,000	10	1.83	18.3	81,967	Slope
375,000	9	2.27	20.4	165,198	0.0250
625,000	17	4.11	69.9	152,068	
875,000	13	4.78	62.1	183,054	Intercept
1,500,000	19	7.52	142.9	199,468	134,304
3,000,000	11	16.00	176.0	187,500	
88,375,000	79		489.6	180,497	264,304
Avg GSF/ Facility	1,118,671			264,304	

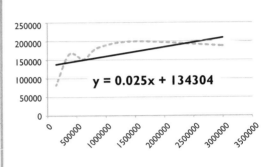

$y = 0.025x + 134304$

Plumbers				873,957	5.9
Facility Size (GSF)	N	# FTE	Actual # FTEs	GSF/FTE	
150,000	8	0.72	5.8	208,333	Slope
375,000	7	0.83	5.8	451,807	0.1017
625,000	16	1.28	20.5	488,281	
875,000	13	2.15	28.0	406,977	Intercept
1,500,000	16	2.59	41.4	579,151	345,117
3,000,000	11	5	55.0	600,000	
82,200,000	71		156.4	525,441	873,957
Avg GSF/ Facility	1,157,746			873,957	

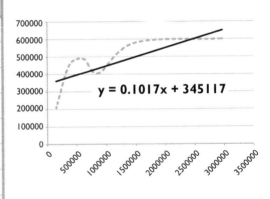

$y = 0.1017x + 345117$

Controls				1,076,484	4.8
Facility Size (GSF)	N	# FTE	Actual # FTEs	GSF/FTE	
150,000	5	0.55	2.8	272,727	Slope
375,000	5	0.91	4.6	412,088	0.1296
625,000	6	1.15	6.9	543,478	
875,000	11	1.61	17.7	543,478	Intercept
1,500,000	9	1.84	16.6	815,217	402,564
3,000,000	7	4.45	31.2	674,157	
50,500,000	43		79.6	634,263	1,076,484
Avg GSF/ Facility	1,174,419			1,076,484	

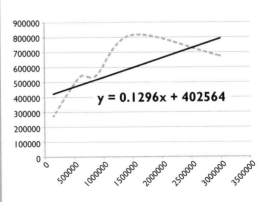

$y = 0.1296x + 402564$

HVAC				497,891	10.4
Facility Size (GSF)	N	# FTE	Actual # FTEs	GSF/FTE	
150,000	9	1.04	9.4	144,231	Slope
375,000	10	1.92	19.2	195,313	0.0592
625,000	18	2.41	43.4	259,336	
875,000	12	3.33	40.0	262,763	Intercept
1,500,000	18	4.52	81.4	331,858	190,051
3,000,000	11	9	99.0	333,333	
86,850,000	78		292.3	297,167	497,891
Avg GSF/ Facility	1,113,462			497,891	

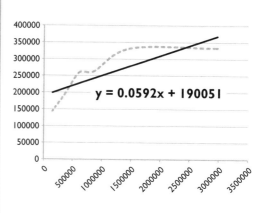

Stationary Engineers				344,624	15.1
Facility Size (GSF)	N	# FTE	Actual # FTEs	GSF/FTE	
150,000	12	2.4	28.8	62,500	Slope
375,000	12	3.77	45.2	99,469	0.0481
625,000	21	4.93	103.5	126,775	
875,000	8	5.5	44.0	159,091	Intercept
1,500,000	16	6.56	105.0	228,659	94,504
3,000,000	11	14.68	161.5	204,360	
83,425,000	80		488.0	170,949	344,624
Avg GSF/ Facility	1,042,813			344,624	

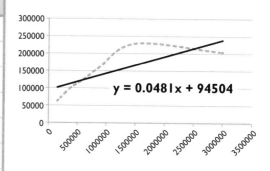

Carpenters				624,398	8.3
Facility Size (GSF)	N	# FTE	Actual # FTEs	GSF/FTE	
150,000	11	0.84	9.2	178,571	Slope
375,000	8	1.05	8.4	357,143	0.0642
625,000	16	1.59	25.4	393,082	
875,000	13	2.63	34.2	332,700	Intercept
1,500,000	17	3.23	54.9	464,396	290,558
3,000,000	10	6.88	68.8	436,047	
81,525,000	75		201.0	405,637	624,398
Avg GSF/ Facility	1,087,000			624,398	

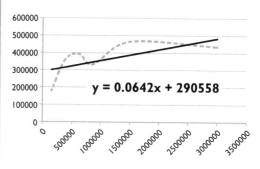

General Mechanics				297,885	17.5
Facility Size (GSF)	N	# FTE	Actual # FTEs	GSF/FTE	
150,000	24	2.15	51.6	69,767	Slope
375,000	14	4.37	61.2	85,812	0.0426
625,000	22	5.21	114.6	119,962	
875,000	12	8.16	97.9	107,230	Intercept
1,500,000	18	9.46	170.3	158,562	76,365
3,000,000	10	15.4	154.0	194,805	
90,100,000	100		649.6	138,701	297,885
Avg GSF/ Facility	901,000			297,885	

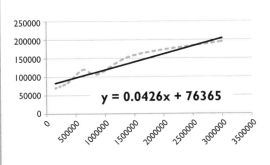

$y = 0.0426x + 76365$

Locksmiths				2,727,952	1.9
Facility Size (GSF)	N	# FTE	Actual # FTEs	GSF/FTE	
150,000	6	0.25	1.5	600,000	Slope
375,000	7	0.45	3.2	833,333	0.4227
625,000	8	0.75	6.0	833,333	
875,000	6	1.16	7.0	754,310	Intercept
1,500,000	12	1.44	17.3	1,041,667	529,912
3,000,000	9	1.6	14.4	1,875,000	
58,775,000	48		49.3	1,192,433	2,727,952
Avg GSF/ Facility	1,224,479			2,727,952	

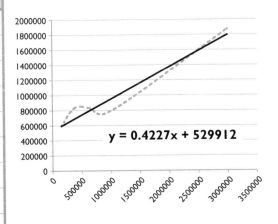

$y = 0.4227x + 529912$

Painters				828,482	6.3
Facility Size (GSF)	N	# FTE	Actual # FTEs	GSF/FTE	
150,000	14	0.85	11.9	176,471	Slope
375,000	11	1.1	12.1	340,909	0.1088
625,000	19	1.78	33.8	351,124	
875,000	12	2.17	26.0	403,226	Intercept
1,500,000	18	3.27	58.9	458,716	262,722
3,000,000	11	5.4	59.4	555,556	
88,600,000	85		202.1	438,353	828,482
Avg GSF/ Facility	1,042,353			828,482	

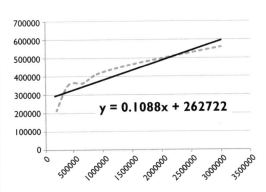

$y = 0.1088x + 262722$

Supervisors				743,332	7.0
Facility Size (GSF)	N	# FTE	Actual # FTEs	GSF/FTE	
150,000	9	0.97	8.7	154,639	Slope
375,000	11	1	11.0	375,000	0.0808
625,000	17	1.26	21.4	496,032	
875,000	13	1.92	25.0	455,729	Intercept
1,500,000	15	3.2	48.0	468,750	323,172
3,000,000	11	5.81	63.9	516,351	
82,975,000	76		178.0	466,099	743,332
Avg GSF/ Facility	1,091,776			743,332	

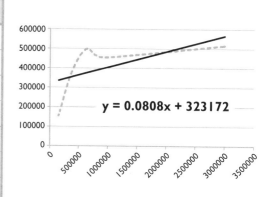

y = 0.0808x + 323172

Managers				1,749,537	3.0
Facility Size (GSF)	N	# FTE	Actual # FTEs	GSF/FTE	
150,000	23	1	23.0	150,000	Slope
375,000	17	1	17.0	375,000	0.2809
625,000	21	1.23	25.8	508,130	
875,000	14	1.5	21.0	583,333	Intercept
1,500,000	17	1.58	26.9	949,367	288,857
3,000,000	11	3	33.0	1,000,000	
93,700,000	103		146.7	638,762	1,749,537
Avg GSF/ Facility	909,709			1,749,537	

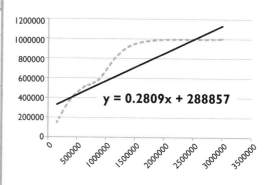

y = 0.2809x + 288857

Help Desk				828,482	6.3
Facility Size (GSF)	N	# FTE	Actual # FTEs	GSF/FTE	
150,000	14	0.85	11.9	176,471	Slope
375,000	11	1.1	12.1	340,909	0.1088
625,000	19	1.78	33.8	351,124	
875,000	12	2.17	26.0	403,226	Intercept
1,500,000	18	3.27	58.9	458,716	262,722
3,000,000	11	5.4	59.4	555,556	
88,600,000	85		202.1	438,353	828,482
Avg GSF/ Facility	1,042,353			828,482	

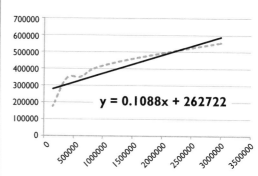

y = 0.1088x + 262722

Administrative Assistants				1,778,919	2.9
Facility Size (GSF)	N	# FTE	Actual # FTEs	GSF/FTE	
150,000	4	0.93	3.7	161,290	Slope
375,000	5	0.96	4.8	390,625	0.2789
625,000	5	1.19	6.0	525,210	
875,000	9	1.3	11.7	673,077	Intercept
1,500,000	9	1.44	13.0	1,041,667	328,639
3,000,000	6	3	18.0	1,000,000	
44,975,000	38		57.1	787,240	1,778,919
Avg GSF/ Facility	1,183,553			1,778,919	

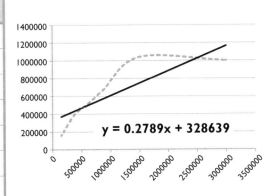

$$y = 0.2789x + 328639$$

Construction Support					0.0

TOTAL				50,561	109.1

Floor Area	Original Tool		Revised Tool	
(SF)	SF/FTE	FTE's	SF/FTE	FTE's
100,000	25,608	4	16,258	6
500,000	25,608	20	18,984	26
1,000,000	25,608	39	22,245	45
1,500,000	25,608	59	25,408	59
2,000,000	25,608	78	28,507	70
2,500,000	25,608	98	31,561	79
3,000,000	25,608	117	34,583	87
3,500,000	25,608	137	37,581	93
4,000,000	25,608	156	40,560	99
4,500,000	25,608	176	43,524	103
5,000,000	25,608	195	46,475	108
5,500,000	25,608	215	49,417	111
6,000,000	25,608	234	52,350	115
6,500,000	25,608	254	55,276	118
7,000,000	25,608	273	58,196	120
7,500,000	25,608	293	61,110	123
8,000,000	25,608	312	64,021	125
8,500,000	25,608	332	66,927	127
9,000,000	25,608	351	69,830	129
9,500,000	25,608	371	72,730	131
10,000,000	25,608	391	75,628	132
10,000,000	49,246	203.06	91,640	109.12

ASHE Facility Management Tool		
Floor Area (SF)	SF/FTE	FTE's
35,000	12,787	2.74
700,000	23,790	29.42
1,105,000	29,431	37.55
4,100,000	42,619	96.20

Sample Lighting
Audit Spreadsheet

BUILDING SUMMARY

Assumptions

Cooling unit cost (cents/ton-hour)	$0.21
Heating unit cost ($/MMBtu)	$24.00
Electricity unit cost (cents/kWh)	$0.09
Fixture retrofit cost	$110.00
Occupancy sensor cost	$100.00

Building Totals (part 1)

Floor	Floor Area (SF)	Cooling Load Reduction (tons)	Cooling Consumption Reduction (ton-hours)	Cooling Savings ($/year)	Heating Consumption Reduction (MMBtu)	Heating Savings ($/year)	Existing Lighting Power (kW)	Existing Lighting Power (watts/SF)
Floor 1	2,420	1.44	2,828	6	(17.0)	(407)	7.3	3.0
Floor 2	2,420	1.44	2,828	6	(17.0)	(407)	7.3	3.0
Floor 3	2,420	1.44	2,828	6	(17.0)	(407)	7.3	3.0
Building total	7,260	4.33	8,485	18	(50.9)	(1,222)	21.9	3.0

Building Totals (part 2)

Floor	Proposed Lighting Power (kW)	Proposed Lighting Power (watts/SF)	Electrical Demand Savings (kW)	Electrical Demand Savings (watts/SF)	Electrical Consumption Savings (kWh)	Electricity Savings ($/year)	Retrofit Cost ($)	Annual Savings ($/year)	Simple Payback (years)
Floor 1	2.2	0.9	5.1	2.1	14,916	13	7,340	146	50.1
Floor 2	2.2	0.9	5.1	2.1	14,916	13	7,340	146	50.1
Floor 3	2.2	0.9	5.1	2.1	14,916	13	7,340	146	50.1
Building total	6.6	0.9	15.2	2.1	44,747	40	22,020	439	50.1

FLOOR I

Room Number	Room Name	Annual Lighting Operation (hours/year)	Annual Room Occupancy (hours/year)	Room Width (feet)	Room Length (feet)	Room Floor Area (SF)	Ceiling Height (feet)	Room Cavity Ratio	Reflectances			IES Room Function	IES Recommended Illumination Level (footcandles)	Measured Illumination Level (footcandles)
									Wall	Ceiling	Floor			
100	Office	2,600	1,824	15	12	180	8	4.13	50	80	20	Office	50	80
101	Office	2,600	1,824	15	12	180	8	4.13	50	80	20	Office	50	80
102	Office	2,600	1,824	15	12	180	8	4.13	50	80	20	Office	50	80
103	Office	2,600	1,824	15	12	180	8	4.13	50	80	20	Office	50	80
104	Office	2,600	1,824	15	12	180	8	4.13	50	80	20	Office	50	80
105	Office	2,600	1,824	15	12	180	8	4.13	50	80	20	Office	50	80
106	Office	2,600	1,824	15	12	180	8	4.13	50	80	20	Office	50	80
107	Office	2,600	1,824	15	12	180	8	4.13	50	80	20	Office	50	80
108	Office	2,600	1,824	15	12	180	8	4.13	50	80	20	Office	50	80
109	Office	2,600	1,824	15	12	180	8	4.13	50	80	20	Office	50	80
110	Office	2,600	1,824	15	12	180	8	4.13	50	80	20	Office	50	80
111	Office	2,600	1,824	15	12	180	8	4.13	50	80	20	Office	50	80
112	Office	2,600	1,824	15	12	180	8	4.13	50	80	20	Office	50	80
113	Office	2,600	1,824	10	8	80	8	6.19	50	80	20	Office	50	75

2,420

Room Number	Room Name	Existing Light Fixtures									
		Fixture Type	Lens Type	Number Fixtures	Lamp Type	Lamp Replacement Cost ($)	Average Lamp Life (hours)	Lamp Temperature (K)	Lamp CRI	Lumens per Lamp	Lamps per Fixture
100	Office	2 x 4 Flourescent Troffer	Prismatic	4	34 watt - T12	2.00	20,000	4200	62	2,650	4
101	Office	2 x 4 Flourescent Troffer	Prismatic	4	34 watt - T12	2.00	20,000	4200	62	2,650	4
102	Office	2 x 4 Flourescent Troffer	Prismatic	4	34 watt - T12	2.00	20,000	4200	62	2,650	4
103	Office	2 x 4 Flourescent Troffer	Prismatic	4	34 watt - T12	2.00	20,000	4200	62	2,650	4
104	Office	2 x 4 Flourescent Troffer	Prismatic	4	34 watt - T12	2.00	20,000	4200	62	2,650	4
105	Office	2 x 4 Flourescent Troffer	Prismatic	4	34 watt - T12	2.00	20,000	4200	62	2,650	4
106	Office	2 x 4 Flourescent Troffer	Prismatic	4	34 watt - T12	2.00	20,000	4200	62	2,650	4
107	Office	2 x 4 Flourescent Troffer	Prismatic	4	34 watt - T12	2.00	20,000	4200	62	2,650	4
108	Office	2 x 4 Flourescent Troffer	Prismatic	4	34 watt - T12	2.00	20,000	4200	62	2,650	4
109	Office	2 x 4 Flourescent Troffer	Prismatic	4	34 watt - T12	2.00	20,000	4200	62	2,650	4
110	Office	2 x 4 Flourescent Troffer	Prismatic	4	34 watt - T12	2.00	20,000	4200	62	2,650	4
111	Office	2 x 4 Flourescent Troffer	Prismatic	4	34 watt - T12	2.00	20,000	4200	62	2,650	4
112	Office	2 x 4 Flourescent Troffer	Prismatic	4	34 watt - T12	2.00	20,000	4200	62	2,650	4
113	Office	2 x 4 Flourescent Troffer	Prismatic	2	34 watt - T12	2.00	20,000	4200	62	2,650	4

		Existing Light Fixtures									
Room Number	Room Name	Ballast Type	Ballast Factor (%)	Ballast Replacement Cost ($)	Average Ballast Life (hours)	Ballasts per Fixture	Assumed Maintenance Factor (%)	Calculated Coefficient of Utiliza-tion (%)	Room Efficacy (Lumens per Watt)	Lighting Power Requirement (watts/SF)	Fixture Power Requirement (watts)
100	Office	Magnetic	87	20.00	40,000	2	80	48.8	26.7	3.0	135
101	Office	Magnetic	87	20.00	40,000	2	80	48.8	26.7	3.0	135
102	Office	Magnetic	87	20.00	40,000	2	80	48.8	26.7	3.0	135
103	Office	Magnetic	87	20.00	40,000	2	80	48.8	26.7	3.0	135
104	Office	Magnetic	87	20.00	40,000	2	80	48.8	26.7	3.0	135
105	Office	Magnetic	87	20.00	40,000	2	80	48.8	26.7	3.0	135
106	Office	Magnetic	87	20.00	40,000	2	80	48.8	26.7	3.0	135
107	Office	Magnetic	87	20.00	40,000	2	80	48.8	26.7	3.0	135
108	Office	Magnetic	87	20.00	40,000	2	80	48.8	26.7	3.0	135
109	Office	Magnetic	87	20.00	40,000	2	80	48.8	26.7	3.0	135
110	Office	Magnetic	87	20.00	40,000	2	80	48.8	26.7	3.0	135
111	Office	Magnetic	87	20.00	40,000	2	80	48.8	26.7	3.0	135
112	Office	Magnetic	87	20.00	40,000	2	80	48.8	26.7	3.0	135
113	Office	Magnetic	87	20.00	40,000	2	80	40.7	22.2	3.4	135

		Proposed Light Fixtures							
Room Number	Room Name	Fixture Type	Occupancy Sensor	Occupancy Sensor Cost ($)	Fixture Retrofit Cost ($/Fixture)	Lens Type	Number Fixtures	Lamp Type	Lamp Replacement Cost ($)
100	Office	2 x 4 Flourescent Troffer	Yes	100	110	Parabolic	4	28 watt - T8	2.00
101	Office	2 x 4 Flourescent Troffer	Yes	100	110	Parabolic	4	28 watt - T8	2.00
102	Office	2 x 4 Flourescent Troffer	Yes	100	110	Parabolic	4	28 watt - T8	2.00
103	Office	2 x 4 Flourescent Troffer	Yes	100	110	Parabolic	4	28 watt - T8	2.00
104	Office	2 x 4 Flourescent Troffer	Yes	100	110	Parabolic	4	28 watt - T8	2.00
105	Office	2 x 4 Flourescent Troffer	Yes	100	110	Parabolic	4	28 watt - T8	2.00
106	Office	2 x 4 Flourescent Troffer	Yes	100	110	Parabolic	4	28 watt - T8	2.00
107	Office	2 x 4 Flourescent Troffer	Yes	100	110	Parabolic	4	28 watt - T8	2.00
108	Office	2 x 4 Flourescent Troffer	Yes	100	110	Parabolic	4	28 watt - T8	2.00
109	Office	2 x 4 Flourescent Troffer	Yes	100	110	Parabolic	4	28 watt - T8	2.00
110	Office	2 x 4 Flourescent Troffer	Yes	100	110	Parabolic	4	28 watt - T8	2.00
111	Office	2 x 4 Flourescent Troffer	Yes	100	110	Parabolic	4	28 watt - T8	2.00
112	Office	2 x 4 Flourescent Troffer	Yes	100	110	Parabolic	4	28 watt - T8	2.00
113	Office	2 x 4 Flourescent Troffer	Yes	100	110	Parabolic	2	28 watt - T8	2.00

Room Number	Room Name	Proposed Light Fixtures								
		Lamp Life (hours)	Lumens per Lamp	Lamp Temperature (K)	Lamp CRI	Lamps per Fixture	Ballast Type	Ballast Factor (%)	Ballast Replacement Cost ($)	Average Ballast Life
100	Office	30,000	2,725	4,100	80	2	Programmed Start Electronic Ballast	71	20	50,000
101	Office	30,000	2,725	4,100	80	2	Programmed Start Electronic Ballast	71	20	50,000
102	Office	30,000	2,725	4,100	80	2	Programmed Start Electronic Ballast	71	20	50,000
103	Office	30,000	2,725	4,100	80	2	Programmed Start Electronic Ballast	71	20	50,000
104	Office	30,000	2,725	4,100	80	2	Programmed Start Electronic Ballast	71	20	50,000
105	Office	30,000	2,725	4,100	80	2	Programmed Start Electronic Ballast	71	20	50,000
106	Office	30,000	2,725	4,100	80	2	Programmed Start Electronic Ballast	71	20	50,000
107	Office	30,000	2,725	4,100	80	2	Programmed Start Electronic Ballast	71	20	50,000
108	Office	30,000	2,725	4,100	80	2	Programmed Start Electronic Ballast	71	20	50,000
109	Office	30,000	2,725	4,100	80	2	Programmed Start Electronic Ballast	71	20	50,000
110	Office	30,000	2,725	4,100	80	2	Programmed Start Electronic Ballast	71	20	50,000
111	Office	30,000	2,725	4,100	80	2	Programmed Start Electronic Ballast	71	20	50,000
112	Office	30,000	2,725	4,100	80	2	Programmed Start Electronic Ballast	71	20	50,000
113	Office	30,000	2,725	4,100	80	2	Programmed Start Electronic Ballast	71	20	50,000

Room Number	Room Name	Proposed Light Fixtures							
		Ballasts per Fixture	Fixture Power Requirement (watts)	Fixture Coefficient of Utilization (%)	Lamp Lumen Depreciation Factor	Lamp Dirt Depreciation Factor	Fixture Maintenance Factor (%)	Lighting Power Requirement (watts/SF)	Calculated Illumination Level (footcandles)
100	Office	1	41	70	0.9	0.9	81	0.91	49
101	Office	1	41	70	0.9	0.9	81	0.91	49
102	Office	1	41	70	0.9	0.9	81	0.91	49
103	Office	1	41	70	0.9	0.9	81	0.91	49
104	Office	1	41	70	0.9	0.9	81	0.91	49
105	Office	1	41	70	0.9	0.9	81	0.91	49
106	Office	1	41	70	0.9	0.9	81	0.91	49
107	Office	1	41	70	0.9	0.9	81	0.91	49
108	Office	1	41	70	0.9	0.9	81	0.91	49
109	Office	1	41	70	0.9	0.9	81	0.91	49
110	Office	1	41	70	0.9	0.9	81	0.91	49
111	Office	1	41	70	0.9	0.9	81	0.91	49
112	Office	1	41	70	0.9	0.9	81	0.91	49
113	Office	1	41	65	0.9	0.9	81	1.03	51

Room Number	Room Name	Savings Calculations							
		Cooling Load Reduction (tons)	Cooling Consumption Reduction (ton-hours)	Cooling Unit Cost (cents/TH)	Cooling Savings ($/year)	Heating Consumption Reduction (MMBtu)	Heating Unit Cost ($/MMBtu)	Heating Savings ($/year)	Existing Lighting Electrical Demand (kW)
100	Office	0.11	209	0.2	0	(1.3)	24.00	(30)	0.540
101	Office	0.11	209	0.2	0	(1.3)	24.00	(30)	0.540
102	Office	0.11	209	0.2	0	(1.3)	24.00	(30)	0.540
103	Office	0.11	209	0.2	0	(1.3)	24.00	(30)	0.540
104	Office	0.11	209	0.2	0	(1.3)	24.00	(30)	0.540
105	Office	0.11	209	0.2	0	(1.3)	24.00	(30)	0.540
106	Office	0.11	209	0.2	0	(1.3)	24.00	(30)	0.540
107	Office	0.11	209	0.2	0	(1.3)	24.00	(30)	0.540
108	Office	0.11	209	0.2	0	(1.3)	24.00	(30)	0.540
109	Office	0.11	209	0.2	0	(1.3)	24.00	(30)	0.540
110	Office	0.11	209	0.2	0	(1.3)	24.00	(30)	0.540
111	Office	0.11	209	0.2	0	(1.3)	24.00	(30)	0.540
112	Office	0.11	209	0.2	0	(1.3)	24.00	(30)	0.540
113	Office	0.05	105	0.2	0	(0.6)	24.00	(15)	0.270
		1.44	2828		6	(17.0)		(407)	7.3

Room Number	Room Name	Savings Calculations								
		Proposed Lighting Electrical Demand (kW)	Electrical Demand Savings (kW)	Electrical Consumption Savings (kWh)	Electricity Unit Cost (cents/kWh)	Electricity Savings ($/year)	Lamp and Ballast Replacement Savings ($/year)	Retrofit Cost ($)	Annual Savings ($/year)	Simple Payback (years)
100	Office	0.164	0.376	1,105	0.1	1	11	540	11	49.8
101	Office	0.164	0.376	1,105	0.1	1	11	540	11	49.8
102	Office	0.164	0.376	1,105	0.1	1	11	540	11	49.8
103	Office	0.164	0.376	1,105	0.1	1	11	540	11	49.8
104	Office	0.164	0.376	1,105	0.1	1	11	540	11	49.8
105	Office	0.164	0.376	1,105	0.1	1	11	540	11	49.8
106	Office	0.164	0.376	1,105	0.1	1	11	540	11	49.8
107	Office	0.164	0.376	1,105	0.1	1	11	540	11	49.8
108	Office	0.164	0.376	1,105	0.1	1	11	540	11	49.8
109	Office	0.164	0.376	1,105	0.1	1	11	540	11	49.8
110	Office	0.164	0.376	1,105	0.1	1	11	540	11	49.8
111	Office	0.164	0.376	1,105	0.1	1	11	540	11	49.8
112	Office	0.164	0.376	1,105	0.1	1	11	540	11	49.8
113	Office	0.082	0.188	552	0.1	0	5	320	5	59.0
		2.2	5.076	14,916		13	144	7340	146	50.1

FLOOR 2

Room Number	Room Name	Annual Lighting Operation (hours/year)	Annual Room Occupancy (hours/year)	Room Width (feet)	Room Length (feet)	Room Floor Area (SF)	Ceiling Height (feet)	Room Cavity Ratio	Reflectances			IES Room Function	IES Recommended Illumination Level (footcandles)	Measured Illumination Level (footcandles)
									Wall	Ceiling	Floor			
200	Office	2,600	1,824	15	12	180	8	4.13	50	80	20	Office	50	80
201	Office	2,600	1,824	15	12	180	8	4.13	50	80	20	Office	50	80
202	Office	2,600	1,824	15	12	180	8	4.13	50	80	20	Office	50	80
203	Office	2,600	1,824	15	12	180	8	4.13	50	80	20	Office	50	80
204	Office	2,600	1,824	15	12	180	8	4.13	50	80	20	Office	50	80
205	Office	2,600	1,824	15	12	180	8	4.13	50	80	20	Office	50	80
206	Office	2,600	1,824	15	12	180	8	4.13	50	80	20	Office	50	80
207	Office	2,600	1,824	15	12	180	8	4.13	50	80	20	Office	50	80
208	Office	2,600	1,824	15	12	180	8	4.13	50	80	20	Office	50	80
209	Office	2,600	1,824	15	12	180	8	4.13	50	80	20	Office	50	80
210	Office	2,600	1,824	15	12	180	8	4.13	50	80	20	Office	50	80
211	Office	2,600	1,824	15	12	180	8	4.13	50	80	20	Office	50	80
212	Office	2,600	1,824	15	12	180	8	4.13	50	80	20	Office	50	80
213	Office	2,600	1,824	10	8	80	8	6.19	50	80	20	Office	50	75

2,420

Sample Forms for Water Chiller Testing

CHILLER SYSTEM TESTING

Air-Cooled Chiller

1. Measure pressure drop across condenser coils and compare to the manufacturer's design pressure drop to determine if the condenser coils could be clogged.

2. Measure pressure drop across evaporator and compare to manufacturer's design pressure drop to determine if the chiller is handling design chill waterflow.

   - Calculate GPM from pressure drop (Sqrt of actual PD ÷ by design PD × design GPM = calculated actual GPM) and compare to pump curve GPM, addition of GPMs at air units (using same method as noted above), or flow meters if available. If the calculated GPM is not within 10% of the comparison to other flow measurement methods, consider water treatment analysis to determine if the evaporator tubes could be clogged.

Water-Cooled Chiller

1. Measure pressure drop across evaporator and compare to manufacturer's design pressure drop to determine if the chiller is handling design chill waterflow.

   - Calculate GPM from pressure drop (Sqrt of actual PD ÷ design PD × design GPM = calculated actual GPM) and compare to pump curve GPM, addition of GPMs at air units (using same method as noted above), or flow meters if available. If the calculated GPM is not within 10% of the comparison to other methods of flow measurement, consider water treatment analysis to determine if evaporator tubes could be clogged.

2. Measure pressure drop across condenser and compare to manufacturer's design pressure drop to determine if the chiller is handling design condenser waterflow.

- Calculate GPM from pressure drop (Sqrt of actual PD ÷ by design PD × design GPM = calculated actual GPM) and compare to pump curve GPM or flow meters if available. If the calculated GPM is not within 10% of the comparison to other flow measurement methods, consider water treatment analysis to determine if the condenser tubes could be clogged.

- Also review head pressure to determine if it is staying within recommended ranges for the chiller. If the head pressure is higher than recommended by the manufacturer, reconsider the possibility that tubes could be clogged/scaled or the cooling tower is not providing proper water temperature.

Chiller Test Report

Project: System:

UNIT DATA		
Unit no.		
Chiller type		
Manufacturer		
Model no.		
Serial no.		
Nominal capacity		
Refrigerant type		

TEST DATA	DESIGN	ACTUAL
Evaporator:		
GPM		
Water pressure drop (ft wg)		
Entering water press. (ft wg)	---	
Leaving water press. (ft wg)	---	
Water temp. drop (°F)		
Ent / lvg water temp. (°F)		
Condenser:		
GPM		
Water pressure drop (ft wg)		
Entering water press. (ft wg)		
Leaving water press. (ft wg)		
Water temp. rise (°F)		
Ent / lvg water temp. (°F)		
Compressors:		
No. compressors	---	
Voltage (avg.)		
Amperage T1		
Amperage T2		
Amperage T3		

UNIT DATA		
Unit no.	Ch-2	
Chiller type		
Manufacturer		
Model no.		
Serial no.		
Nominal capacity		
Refrigerant type		

TEST DATA	DESIGN	ACTUAL
Evaporator:		
GPM		
Water pressure drop (ft wg)		
Entering water press. (ft wg)	---	
Leaving water press. (ft wg)	---	
Water temp. drop (°F)		
Ent / lvg water temp. (°F)		
Condenser:		
GPM		
Water pressure drop (ft wg)		
Entering water press. (ft wg)		
Leaving water press. (ft wg)		
Water temp. rise (°F)		
Ent / lvg water temp. (°F)		
Compressors:		
No. compressors	---	
Voltage (avg.)		
Amperage T1		
Amperage T2		
Amperage T3		

Remarks:

Technician: Date completed:

Cooling Tower Test Form

Project: System:

UNIT DATA	
Unit no.	
Manufacturer	
Model no.	
Serial no.	
Fan type / no. / size	
Motor manuf. / frame	
HP / RPM	
Volts / PH / HZ	
FL amps / SF	
Fan sheave make	
Fan sheave dia / bore	
Motor sheave make	
Motor sheave dia / bore	
Sheave setting	
No. belts / size	

Volts / PH / HZ	DESIGN	ACTUAL
Entering air WB temp (°F)		
Water pressure drop (ft wg)		
Water temp. drop (°F)		
Sump water temp. (°F)		
Fan RPM		
Voltage (avg.)		
Amperage T1		
Amperage T2		
Amperage T3		
Recirc. Pump:		
Voltage (avg.)	N/A	N/A
Amperage T1	N/A	N/A
Amperage T2	N/A	N/A
Amperage T3	**N/A**	**N/A**
BHP	N/A	N/A

UNIT DATA	
Unit no.	Ch-2
Manufacturer	
Model no.	
Serial no.	
Fan type / no. / size	
Motor manuf. / frame	
HP / RPM	
Volts / PH / HZ	
FL amps / SF	
Fan sheave make	
Fan sheave dia / bore	
Motor sheave make	
Motor sheave dia / bore	
Sheave setting	
No. belts / size	

TEST DATA	DESIGN	ACTUAL
Entering air WB temp (°F)		
Water pressure drop (ft wg)		
Water temp. drop (°F)		
Sump water temp. (°F)		
Fan RPM		
Voltage (avg.)		
Amperage T1		
Amperage T2		
Amperage T3		
Recirc. Pump:		
Voltage (avg.)	N/A	N/A
Amperage T1	N/A	N/A
Amperage T2	N/A	N/A
Amperage T3	**N/A**	**N/A**
BHP	N/A	N/A

Remarks:

Technician: Date completed:

Pump Test Form

1. Measure block-off pressures on pump and compare to manufacturer's pump curve to verify impeller is in good condition and is the correct impeller to match the pump performance data on the nameplate.

2. If pump is on a VFD, make sure any balance valves at the pump are fully open.

Pump Test Report

Project: System:

Design Data			
Pump no.			
Location / print no.			
Type			
Manufacturer			
Model No.			
Series / size			
GPM			
Head / NPSHR (ft wg)			
Pump RPM / impeller dia.			
Motor manufacturer			
Motor frame			
Motor horsepower / RPM			
Volts / phase			
Full load amps / SF			
Brake horsepower			
Test Data			
Shut off differential pressure			
Shut off head			
Open diff press			
Open head			
Open GPM			
Voltage (avg.)			
Amperage T1			
Amperage T2			
Amperage T3			
Brake horsepower			
Remarks			

Technician: Date completed:

Sample Boiler Test Forms

WATER BOILER

1. On water tube boilers, measure pressure drop across boiler water side; compare to manufacturer's design pressure drop to determine if boiler tubes could be clogged/ scaled and restricting flow.

2. On water tube or fire tube boiler, have combustion efficiency test performed to determine if boiler firing system needs tuning.

STEAM BOILER

1. Verify that deaerator is working properly.

2. Perform combustion efficiency test to determine if boiler firing system needs to be tuned up.

ELECTRICAL BOILER

1. Verify amperage of elements vs. KW rating.

2. Calculate GPM × temperature differential × 500 ÷ by 3413 = KW to determine if elements might need repair or descaling.

Boiler Test Report

Project: _____   System: _____

Unit Data			

Unit no.	B-1
Boiler type	
Manufacturer	
Model no.	
Serial no.	
Fuel type	
MBH input / output	

Test Data	Design	Actual
GPM		
Water pressure drop (ft wg)		
Entering water press. (ft wg)		
Leaving water press. (ft wg)		
Water temp rise (°F)		
Entering water temp. (°F)		
Leaving water temp. (°F)		

ELECTRIC BOILER:

		Design	Actual
Kilowatts		N/A	N/A
Voltage (avg)	N/A	N/A	
Amperage t1		N/A	N/A
Amperage t2		N/A	N/A
Amperage t3		N/A	N/A

Unit no.	B-2
Boiler type	
Manufacturer	
Model no.	
Serial no.	
Fuel type	
MBH input / output	

Test Data	Design	Actual
GPM		
Water pressure drop (ft wg)		
Entering water press. (ft wg)		
Leaving water press. (ft wg)		
Water temp rise (°f)		
Entering water temp. (°f)		
Leaving water temp. (°f)		

ELECTRIC BOILER:

		Design	Actual
Kilowatts		N/A	N/A
Voltage (avg)		N/A	N/A
	Amperage t1	N/A	N/A
	Amperage t2	N/A	N/A
	Amperage t3	N/A	N/A

Remarks:

Technician: _____   Date completed: _____

Sample Exhaust Fan
Test Form

1. **Measure exhaust in all locations.** *Note:* Turn exhaust fan on/off, as necessary, to verify if a specific grille is really exhaust or return and to determine which grilles are connected to which exhaust fans.

2. **Verify that each area served by an exhaust grille really requires exhaust.** Obvious areas that require exhaust include restrooms, most lab areas, and negative pressure isolation rooms. (Refer to the 2010 FGI *Guidelines for Design and Construction of Health Care Facilities* for areas that require 100% exhaust.)

3. **Measure the cubic footage of each area exhausted to ensure that exhaust does not exceed code requirements unless necessary for proper pressurization in an area.** (Refer to the 2010 FGI *Guidelines* and local building codes for required air change rates.)

4. **Determine the required exhaust CFM for each area using the following formula:**

   Area (SF) served by exhaust × height to ceiling of the area × required ACH ÷ by 60 = required exhaust CFM

   Note: Any reduction in exhaust can typically be matched with an equal reduction in the amount of outside air introduced into the air unit that serves the area exhausted.

* Always verify that any required pressurization is properly maintained after any changes are made in exhaust or outside airflow.

Fan Test Report

Project: Unit No.:

Unit Data	
Location / print no.	
Manufacturer	
Model no.	
Fan type / no. / size	
Motor Data	
Motor manf. / frame	
H.p. / rpm	
Volts / phase / hz	
F.l. amps / s.f.	
Drive Data	
Motor sheave model	
Motor shv. Dia. / bore	
Motor shv setting	
Fan sheave model	
Fan shv. Dia. / bore	
Centerline distance	
No. Belts / size	

Test Data	Design	Actual
Total CFM		
Outlet CFM		
External sp (in wc)		
Discharge sp (in wc)	---	
Suction sp (in wc)	---	
Fan speed setting	---	
Fan RPM		
Voltage (avg.)		
Amperage t1		
Amperage t2		
Amperage t3		

Air Outlet Test Data									
Area Served		Outlet			Design CFM	Preliminary		Final CFM	% of
		No.	Type	Size		CFM	CFM		Design
		1							
		2							
		3							
		4							
		5							
		6							
		7							
		8							
		9							
		10							

Remarks:

Technician(s):   Date completed:

Sample Room
Ventilation Schedule

Appendix

6.5

Room Ventilation Schedule

PROJECT: Sample

JOB #: 01-09-0055

DATEL 30-Sep-09

ROOM NUMBER	ROOM NAME	AIR HANDLING UNIT #	TERMINAL BOX #	FLOOR AREA SQ. FT
Level 1				
5705	OPERATING ROOM	8	501	630
5705A	EQUIPMENT	8	502	200
5706	OPERATING ROOM	8	503	630
5799B	CORRIDOR	8	504	2,180
5707	OPERATING ROOM	8	505	630
5708	OPERATING ROOM	8	506	630
5707A	EQUIPMENT	8	507	200
5708B	SUPPLY	8	508	710
5799C	CORRIDOR	8	509	660
5799A	CORRIDOR	8	510	820
5704	OPERATING ROOM	8	511	630
5705X	DECONTAMINATION	8	512	110
5703A	EQUIPMENT	8	513	200
5799X	SUPPLY	8	514	770
5703	OPERATING ROOM	8	515	630
5702	OPERATING ROOM	8	516	630
5799	CORRIDOR	8	517	1,960
5701A	EQUIPMENT	8	518	200
5701	OPERATING ROOM	8	519	630

(continued)

Room Ventilation Schedule *(continued)*

ROOM NUMBER	ROOM NAME	AIR HANDLING UNIT #	TERMINAL BOX #	FLOOR AREA SQ. FT
Level 1				
5700	PRESSURE SETUP	8	520	700
5799AX	SUPPLY	8	521	1,190
5700C	PREP	8	522	300
5700A	PUMP	8	524	1,020
5709	OPERATING ROOM	9	525	610
5710	OPERATING ROOM	9	526	610
5710B	OFFICE	9	527	428
5799E	CORRIDOR	9	528	1,900
5799BX	SUPPLY	9	529	830
5711	OPERATING ROOM	9	530	610
5711A	OFFICE	9	531	122
5712	OPERATING ROOM	9	532	610
5713	OPERATING ROOM	9	533	610
5712A	EQUIPMENT	9	534	200
5799F	CORRIDOR	9	535	960
5710A	EQUIPMENT	9	536	200
5799D	CORRIDOR	9	537	1,030
5718	OPERATING ROOM	9	538	610
5717	OPERATING ROOM	9	539	610
5716A	EQUIPMENT	9	540	200
5799G	CORRIDOR	9	541	1,950
5716	OPERATING ROOM	9	542	610
5715	OPERATING ROOM	9	543	610
5714A	EQUIPMENT	9	544	200
5714X	DECONTAMINATION	9	545	130
5799CX	SUPPLY	9	545	1,550
5714	OPERATING ROOM	9	546	610
5707B	OFFICE	8	547	122
5707C	OFFICE	8	548	428
7499A	CORRIDOR	14	701	840
7406	OPERATING ROOM	14	702	610
7406A	STERILE	14	703	100
7407A	EQUIPMENT	14	703	130

(continued)

Room Ventilation Schedule *(continued)*

ROOM NUMBER	ROOM NAME	AIR HANDLING UNIT #	TERMINAL BOX #	FLOOR AREA SQ. FT
Level 1				
7408A	EQUIPMENT	14	704	240
7408B	OFFICE	14	705	122
7407	OPERATING ROOM	14	706	610
7408	OPERATING ROOM	14	707	610
7460	SUPPLY	15	708	1,010
7409X	OFFICE	14	709	428
7499B	CORRIDOR	14	710	2,100
7409	OPERATING ROOM	14	711	610
7410	OPERATING ROOM	14	712	610
7405	OPERATING ROOM	14	713	610
7406X	DECONTAMINATION	14	714	100
7460A	SUPPLY	15	714	1,010
7404A	EQUIPMENT	14	715	200
7405A	STERILE	14	715	65
7404	OPERATING ROOM	14	716	610
7403	OPERATING ROOM	14	717	610
7499F	CORRIDOR	14	718	1,900
7402A	EQUIPMENT	14	719	200
7402	OPERATING ROOM	14	720	610
7401	OPERATING ROOM	14	721	610
7411X	DECONTAMINATION	15	722	130
7422	OPERATING ROOM	15	723	610
7400	CONTROL	15	724	200
7,499.00	STAGING	15	724	800
7499C	CORRIDOR	15	724	800
7499D	CORRIDOR	15	725	600
7411A	EQUIPMENT	15	726	270
7411	OPERATING ROOM	15	727	610
7413X	OFFICE	15	728	428
7412	OPERATING ROOM	15	729	610
7413	OPERATING ROOM	15	730	610
7499E	CORRIDOR	15	731	1,900
7413A	EQUIPMENT	15	732	270

Room Ventilation Schedule *(continued)*

ROOM NUMBER	ROOM NAME	AIR HANDLING UNIT #	TERMINAL BOX #	FLOOR AREA SQ. FT
Level 1				
7414A	OFFICE	15	733	122
7414	OPERATING ROOM	15	734	610
7415	OPERATING ROOM	15	735	610
7415A	EQUIPMENT	15	736	200
7416	OPERATING ROOM	15	737	610
7422A	INDUCTION	15	738	260
7470	CORRIDOR	15	739	600
7421	OPERATING ROOM	15	740	610
7420	OPERATING ROOM	15	741	610
7419A	INDUCTION	15	742	260
7499H	CORRIDOR	15	743	2,500
7419	OPERATING ROOM	15	744	610
7418	OPERATING ROOM	15	745	610
7417A	EQUIPMENT	15	746	200
7480	SUPPLY	15	747	1,950
7417	OPERATING ROOM	15	748	610
7499G	CORRIDOR	15	749	840
5700B1	WASH	8	0	10
5700D	JANITOR'S CLOSET	8	0	70
5708A	JANITOR'S CLOSET	8	0	50
5709A	JANITOR'S CLOSET	9	0	50
7411B	JANITOR'S CLOSET	15		30

(continued)

Room Ventilation Schedule *(continued)*

ROOM NAME	AIR HANDLING UNIT #	TERMINAL BOX #	FLOOR AREA SQ. FT
Non-Medical Area	N/A	N/A	N/A
Airborn Infectious Isolation	2	12	In
Anesthesia Storage	N/A	8	In
Autopsy	N/A	12	In
Bath Room	N/A	10	In
Bed Pan Room	N/A	10	In
Bronchoscopy	2	12	In
Central Clean Supply	N/A	4	Out
Central Supply Soiled	N/A	6	In
Clean Holding	N/A	4	Out
Clean Linen Storage	N/A	2	Out
Clean Workroom	N/A	4	Out
Critical Care	2	6	N/A
Decontamination Room	N/A	6	In
Delivery Room	3	15	Out
Dietary Day Storage	N/A	2	In
Endoscopy	2	6	In
ER Waiting Exh	2	12	In
ER Waiting Ret	2	12	In
ETO Sterilizer Room	N/A	10	In
Exam Room	N/A	6	N/A
Food Prep Center	N/A	10	N/A
Hydrotherapy	N/A	6	In
Intensive Care	2	6	N/A
Isolation Anteroom	0	10	In/Out
Janitor's Closet	N/A	10	In
Lab - Biochemistry	N/A	6	Out
Lab - Cytology	N/A	6	In
Lab - General	N/A	6	N/A
Lab - Glass Washing	N/A	10	In
Lab - Histology	N/A	6	In
Lab - Microbiology	N/A	6	In
Lab - Nuclear Med.	N/A	6	In
Lab - Pathology	N/A	6	In
Lab - Serology	N/A	6	Out
Lab - Sterilizing	N/A	10	In
Laundry General	N/A	10	N/A
LDRP	2	6	N/A
Medication Room	N/A	4	Out
Non-Refrig. Body Holding	N/A	10	In

(continued)

Room Ventilation Schedule *(continued)*

ROOM NAME	AIR HANDLING UNIT #	TERMINAL BOX #	FLOOR AREA SQ. FT
Newborn Intensive Care	2	6	N/A
Newborn Nursery Suite	2	6	N/A
Operating Room	3	15	Out
Patient Corridor	N/A	2	N/A
Patient Room	2	6	N/A
Pharmacy	N/A	4	Out
Physical Therapy	N/A	6	In
Procedure Room	3	15	Out
Protective Environment Room	2	12	Out
Rad./Surgery/CCU	3	15	Out
Rad./Treatment/Diag.	N/A	6	N/A
Rad./Treatment/Diag. Exh.	N/A	6	N/A
Radiology Darkroom	N/A	10	In
Radiology Waiting Exh.	2	12	In
Radiology Waiting Ret.	2	12	In
Recovery Room	2	6	N/A
Soiled Holding	N/A	10	In
Soiled Linen	N/A	10	In
Soiled Linen Storage	N/A	10	In
Soiled Workroom	N/A	10	In
Sterile Storage	N/A	4	Out
Sterilizer Equipment	N/A	10	In
Toilet Room	N/A	10	In
Trash Chute	N/A	10	In
Trauma Room	3	15	Out
Treatment Room	N/A	6	N/A
Triage Exh.	N/A	12	In
Triage Ret.	N/A	12	In
Warewashing	N/A	10	In